Lippincott's Pathophysiology Series

PULMONARY PATHOPHYSIOLOGY

Lippincott's Pathophysiology Series

PULMONARY PATHOPHYSIOLOGY

Michael A. Grippi, M.D.
Associate Professor of Medicine
Pulmonary and Critical Care Division
Vice Chairman, Clinical Affairs
Department of Medicine
University of Pennsylvania Medical Center
Philadelphia, Pennsylvania

With 11 additional contributors

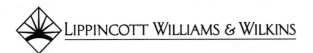
LIPPINCOTT WILLIAMS & WILKINS

Acquisitions Editor: Richard Winters
Sponsoring Editor: Mary Beth Murphy
Production Editor: Virginia Barishek
Indexer: M. L. Coughlin
Interior Designer: Larry Pezzato
Cover Designer: Larry Pezzato
Production: P. M. Gordon Associates
Compositor: Achorn Graphic Services
Printer/Binder: Courier Book Company—Kendallville

6 5 4

Library of Congress Cataloging-in-Publication Data

Grippi, Michael A.
    Pulmonary pathophysiology / Michael A. Grippi ; with 11 additional
  contributors.
      p. cm. — (Lippincott's pathophysiology series)
    Includes bibliographical references and index.
    ISBN 0–397–51329–1
    1. Lungs–Pathophysiology.   I. Title.   II. Series.
    [DNLM: 1. Lung Diseases—physiopathology.   2. Lung—physiology.
  WF 600 G868p 1995]
  RC711.G75   1995
  616.2'407—dc20
  DNLM/DLC
  for Library of Congress   94–41688
                                                                   CIP

♾ This paper meets the requirements of ANSI/NISO Z39.48–1992 (Permanence of Paper).

The authors and publisher have exerted every effort to ensure that drug selection and dosage set forth in this text are in accord with current recommendations and practice at the time of publication. However, in view of ongoing research, changes in government regulations, and the constant flow of information relating to drug therapy and drug reactions, the reader is urged to check the package insert for each drug for any change in indications and dosage and for added warnings and precautions. This is particularly important when the recommended agent is a new or infrequently employed drug.

. . . To Barbara, Kristen, and Amy
. . . To Joseph, Catherine, and Jean
. . . To my family

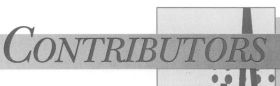

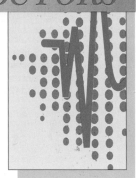

Michael A. Grippi, M.D.

Associate Professor of Medicine
Pulmonary and Critical Care Division
Vice Chairman, Clinical Affairs
Department of Medicine
University of Pennsylvania Medical
 Center
Philadelphia, Pennsylvania

John Hansen-Flaschen, M.D.

Associate Professor of Medicine
Chief, Pulmonary and Critical Care
 Division
Department of Medicine
University of Pennsylvania Medical
 Center
Philadelphia, Pennsylvania

Mark A. Kelley, M.D.

Professor of Medicine
Pulmonary and Critical Care Division
Department of Medicine
Vice Dean, Clinical Affairs
University of Pennsylvania Medical
 Center
Philadelphia, Pennsylvania

Paul N. Lanken, M.D.

Associate Professor of Medicine
Pulmonary and Critical Care Division
Department of Medicine
Medical Director, Medical Intensive
 Care Unit
University of Pennsylvania Medical
 Center
Philadelphia, Pennsylvania

Scott Manaker, M.D., Ph.D.

Assistant Professor of Medicine
Pulmonary and Critical Care Division
Department of Medicine
University of Pennsylvania Medical
 Center
Philadelphia, Pennsylvania

Richard K. Murray, M.D.

Assistant Professor of Medicine
Pulmonary and Critical Care Division
Department of Medicine
University of Pennsylvania Medical
 Center
Philadelphia, Pennsylvania

Harold I. Palevsky, M.D.

Associate Professor of Medicine
Pulmonary and Critical Care Division
Department of Medicine
Medical Director, Respiratory Care
 Services
University of Pennsylvania Medical
 Center
Philadelphia, Pennsylvania

Reynold A. Panettieri, Jr., M.D.

Assistant Professor of Medicine
Pulmonary and Critical Care Division
Department of Medicine
University of Pennsylvania Medical
 Center
Philadelphia, Pennsylvania

Basil J. Petrof, M.D.

Assistant Professor of Medicine
Respiratory Division
Royal Victoria Hospital
Montreal, Quebec, Canada

Milton D. Rossman, M.D.

Associate Professor of Medicine
Pulmonary and Critical Care Division
Department of Medicine
University of Pennsylvania Medical
 Center
Philadelphia, Pennsylvania

Richard J. Schwab, M.D.
Assistant Professor of Medicine
Pulmonary and Critical Care Division
Department of Medicine
Clinical Director, Penn Center for
 Sleep Disorders
University of Pennsylvania Medical
 Center
Philadelphia, Pennsylvania

Gregory Tino, M.D.
Assistant Professor of Medicine
Pulmonary and Critical Care Division
Department of Medicine
University of Pennsylvania Medical
 Center
Philadelphia, Pennsylvania

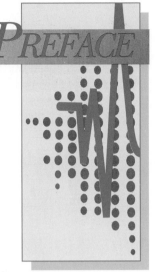

This book is an outgrowth of a core course in pathophysiology designed for second-year medical students at the University of Pennsylvania School of Medicine. It has been written with several goals in mind: (1) to review normal respiratory physiology as the basis for understanding pathophysiologic alterations important in disease states; (2) to provide a framework for understanding commonly used pulmonary diagnostic tests; (3) to develop a rational basis for various therapeutic strategies used in treating respiratory diseases; and (4) to demonstrate the clinical relevance of pathophysiology by anchoring concepts in case presentations grouped along thematic lines.

The audience to whom the book is addressed includes medical students, residents and fellows in training, and practicing physicians. The authors' experience has been that although students learn many of the fundamental concepts during their undergraduate medical education, these concepts are not rediscovered or fully understood until later in training, for example, during residency or fellowship. Therefore, although the book is targeted primarily to medical students, it should prove useful to all physicians interested in pulmonary physiology.

The volume is organized in four parts. Part I deals with the structure and mechanical properties of the lungs, chest wall, and airways. Included are respiratory mechanics, obstructive and restrictive pulmonary diseases, and the physiologic basis of pulmonary function testing. Part II addresses gas exchange in the lungs and gas transport to and from peripheral tissues. Part III focuses on the pulmonary circulation and its interface with ventilation. Part IV covers integrated respiratory functions, including control of breathing, respiratory failure, and pulmonary exercise physiology. Each part concludes with a series of clinical presentations, designed to highlight pathophysiologic principles addressed in the preceding chapters. Brief case scenarios are given, along with supporting laboratory studies; an analysis of the information is provided at strategic points.

This book is not an exhaustive review of pulmonary medicine or pathophysiology. Rather, it is a presentation of essential material and is based on the development of important pathophysiologic concepts. Additional information can be found in a number of other publications on the subject, as well as in comprehensive textbooks of pulmonary medicine.

Michael A. Grippi, M.D.

CONTENTS

PART I:

STRUCTURAL–FUNCTIONAL CORRELATES OF THE LUNGS, AIRWAYS, AND CHEST WALL

PART II:

GAS EXCHANGE AND TRANSPORT

PART III:

THE PULMONARY CIRCULATION AND ITS RELATIONSHIP TO VENTILATION

PART IV:

INTEGRATED RESPIRATORY FUNCTIONS: CONTROL OF BREATHING, RESPIRATORY FAILURE, AND EXERCISE

APPENDICES

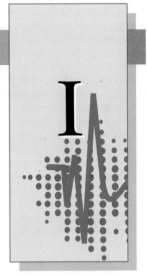

STRUCTURAL–FUNCTIONAL CORRELATES OF THE LUNGS, AIRWAYS, AND CHEST WALL

Lippincott's Pathophysiology Series: Pulmonary Pathophysiology, edited by Michael A. Grippi. J. B. Lippincott Company, Philadelphia © 1995.

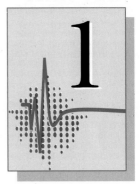

Structure of the Airways and Lung Parenchyma

Michael A. Grippi

The role of the lung is gas exchange—the extraction of oxygen from the environment and elimination of carbon dioxide. These processes are necessary for cellular metabolism. Multiple organ functions must be integrated and coordinated for successful gas exchange. Ambient gas is pumped to the gas exchanging surfaces of the lung, while carbon dioxide–laden alveolar gas is eliminated by the same pumping mechanism. The pulmonary circulation provides blood flow through the lungs for continuous uptake and delivery of oxygen and, at the same time, unloads carbon dioxide into the alveoli. Furthermore, exquisite coupling between ventilation and circulation is essential for maximal efficiency of gas exchange. Finally, the gas exchange system must be monitored, controlled, and continuously fine tuned to cope with wide variations in metabolic demand, such as during exercise and in a variety of disease states.

In addition to its primary role in gas exchange, the lung serves a number of metabolic functions. These include production of surfactant and other compounds and metabolism of a variety of chemical mediators. Derangements in these functions can have a profound impact on the lung's ability to carry out gas exchange.

Normally, the lung is remarkably able to maintain appropriate levels of oxygen uptake and carbon dioxide elimination in a variety of circumstances. Lung disease, however, can selectively or universally affect the individual physiologic steps involved in gas exchange. For example, the obstructive airway diseases (see Chaps. 5 and 6) impede gas flow into and out of the alveoli, whereas the restrictive lung diseases (see Chap. 7) disturb the relationship between ventilation and blood flow or create a barrier for diffusion of gas.

The function of the lung is closely coupled to its structure; that is, form follows function. This chapter provides an overview of lung structure. The configuration of the thorax and its contents are described before airway and alveolar structure is considered. Anatomic relationships among the airways, alveoli, and pulmonary circulation are then reviewed. Finally, brief mention is made of the pulmonary lymphatic system and lung and airway innervation.

OVERALL CONFIGURATION OF THE THORAX AND ITS CONTENTS

The lungs are encompassed by the chest wall on all sides and by the diaphragm inferiorly (Fig. 1-1). The gas-exchanging function of the lungs is profoundly affected by the mechanical properties of the chest wall and diaphragm, as discussed in Chapter 2. Movement of the lungs within the thoracic cavity during inspiration and expiration is facilitated by a space between the two structures—the *pleural space*—created by apposition of the inner lining surface of the chest wall, the *parietal pleura,* and the outer lining surface of the lung, the *visceral pleura.* A thin film of fluid separates the parietal and visceral pleurae and serves as a lubricant. The precise mechanism for pleural fluid formation remains unknown. Removal of the fluid depends, in part, on the pulmonary lymphatic system. Changes in pressure within the pleural space help to determine inspiratory and expiratory airflow in healthy and diseased lungs (see Chap. 2).

The pleural "envelopes" surrounding each lung extend medially to create the *mediastinum,* a centrally located anatomic compartment containing the major

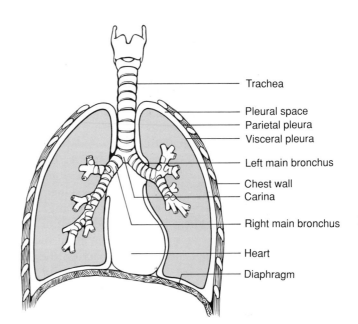

Figure 1-1. Anatomic relationships of the lungs, chest wall, diaphragm, pleural space, and central airways. The pleural space is created by apposition of the visceral and parietal pleurae.

airways and great vessels, including the pulmonary arteries and veins. The main bronchi and pulmonary arteries and veins penetrate each lung at the *hila* (Fig. 1-2). The point of bifurcation of the trachea into left and right main bronchi—the *carina*—lies in close proximity to the aortic arch and the division of the main pulmonary artery into branches supplying the left and right lungs. The *phrenic nerves,* derived from the third, fourth, and fifth cervical nerve roots, innervate the diaphragm and lie along the lateral aspects of the trachea.

AIRWAY STRUCTURE AS RELATED TO FUNCTION

The airways may be viewed as a series of dichotomously branching tubes; each "parent" airway gives rise to two "daughter" branches (Fig. 1-3). On average, there are 23 generations of airways in the human lung. The first 16 are known as *conducting* airways because they provide a conduit for gas flow to and from the gas-exchanging regions of the lung. These airways include bronchi, bronchioles, and terminal bronchioles. The last seven generations include the respiratory bronchioles, alveolar ducts, and alveolar sacs, all of which give rise to alveoli. The first-order respiratory bronchiole ($z = 17$ in Fig. 1-3) and all its distal gas-exchanging airways constitute a pulmonary *acinus.*

The structure of the walls of the conducting airways is quite different from that of the gas-exchanging regions (Fig. 1-4). The walls of the conducting airways are made up of three principal areas: the inner mucosal surface; the smooth muscle layer, separated from the mucosa by submucosal connective tissue; and the outer connective tissue layer, which, in large bronchi, contains cartilage. There are important functional correlates of this airway wall structure, and common clinical disorders are characterized by alterations in one or more components, as discussed in Chapters 5 and 6.

The bronchial epithelium is *pseudostratified,* containing tall cells and shorter

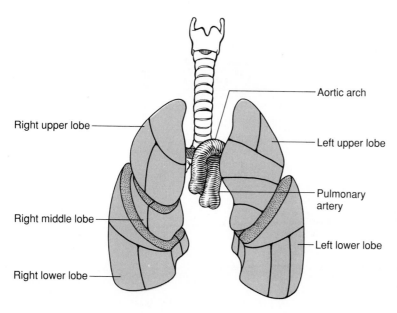

Right upper lobe

Right middle lobe

Right lower lobe

Aortic arch

Left upper lobe

Pulmonary artery

Left lower lobe

Figure 1-2. Relationship between major airways and great vessels in the chest. In the mediastinum, the trachea divides at the carina into left and right main bronchi, which lie near the aortic arch and pulmonary artery. The phrenic nerves, not shown in the figure, descend along both sides of the trachea and continue in a caudal direction, innervating the two hemidiaphragms. Three lobes constitute the right lung and two the left, including a subdivision of the left upper lobe, the lingula. Each lobe is completely or partially enveloped by visceral pleura and contains two to five segments, the borders of which are shown schematically by the thick lines within each lobe.

Figure 1-3. The tracheobronchial tree as a system of dichotomously branching tubes. The conducting zone, made up of the first 16 generations of airways to the level of the terminal bronchioles (z = 0–16), does not participate in gas exchange. The transitional and respiratory zones, in which gas exchange occurs, include the respiratory bronchioles, alveolar ducts, alveolar sacs, and alveoli (z = 17–23). (From Weibel ER. Geometry and dimensions of airways of conductive and transitory zones. In: Morphometry of the Human Lung. New York: Springer-Verlag, 1963:111.)

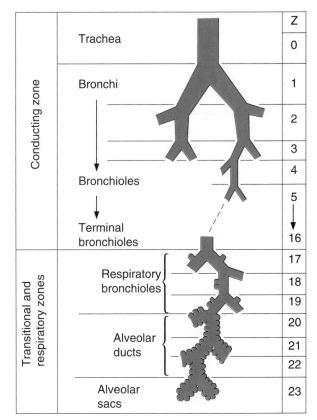

Figure 1-4. Airway wall structure: bronchus, bronchiole, alveolus. The bronchial wall contains ciliated pseudostratified epithelium, smooth muscle cells, mucus glands, connective tissue, and cartilage. In smaller bronchioles, a simple epithelium is found; cartilage is absent, and the wall is thinner. The alveolar wall is designed primarily for gas exchange, rather than structural support. (From Weibel ER, Taylor RC. Design and structure of the human lung. In: Fishman AP, ed. Pulmonary Diseases and Disorders, Vol. 1. New York: McGraw-Hill, 1988:14.)

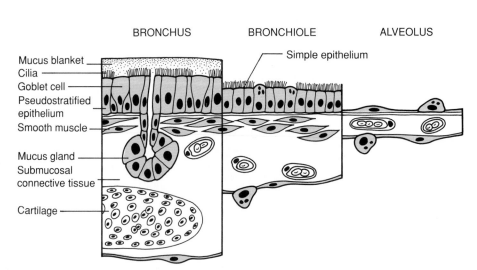

basal cells, each of which is attached to the basement membrane. In the bronchioles, a *simple epithelium* is present. Airway epithelial cells have cilia at their apical surfaces; the cilia are important elements of the *mucociliary escalator*. The cilia beat in the direction of the airway opening, propelling a blanket of mucus secreted by goblet cells, which are interposed between ciliated epithelial cells. The mucociliary escalator is an important airway clearance mechanism and part of the respiratory host defense system.

Airway smooth muscle lies in continuous bundles within the submucosal connective tissue, extending from the major bronchi to the respiratory bronchioles. Muscle bundles extend into the gas-exchanging regions as well, lying in the walls at the openings of alveoli.

STRUCTURE OF THE GAS-EXCHANGING REGION

The gas-exchanging region must permit efficient diffusion of oxygen and carbon dioxide across alveolar and capillary walls. At the same time, it must support gas exchange over a lifetime and withstand the mechanical forces of lung inflation, deflation, and pulmonary blood flow. The apposition of vascular endothelium and alveolar epithelium in a supportive connective tissue stroma appears ideally suited to fulfill these requirements (Fig. 1-5).

The alveolar epithelium consists of two types of cells: squamous lining cells (type I cells) and secretory cells (type II cells). Type I cells, although significantly fewer in number than type II cells, account for 95% of the alveolar surface area. Type II cells produce and secrete *surfactant*, a substance composed of proteins and phospholipids, which spreads along the alveolar surface and lowers surface tension (see Chap. 2).

The capillary endothelium also consists of a layer of squamous lining cells that rest on the endothelial basement membrane. In parts of the alveoli, the basement membranes of the epithelium and endothelium are fused, creating an ultrathin barrier for gas exchange (see Chap. 9). Unlike the "tight" junctions between adjacent epithelial cells, which constitute a tight seal, the junctions between endothelial cells are "leaky," allowing water and solutes to move back and

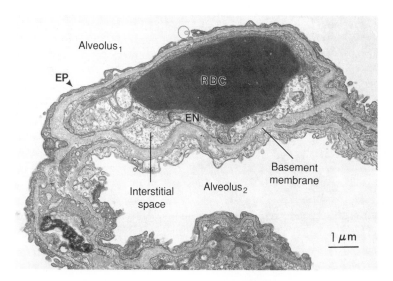

Figure 1-5. The alveolar–capillary membrane. Two adjacent alveoli are shown. Fusion of the basement membranes of the epithelial, type I cell (EP), and endothelial cell (EN) near Alveolus$_1$ creates an ultrathin barrier to diffusion of oxygen and carbon dioxide between the alveolar space and capillary. Near Alveolus$_2$, the epithelial and endothelial cells are separated by the interstitial space. The interstitial space is a potential site for collection of fluid. RBC, red blood cell. (Photomicrograph courtesy of Giuseppe G. Pietra, M.D.)

forth between plasma and the *interstitial space,* the region between epithelial and endothelial basement membranes (see Chap. 14).

Additional cell types exist within the interstitium, including macrophages and lymphocytes, cells important in host defense. These cells are discussed in more detail in Chapter 7.

GAS FLOW IN AIRWAYS

As a series of dichotomously branching tubes, the airways present a somewhat complex route for gas movement to and from the gas-exchanging regions. Although the diameter of each daughter branch is less than the diameter of the parent airway from which it is derived, the total cross-sectional area of each successive airway generation *increases* because of a marked increase in the number of airways (Fig. 1-6).

In the human lung, the airway diameter for each airway generation (z) can be estimated according to the following equation:

$$d(z) = d_0 \cdot 2^{-z/3} \qquad\qquad [1\text{-}1]$$

where

$$d(z) = \text{diameter of airway generation z}$$
$$d_0 = \text{diameter of the trachea (airway generation ''0'')}$$

Figure 1-7 shows the average diameter of each generation of human airways.

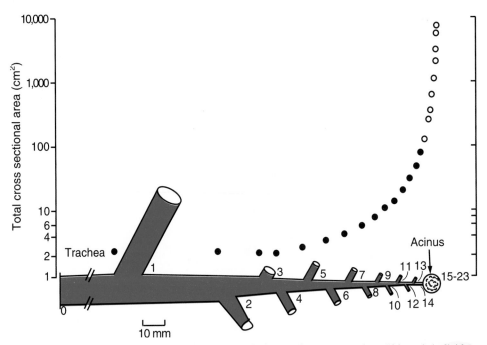

Figure 1-6. Total airway cross-sectional area in relation to airway generation. Although individual airway cross-sectional area decreases in successive airway generations, total cross-sectional area increases markedly because of an increase in the number of airways. (From Weibel ER. Design of the airways and blood vessels considered as branching trees. In: Crystal RG, West JB, eds. The Lung: Scientific Foundations. New York: Raven Press, 1991:717.)

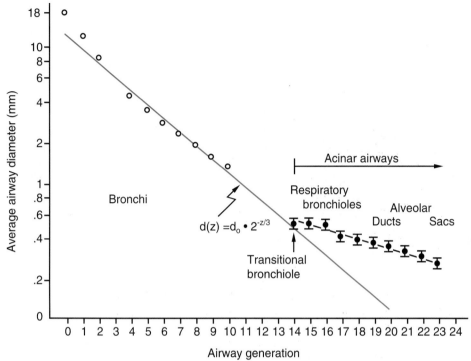

Figure 1-7. Average airway diameter as a function of airway generation. Individual airway diameter decreases in each successive generation of airways. For larger airways, to the level of the terminal bronchioles, airway diameter in a given generation (z) can be predicted if the diameter of the trachea (d_0) is known. (From Haefeli-Bleuer B, Weibel ER. Morphometry of the human pulmonary acinus. Anat Rec 220:413, 1988.)

The factors determining rates and patterns of airflow in the conducting airways, including airway diameter, are discussed in Chapter 2. As the total cross-sectional area of the airways increases in successive airway generations, gas flow rates actually decrease. Eventually, at the level of the respiratory bronchioles, gas movement occurs primarily by diffusion (see Chap. 9), rather than by "bulk flow."

PULMONARY CIRCULATION IN RELATION TO AIRWAYS

In general, the overall distribution of the pulmonary arteries and veins follows a pattern similar to that of the airways (Fig. 1-8). Pulmonary arteries tend to be paired with bronchi of similar size; the parallels are less evident for pulmonary veins. In addition to pulmonary arteries and veins, the lungs possess a *bronchial circulation,* with bronchial arteries arising from the aorta and intercostal arteries. The pulmonary circulation is described in Chapter 12, and important functional relationships between the pulmonary circulation and distal airways are discussed in Chapter 13.

PULMONARY LYMPHATICS

Pulmonary lymphatics constitute an important system for coping with extravascular fluid in the lung, in both health and disease states (see Chap. 14).

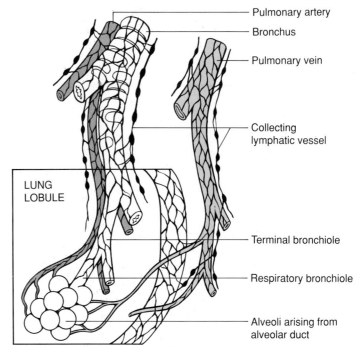

Figure 1-8. Anatomic relationship of airways, pulmonary arteries, pulmonary veins, and lymphatics. Arteries and airways of similar size are "paired." The relationship between airways and pulmonary veins is not as close. (From Nagaishe C, Nagasawa N, Okado Y, Yamashita M, Inaba N. Functional Anatomy and Histology of the Lung. Baltimore: University Park Press, 1972:148.)

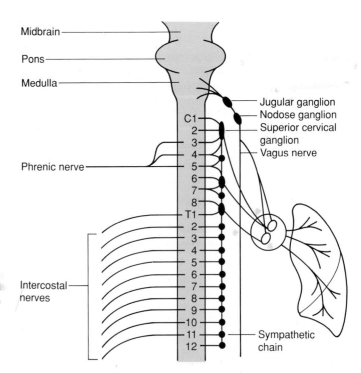

Figure 1-9. Innervation of the lungs. The phrenic and intercostal nerves provide motoneuron output to the principal muscles of respiration. Sympathetic and parasympathetic nerves innervate the lung, playing important roles in control of airway diameter and rates of airflow, and in conveying information about lung inflation.

The lymphatics lie along the visceral pleural surface and within the pulmonary parenchyma, where they are in close approximation to the pulmonary arteries, veins, and airways (see Fig. 1-8). The lymphatic channels contain numerous valves that promote unidirectional flow of lymph toward the lung hilum. Pulmonary lymphatics drain into lymph nodes that lie around major airways and within the mediastinum.

In addition to maintaining lung fluid balance, the lymphatic system is a key part of the host defense system. Lymphoid tissue is found within airway walls, constituting the bronchus-associated lymphoid tissue. The roles of immune effector cells, including those that are part of the lymphatic system, in mediating lung disease are described in Chapter 7.

INNERVATION OF THE LUNGS AND AIRWAYS

Branches of the vagus nerve and the thoracic sympathetic ganglia innervate the lung (Fig. 1-9). Afferent and efferent neurons play important roles in modulating lung function, including control of airway diameter, as discussed in Chapter 5. In addition, afferent fibers are important in sensing airflow and the degree of lung inflation (see Chap. 16).

SELECTED READING

Haefeli-Bleuer B, Weibel ER. Morphometry of the human pulmonary acinus. Anat Rec 220:401–414, 1988.

Murray JF. The Normal Lung: The Basis for Diagnosis and Treatment of Pulmonary Disease. Philadelphia: WB Saunders, 1986:23–82.

Osmond DG. Functional anatomy of the chest wall. In: Roussos C, Macklem PT, eds. The Thorax (Part A). New York: Marcel Dekker, 1985:199–233.

Weibel ER. Design of the airways and blood vessels considered as branching trees. In: Crystal RG, West JB, eds. The Lung: Scientific Foundations. New York: Raven Press, 1991:711–720.

Lippincott's Pathophysiology Series: Pulmonary Pathophysiology, edited by Michael A. Grippi. J. B. Lippincott Company, Philadelphia © 1995.

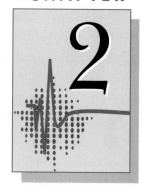

Respiratory Mechanics

Michael A. Grippi

Chapter 1 provides a simple review of thoracic anatomy, including the functional anatomy of the lungs. We now turn our attention to the area of respiratory physiology that deals with the mechanical forces responsible for gas flow into and out of the chest—*pulmonary mechanics.* To accomplish oxygen uptake and carbon dioxide elimination, a fresh supply of gas must be brought repeatedly to the gas-exchanging units (alveoli) by the respiratory pump.

An understanding of the pump mechanism entails a number of considerations:

1. *The respiratory muscles.* Work must be done on the respiratory system to produce gas flow. The respiratory muscles are responsible for performing this work.
2. *The elastic properties of the lung and chest wall.* The lung and chest wall are distensible structures, and their mechanical characteristics are important determinants of the volumes of gas moved and rates of airflow achieved.
3. *The flow-resistive properties of the airways, lung parenchyma, and chest wall.* The resistance to inspiratory and expiratory airflow plays a critical role in determining both the level of ventilation and its pattern. The elastic and flow-resistive properties of the pump constitute the so-called "impedance" of the respiratory system.
4. *The heterogeneity of ventilation.* Ventilation is not uniform throughout the lung, even in healthy subjects. An understanding of this nonuniformity is based on knowledge of the interaction of a variety of mechanical forces operative in the respiratory system.
5. *The work of breathing.* The work performed by the respiratory muscles

is determined by the change in thoracic volume that occurs with each breath and the pressures generated. Work of breathing is an intuitive concept with important clinical implications.

An alteration in the mechanical properties of the respiratory system is a common finding in many clinically important pulmonary disorders. In fact, a change in mechanical properties may be the principal pathophysiologic feature of a patient's illness (e.g., an increase in airway resistance during an episode of acute asthma). On the other hand, a change in the mechanical properties of the respiratory system may be simply one manifestation of a multifaceted disease in which gas exchange, pulmonary blood flow, and other physiologic processes are also affected (e.g., congestive heart failure or pulmonary fibrosis).

The goals of this chapter are (1) to provide a basis for understanding respiratory mechanics in health and disease; (2) to provide a rationale for therapeutic measures used commonly in pulmonary medicine (e.g., use of bronchodilators in asthma and mechanical ventilation in respiratory failure); and (3) to elaborate the substrate on which many clinical tests of lung function are based.

THE RESPIRATORY MUSCLES

In a spontaneously breathing subject, *inspiratory muscle activity* is required to overcome the impedance of the respiratory system. The most important inspiratory muscle is the diaphragm, a dome-shaped skeletal muscle that separates the thoracic and abdominal cavities. The diaphragm consists of two discrete regions: the *costal* portion, which inserts on the ribs, and the *crural* portion, which surrounds central organs (e.g., the esophagus) and has no rib insertions. Under conditions of quiet breathing, the diaphragm is the only operative inspiratory muscle. When additional ventilation is required, such as during exercise or in disease states like asthma, other muscles become active. These include the external intercostals, the scalenes, and the sternocleidomastoids. The latter two muscles are called *accessory muscles of respiration*.

Unlike inspiration, expiration is normally a passive phenomenon; the elastic recoil of the lung and chest wall account for the generation of an expiratory pressure gradient for flow (see sections on Elastic Properties of the Respiratory System and Flow-Resistive Properties of the Respiratory System, later). When airway obstruction develops, expiration becomes an active process, requiring work by expiratory muscles, including the internal intercostals and the abdominals (external and internal oblique, transverse abdominis, and rectus abdominis). Additional expiratory muscles have been recognized: the glottic muscles and the diaphragm. The glottic muscles narrow the glottis during expiration, providing a brake on expiratory airflow; early expiratory contraction of the diaphragm further brakes expiration. This braking action is operative during quiet breathing and opposes the expiratory action of the static elastic recoil pressure generated during the previous inspiration.

DETERMINANTS OF RESPIRATORY MUSCLE TENSION

As with other skeletal muscles, the respiratory muscles are characterized by length–tension, force–frequency, and force–velocity relationships. In addition, because the diaphragm is dome shaped, special consideration must be given to

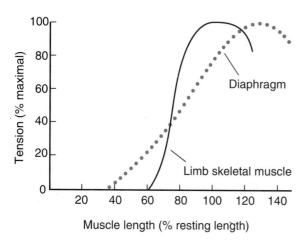

Figure 2-1. Length–tension relationships for limb skeletal muscle and the diaphragm. The limb muscle's maximal tension is generated at its resting length. The diaphragm's maximal tension is generated at approximately 130% of its resting length.

the relationship between pressure and radius of curvature, as described by Laplace's law (see below).

The force generated by a limb skeletal muscle is a function of its length (Fig. 2-1). For a constant level of stimulation, maximal tension is generated at the muscle's resting length. Any shortening or stretching of the muscle before stimulation results in generation of submaximal tension. Unlike limb skeletal muscle, however, the diaphragm generates peak force at approximately 130% of its resting length. The decline in force generated with decreasing muscle length, which corresponds to an increase in resting lung volume, assumes clinical importance. For example, in chronic obstructive pulmonary disease, which includes chronic bronchitis and emphysema (see Chap. 6), hyperinflation of the lung produces flattening of the diaphragm. The flattened diaphragm has a shorter length and, hence, produces less force. It operates at a mechanical disadvantage.

The force of contraction is also a function of the frequency of muscle fiber stimulation and the velocity of fiber shortening (Fig. 2-2). Up to a point, force generation increases with increasing stimulation frequency. Thereafter, force remains constant, despite further increases in stimulus frequency (see Fig. 2-2A). On the other hand, less tension is generated with higher velocities of muscle shortening (see Fig. 2-2B). The clinical implication of the latter relationship is that for a given level of stimulation of the respiratory muscles, less force is generated at higher airflow rates, because higher airflow rates correlate with greater velocities of muscle shortening.

In addition to these fundamental relationships, the unique geometry of the diaphragm as a curved muscle must be considered. Laplace's law describes the relationship between pressure, tension, and radius of curvature:

$$P = 2T/r \qquad\qquad [2\text{-}1]$$

where

P = pressure generated by muscle
T = muscle tension
r = radius of curvature

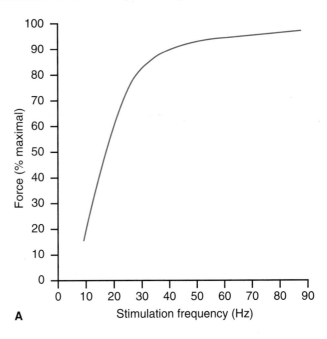

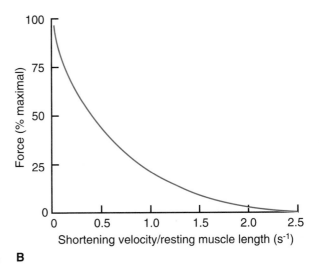

Figure 2-2. Force–frequency and force–velocity relationships of skeletal muscle. **(A)** Force–frequency relationship. Up to a point, force increases as stimulus frequency increases. Thereafter, force remains constant despite increasing stimulation frequency. Force is expressed as a percentage of the maximal force that can be generated. **(B)** Force–velocity relationship. Force declines as the velocity of shortening increases. Velocity is expressed as the ratio of actual velocity to resting muscle length.

As the diaphragm flattens, the radius of curvature increases and pressure generation decreases (Fig. 2-3). This effect, along with muscle shortening, contributes to a decline in diaphragm strength in patients with hyperinflation due to chronic obstructive pulmonary disease.

TRANSDIAPHRAGMATIC PRESSURE

Respiratory muscle activity results in ventilation by producing a conformational change in the chest wall. Specifically, during quiet inspiration, descent of

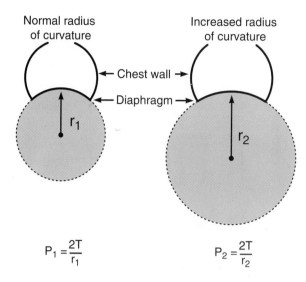

Figure 2-3. Effect of changes in radius of curvature on pressure generation by the diaphragm, according to Laplace's law. Normal radius of curvature on the left. Increased radius of curvature due to flattening of the diaphragm on the right. As the diaphragm flattens, it subtends a greater radius of curvature ($r_2 > r_1$). For equal tension (T), the pressure generated by the flattened muscle is less than that generated by the normally curved muscle ($P_2 < P_1$).

the diaphragm (flattening of its dome) causes the lower rib cage to enlarge transversely and anteroposteriorly. As a result, intrathoracic pressure falls (becomes negative) and the lung expands as air enters the thoracic cavity along the negative pressure gradient created. As intrathoracic pressure falls, abdominal pressure rises, because downward motion of the diaphragm compresses the abdominal contents. Intrathoracic pressure is usually measured as pleural pressure (see section on Pressure Relationships in the Respiratory System). *Transdiaphragmatic pressure*, the difference between abdominal pressure and pleural pressure (Fig. 2-4), is calculated as:

$$Pdi = Pab - Ppl \qquad [2\text{-}2]$$

where

$$Pdi = \text{transdiaphragmatic pressure}$$
$$Pab = \text{abdominal pressure}$$
$$Ppl = \text{pleural pressure}$$

The generation of a positive transdiaphragmatic pressure indicates active contraction of the diaphragm. When the diaphragm is paralyzed or fatigued, it may move upward into the chest cavity during inspiration as other inspiratory muscles contract and create a negative intrathoracic pressure. Consequently, transdiaphragmatic pressure remains at zero. Measurement of transdiaphragmatic pressure is the most definitive way of diagnosing bilateral diaphragm paralysis. Diaphragm paralysis may arise from a number of disorders, including disease of the medulla or phrenic motor nucleus, demyelinating diseases of peripheral nerves (e.g., Guillain-Barré syndrome), diseases of the neuromuscular junction (e.g., myasthenia gravis), or primary diseases of muscle (e.g., muscular dystrophy).

As noted, a low transdiaphragmatic pressure may also be seen with diaphragm fatigue. Under basal conditions, the diaphragm and other muscles of respiration consume less than 5% of the body's total oxygen consumption. When high ventilatory requirements exist (e.g., during exercise or in the clinical setting of pneumonia in a patient with emphysema), the oxygen requirements of the

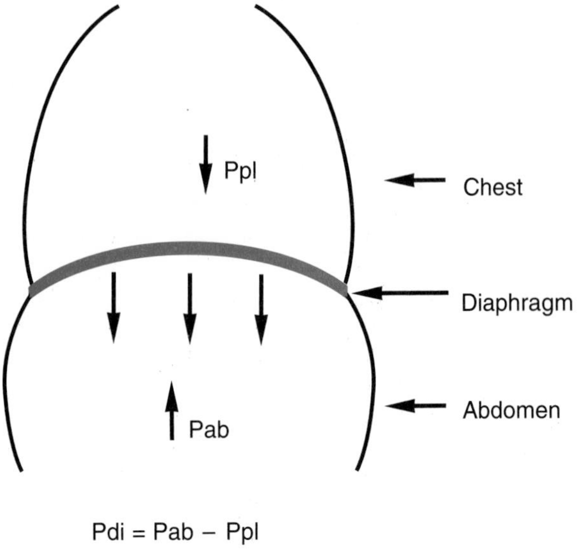

Figure 2-4. Concept of transdiaphragmatic pressure (Pdi). Pdi is the pressure generated across the diaphragm during inspiration. It is calculated as the difference between intraabdominal pressure (Pab) and pleural pressure (Ppl). As the diaphragm contracts and descends into the abdomen, Ppl falls and Pab rises. Pab is measured using an intragastric balloon catheter; Ppl is approximated using an intraesophageal balloon catheter.

Pdi = Pab − Ppl

respiratory muscles represent a substantial component of overall oxygen consumption. The excessive oxygen requirement, in conjunction with less well understood factors, may result in respiratory muscle fatigue (see Chap. 18). This is evident as an increased respiratory rate, paradoxical diaphragm and abdominal wall movement (inward motion of the anterior abdominal wall during inspiration as the diaphragm is drawn upward into the chest cavity by negative pressure), and, eventually, a rise in arterial carbon dioxide tension (Pa_{CO_2}).

PRESSURE RELATIONSHIPS IN THE RESPIRATORY SYSTEM

In the analyses that follow, it is important to have a frame of reference for the various pressures responsible for airflow, or lack thereof. These pressures are depicted schematically in Figure 2-5.

Pao is the pressure at the airway opening (e.g., the mouth). Under normal circumstances, at times of no airflow (at end-inspiration and end-expiration) and when the airway is open to the atmosphere, Pao is zero. Pbs is the pressure at the body surface, normally atmospheric. (Some mechanical ventilators create a negative pressure at the body surface by generating a vacuum around the patient's trunk. Under these circumstances, Pbs is intermittently less than zero.) Ppl is *pleural pressure*, that is, the pressure within the pleural space. Its magnitude depends on the magnitudes and directions of the forces generated by the elastic lung parenchyma and chest wall. Ppl can be measured using a balloon catheter placed within the esophagus because changes in intraesophageal pressure during respiration closely approximate changes in intrapleural pressure. The pressure created by the elastic lung parenchyma is not depicted in Figure 2-5; it is directed inward and is called the *elastic recoil pressure*, Pel. *Alveolar pressure*, Palv, is the pressure within alveoli. It may be negative (during inspiration), positive (during expiration), or zero (at end-inspiration and end-expiration), when there is no airflow and the glottis is open to atmosphere. The alveolar pressure is the sum of elastic recoil pressure and pleural pressure:

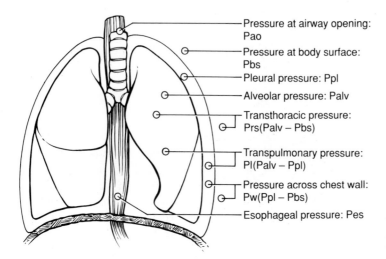

Pressure at airway opening: Pao

Pressure at body surface: Pbs

Pleural pressure: Ppl

Alveolar pressure: Palv

Transthoracic pressure: Prs(Palv – Pbs)

Transpulmonary pressure: Pl(Palv – Ppl)

Pressure across chest wall: Pw(Ppl – Pbs)

Esophageal pressure: Pes

Figure 2-5. Schematic representation of the pressures and pressure gradients responsible for airflow. See text for details.

$$\text{Palv} = \text{Pel} + \text{Ppl} \qquad [2\text{-}3]$$

Pl is pressure across the lung—*transpulmonary pressure*. It represents the pressure necessary to produce airflow and to maintain a given level of lung inflation. Ppl is the difference between alveolar and pleural pressures (Pl = Palv − Ppl). Pw is the *pressure across the chest wall,* that is, the difference between pleural pressure and pressure at the body surface (Pw = Ppl − Pbs). Prs is *transthoracic pressure,* the pressure across the entire respiratory system. It represents the difference between alveolar pressure and pressure at the body surface (Prs = Palv − Pbs).

With this framework at hand, the elastic properties of the lung, chest wall, and respiratory system as a whole will now be examined.

ELASTIC PROPERTIES OF THE RESPIRATORY SYSTEM

When the inspiratory muscles contract, a pressure gradient is created between the atmosphere and alveoli, resulting in airflow. The pressure gradient overcomes: (1) the elastic recoil of the respiratory system, (2) the frictional resistance to flow in the airways, and (3) the inertial resistance of the tracheobronchial air column, lung, and chest wall. These three terms are expressed in the *equation of motion of the lung:*

$$\text{Ptot} = (E \cdot \Delta V) + (R \cdot \dot{V}) + (I \cdot \ddot{V}) \qquad [2\text{-}4]$$

where

Ptot = driving pressure
E   = elastance
ΔV   = change in lung volume
R   = resistance
$\dot{V}$ = airflow rate
I   = inertance
$\ddot{V}$ = rate of change of airflow rate (acceleration)

The individual terms of the equation are considered in the sections that follow.

The first term, $(E \cdot \Delta V)$, represents the pressure necessary to overcome the elastic recoil of the respiratory system. It is simplest to first analyze separately the elastic properties of the lung and the chest wall, and then to integrate these two structures into a single functional unit.

THE LUNG

As an analogy to lung inflation, consider an elastic balloon. To inflate a balloon, a pressure gradient must be developed across its wall (equivalent to transpulmonary pressure). This gradient may be generated by applying a negative pressure around the balloon after placing it in a jar from which air can be removed using a vacuum pump. Alternatively, a positive pressure may be created inside the balloon from a positive pressure source, such as a tank of compressed air. In either case, once the balloon is inflated, removal of the source of negative or positive pressure permits the balloon to deflate rapidly because of its intrinsic elastic recoil.

A more physiologic model is the excised lung (Fig. 2-6). Figure 2-6A shows a lung enclosed in a jar, with the airway opening connected to a *spirometer*, a device that measures changes in lung volume. The (negative) pressure in the jar is measured using a manometer. As air in the jar is evacuated, the lung expands due to an increasing transpulmonary pressure. A series of stepwise increases in inflation pressure (actually, progressive decreases in surrounding pressure) is made and the corresponding lung volumes are noted. After maximal inflation, the vacuum in the jar is released in stepwise fashion and, once again, the corresponding lung volumes are recorded. In this way, a static *pressure–volume curve* is generated; measurements of pressure and volume are made at times of no airflow (see Fig. 2-6B).

A number of important points should be made about these curves. An obvious feature is that there are two distinct curves, one for inspiration and another for expiration. A greater transpulmonary pressure is required to attain a given lung volume during inflation than during deflation. This difference between inspiratory and expiratory pressure–volume curves represents *hysteresis*, a property of all elastic structures. An additional important finding is that the curves do not pass through the origin—the y-intercept is not zero. This indicates that there is a small, but measurable, volume of gas within the lung even when there is no distending pressure applied. Indeed, when a human lung is removed from the thoracic cavity at autopsy or during surgery, the lung is not gasless.

Lung Compliance

Examination of Figure 2-6B also reveals that the relationship between pressure and change in volume is not constant over the entire range of lung volume. At low lung volume, the relationship can be expressed as:

$$P = E \cdot \Delta V \tag{2-5}$$

where

P = distending pressure
E = elastance
ΔV = change in lung volume

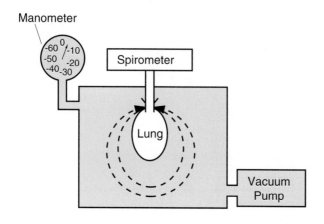

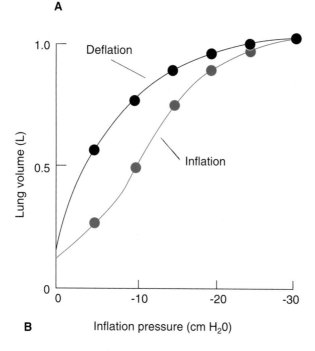

Figure 2-6. Generation of pressure–volume (P–V) curves from an excised lung. **(A)** Inflation is achieved by evacuating air from the container in which the lung is placed. Pressures are noted on the manometer, and lung volumes, or, more precisely, changes in lung volume, are measured with the spirometer. **(B)** Inspiratory and expiratory P–V curves. The points used to construct the curves are determined at times of no airflow. Therefore, these are static P–V curves. The lower curve is generated during stepwise inflation and the upper curve during stepwise deflation. See text for details.

Elastance, a constant, is a measure of tissue elasticity. As elastance increases, the distending pressure required to achieve a given change in volume increases.

At high lung volume, greater distending pressure is required to produce a given change in lung volume. At maximal lung volume, further increments in distending pressure produce no further change in volume; that is, the pressure–volume curve is flat. The change in volume per unit change in pressure—the slope of the pressure-volume curve at any point—is called *static compliance* (Cstat). It is a measure of the distensibility of the lung and is the reciprocal of elastance (E = 1/Cstat). The lung is more compliant at low and moderate volumes than at high volumes.

A number of factors affect static lung compliance, including lung size. A larger lung undergoes a greater change in volume per unit change in pressure than a smaller lung. For comparative purposes, one can "normalize" for the

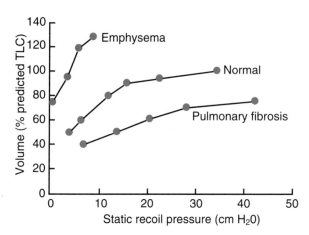

Figure 2-7. Pressure–volume curves in health and disease states. The static recoil pressure of the lung (equal to transpulmonary and pleural pressures under no-flow conditions) is plotted on the abscissa. Lung volume is plotted on the ordinate and is expressed as percent predicted TLC. For the hyperinflated lungs of emphysema, TLC is greater than 100% predicted; for the small lungs of pulmonary fibrosis, TLC is less than 100% predicted. In addition, the slope of the curve for emphysema is increased, whereas that for pulmonary fibrosis is reduced.

effect of lung size on compliance. The normalized compliance is known as *specific compliance,* calculated as the static compliance divided by the lung volume at which it is measured. Clinically, static compliance measurements are made from the expiratory pressure–volume curve over a volume range extending from end-expiratory lung volume *(functional residual capacity,* FRC) to a volume 500 ml above FRC. Normal adult static lung compliance is approximately 200 ml/cm H_2O or 0.2 L/cm H_2O.

Pathologic conditions produce increases or decreases in static lung compliance. Emphysema, characterized by loss of connective tissue components in the lung and loss of alveoli, produces increased static lung compliance (see Chap. 6). Pulmonary fibrosis (see Chap. 7), congestive heart failure (pulmonary edema), lung hemorrhage, and pneumonia produce decreased static lung compliance. Representative pressure–volume curves for the healthy state and selected pathologic conditions are shown in Figure 2-7.

The pressure term in the pressure–volume relationships described thus far is transpulmonary pressure. Under static conditions, with the glottis open to atmosphere, Palv is zero, and Pl = Ppl. Ppl, in turn, equals static elastic recoil pressure (Pel). What are the factors that determine the elastic recoil of the lung? One factor is elastic tissue content. Both elastin and collagen are present in alveolar walls and around bronchi and blood vessels. The geometric arrangement of these fibers imparts elastic properties to the lungs, analogous to the effect of a complicated arrangement of nylon fibers in a stocking. An additional factor important in determining pressure–volume relationships in the lung is surface tension.

Surface Tension

Surface tension is the force generated at the surface of a liquid–gas interface (Fig. 2-8A). Surface tension arises when *cohesive* forces between molecules in the liquid phase exceed *adhesive* forces between molecules in the liquid and gas phases. As a result, the liquid's surface area is minimal.

As an analogy, consider a soap bubble. Surface forces in a soap bubble tend to minimize the bubble's surface area, producing a positive pressure within the bubble (see Fig. 2-8A). Laplace's law can be used to calculate the pressure generated. According to Laplace's law, the smaller the radius of the bubble, the

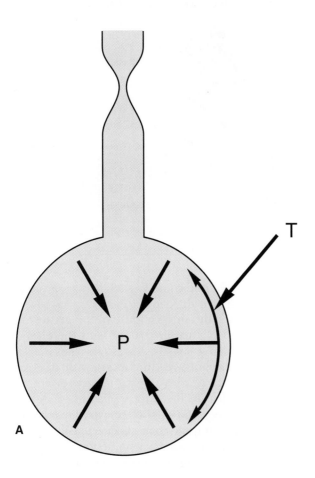

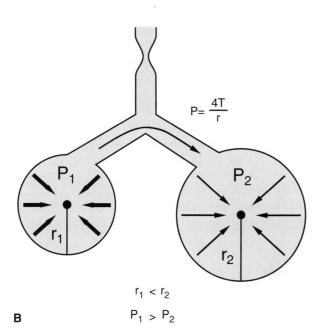

$$P = \frac{4T}{r}$$

Figure 2-8. Surface tension and bubble pressure. **(A)** Surface tension (T) in a soap bubble. Forces active at the surface of the bubble tend to minimize surface area and promote collapse, creating a positive pressure (P) within the bubble. **(B)** Laplace's law. For a given surface tension, a smaller bubble will deflate into a larger one, because the smaller radius of curvature ($r_1 < r_2$) results in a higher pressure ($P_1 > P_2$) in the smaller bubble. (For calculation of P in a structure with a *single* liquid–gas interface, Laplace's law becomes $P = 2T/r$.)

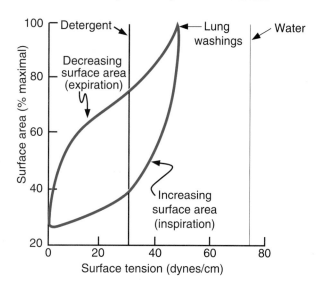

Figure 2-9. The relationship between surface tension and surface area (expressed as percent maximal area) for water, water with a detergent added, and surfactant-containing fluid washed out of the lung. Surface tension is measured using a surface balance. When added to water, the detergent markedly lowers surface tension. However, as for water, surface tension remains constant and independent of surface area. For the surfactant-containing fluid, surface tension varies as a function of surface area. It declines to almost zero when the surface area is small. In addition, surface tension varies according to whether the measurement is made as the surface area is being enlarged (inspiration) or reduced (expiration); that is, it shows hysteresis. (Adapted from Clements JA, Tierney DF. Alveolar instability associated with altered surface tension. In: Handbook of Physiology, Respiration. Section 3, Vol. II. Fenn WO, Rahn H, eds. Bethesda, MD: American Physiological Society, 1988:1568.)

greater is the pressure. Similarly, the greater the surface tension, the greater is the pressure (see Fig. 2-8B). What does all of this have to do with the elastic properties of the lung?

Surface tension forces operative in the lung act in concert with natural tissue elastic recoil to promote alveolar collapse. This surface tension effect is, however, modified by a remarkable substance in the lung, *surfactant,* secreted by type II alveolar epithelial cells. Surfactant, composed of phospholipids and proteins, lines the alveolar surface and lowers intraalveolar surface tension. Surfactant has two unique properties: (1) it produces a greater reduction in surface tension at smaller surface areas (i.e., at smaller lung volumes); and (2) it is more effective in lowering surface tension during expiration than inspiration (Fig. 2-9).

Surfactant serves several important physiologic roles. First, by lowering surface tension, it increases lung compliance. Second, surfactant stabilizes lung units through two effects: (1) by lowering surface tension to a greater degree at low lung volumes than at high volumes, thereby minimizing collapse of alveoli (atelectasis); and (2) by preventing emptying of smaller alveoli into larger ones as a result of lowering surface tension to a greater extent in the smaller units. The latter offsets the effect of a smaller radius of curvature and an increased pressure. Respiratory distress syndrome of the newborn, also known as *hyaline membrane disease,* is characterized by a deficiency of normal surfactant. Affected infants have stiff, noncompliant lungs that are prone to collapse.

Although the discussion thus far has centered on the isolated lung preparation, structural and functional characteristics of the chest wall are important in any analysis of the mechanics of the respiratory system.

THE CHEST WALL

Like the lung, the chest wall, which includes the bony thorax, intercostal muscles, overlying soft tissue, and parietal pleura, is compressible and distensible. At FRC, the inward elastic recoil of the lung is counterbalanced by the outward elastic recoil of the chest wall. As the volume of the thoracic cavity

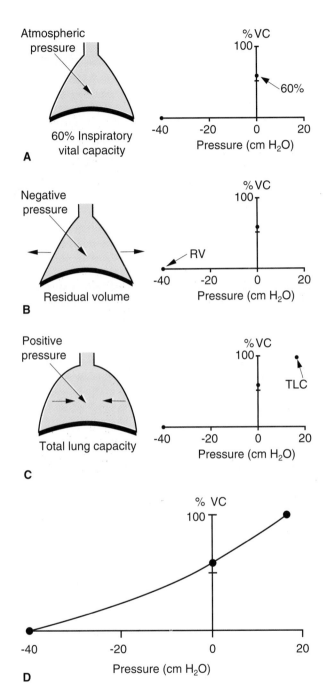

Figure 2-10. Pressure–volume relationship for the isolated chest wall. **(A)** "Resting" position for chest wall. At 60% of the inspired vital capacity (VC), pressure across the chest wall is 0 (atmospheric). **(B)** At volumes between residual volume (RV) and 60% of inspired VC, a negative pressure is generated by the *outward* recoil of the chest wall. **(C)** At volumes between 60% of inspired VC and total lung capacity (TLC), a positive pressure is generated by the *inward* recoil of the chest wall. **(D)** Pressure–volume curve for the chest wall between RV and TLC. See text for details.

enlarges from FRC to its maximal volume (*total lung capacity,* TLC), the outward recoil tendency of the chest wall decreases. At approximately 60% of the inspired vital capacity (the maximal amount of air that can be inspired from the smallest lung volume—residual volume), chest wall recoil becomes zero. Further thoracic expansion is accompanied by the development of an inwardly directed chest wall recoil. The pressure–volume relationship for the isolated chest wall is shown in Figure 2-10. The abscissa denotes pressure across the chest wall (Ppl − Pbs).

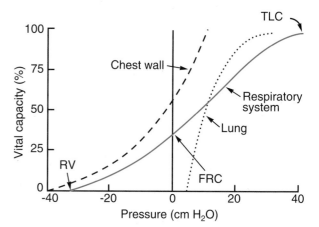

Figure 2-11. Pressure–volume curves for the lung, chest wall, and intact respiratory system. The curve for the intact respiratory system is equivalent to the algebraic sum of the curves for the lung and chest wall. See text for details.

Normal chest wall compliance is approximately 0.2 L/cm H_2O. A number of clinical disorders are characterized by alterations in chest wall compliance, including extreme obesity, extensive pleural fibrosis, and kyphoscoliosis.

THE RESPIRATORY SYSTEM

The lung and chest wall are functionally coupled through the pleural space. As noted, the pressure across the respiratory system, Prs, is the algebraic sum of the pressures across the lung and chest wall:

$$Prs = Pl + Pw \qquad [2\text{-}6]$$

$$= (Palv - Ppl) + (Ppl - Pbs) \qquad [2\text{-}7]$$

$$= Palv - Pbs \qquad [2\text{-}8]$$

The pressure–volume relationships of the lung, chest wall, and total respiratory system are shown in Figure 2-11. The composite curve denotes the pressure that must be generated across the system by respiratory muscles (or a mechanical ventilator) to overcome the static elastic recoil of the lung and chest wall at a particular lung volume. The static compliance of the respiratory system (Crs), normally about 0.1 L/cm H_2O, is calculated as:

$$Crs = \Delta V/Prs = \Delta V/(Pl + Pw) \qquad [2\text{-}9]$$

where

$$\Delta V = \text{change in thoracic volume}$$

At TLC, the inwardly directed elastic recoils of the lung and chest wall sum to generate a large, inwardly directed recoil pressure for the respiratory system. At *residual volume* (RV)—the lung volume after forced expiration from TLC—the outwardly directed elastic recoil of the chest wall far outweighs the small, inwardly directed recoil of the lung, resulting in an outwardly directed recoil pressure for the respiratory system. Of particular note is the relationship between lung and chest wall elastic recoils at FRC. At FRC, lung elastic recoil is equal in magnitude to chest wall recoil, and the two are in opposite directions. The respiratory system therefore "comes to rest" at this volume and remains there until inspiratory or expiratory muscles contract to inflate or deflate the system.

Thus far, emphasis has been placed on the "static" nature of the measurements. Relationships between pressure and volume have been determined at times of no airflow. Obviously, with inspiration and expiration, airflow occurs. Therefore, any analysis of respiratory mechanics must take into account the flow-resistive properties of the respiratory system.

FLOW-RESISTIVE PROPERTIES OF THE RESPIRATORY SYSTEM

In the equation of motion of the lung,

$$Ptot = (E \cdot \Delta V) + (R \cdot \dot{V}) + (I \cdot \ddot{V})$$

the static component, $(E \cdot \Delta V)$, is only one of three terms. The last term, $(I \cdot \ddot{V})$, the pressure required to overcome inertial resistance, is quantitatively small and, for practical purposes, can be neglected (it refers to the force required to accelerate the tracheobronchial air column and lung and chest wall tissues from their resting, motionless state). The middle term, $(R \cdot \dot{V})$, denotes the pressure necessary to overcome the resistance to airflow. The following discussion centers on the flow-resistive properties of the respiratory system, as summarized in this term. First, patterns of airflow in the tracheobronchial tree are reviewed; airflow resistance is considered subsequently.

TYPES OF AIRFLOW

Analogous to Ohm's law for electrical circuits, the rate of gas flow through a tube is determined by pressure and resistance:

$$\dot{V} = P/R \qquad [2\text{-}10]$$

where

$\dot{V}$ = flow rate
P = driving pressure
R = resistance

Flow through a system of tubes may assume one of three patterns (Fig. 2-12). *Laminar flow* is characterized by streamlines of gas moving parallel to one another and the sides of the tube (see Fig. 2-12A). Laminar flow prevails at low flow rates and is described by Poiseuille's law:

$$\dot{V} = \frac{P\pi r^4}{8\eta l} \qquad [2\text{-}11]$$

where

$\dot{V}$ = flow rate
P = pressure
r = tube radius
η = gas viscosity
l = tube length

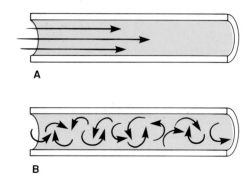

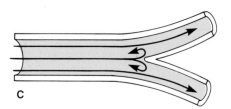

Figure 2-12. Types of airflow in tubes.
(A) Laminar. **(B)** Turbulent. **(C)** Transitional.
(Adapted from West JB. Airway resistance. In:
Respiratory Physiology: The Essentials. 4th ed.
Baltimore: Williams & Wilkins, 1990:102.)

Rearranging equation [2-11] yields:

$$P = \frac{8\eta l \dot{V}}{\pi r^4} \qquad\qquad\qquad [2\text{-}12]$$

Substituting K (a constant) for the term, $8\,\eta l/\pi r^4$, yields:

$$P = K \cdot \dot{V} \qquad\qquad\qquad [2\text{-}13]$$

Examination of equation [2-11] reveals that flow rate varies directly with the fourth power of the radius. Halving the tube's radius reduces flow rate 16-fold.

Turbulent flow, a more random movement of gas along the tube (see Fig. 2-12B), prevails at high flow rates. Gas density is important in determining turbulent flow rates; an increase in density results in a decrease in flow rate. In addition, the driving pressure for turbulent flow is proportional to the square of flow rate ($P = K \cdot \dot{V}^2$). Whether flow through a system is turbulent or laminar can be predicted by calculating the Reynolds number (Re), a unitless number relating mean velocity of flow to gas density, gas viscosity, and tube radius:

$$Re = 2rvd/\eta \qquad\qquad\qquad [2\text{-}14]$$

where

v = mean velocity of flow
d = gas density

When Re exceeds 2000, flow is turbulent; when Re is less than 2000, flow is laminar.

Transitional flow is characterized by eddies that form at tube bifurcations (see Fig. 2-12C). Given the dichotomous branching of the tracheobronchial tree, transitional flow is an important flow pattern in the lung.

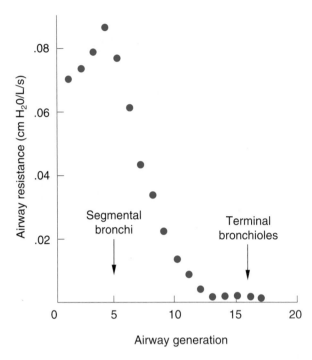

Figure 2-13. Variation of airway resistance with airway generation. Generation "0" is the trachea; higher generations of airways are denoted in moving from central to peripheral airways. (Adapted from Pedley TJ, Schroter RC, Sudlow MF. The prediction of pressure drop and variation of resistance within the human bronchial airways. Respir Physiol 9:391, 1970.)

AIRWAY RESISTANCE

As noted, the driving pressure, calculated as the difference between alveolar pressure and pressure at the airway opening, is one of the two primary variables determining flow rate; the other is airway resistance (Raw). The major component of airway resistance is the frictional resistance offered by the walls of the tracheobronchial tree.

Airway resistance is not distributed evenly throughout the respiratory system. In an adult breathing quietly with mouth closed, the nose offers approximately 50% of the total resistance. During mouth breathing, the pharynx and larynx offer about 25% of overall resistance; during exercise, this figure can increase to 50%. Within the chest, the larger airways—trachea and lobar and segmental bronchi—provide 80% of the remaining airway resistance; small airways, less than 2 mm in diameter, contribute 20%. The distribution of airway resistance is shown in Figure 2-13. Although the individual cross-sectional areas of the peripheral airways are small, their large number generates a large overall cross-sectional area and a lower resistance (see Chap. 1).

Several factors determine airway resistance or, as used clinically, airway *conductance* (Gaw), the reciprocal of resistance. One major determinant is lung volume. At higher lung volume, a greater tethering effect of the lung parenchyma on the airways produces an increase in the cross-sectional area of each airway. A larger cross-sectional area results in reduced resistance. This relationship is depicted in Figure 2-14.

Additional factors that determine airway resistance include airway length, airway smooth muscle tone, and the physical properties of the gases flowing through the airways, such as gas density and viscosity. Clinically, advantage is

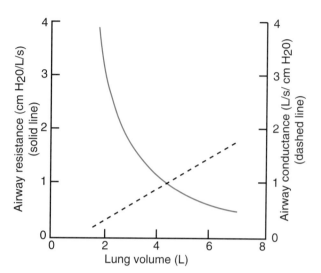

Figure 2-14. Airway resistance and its reciprocal, airway conductance, as functions of lung volume. As lung volume increases, airway diameters increase; resistance falls and conductance increases. (Adapted from Briscoe WA, Dubois AB. The relationship between airway resistance, airway conductance and lung volume in subjects of different age and body size. J Clin Invest 37:1280, 1958.)

taken of the density dependence of resistance by having patients with obstructing lesions of their upper airways breathe an 80% helium–20% oxygen mixture. Because this gas mixture is less dense than air, the resistance of the obstructed upper airway is reduced (see Chap. 4).

Normal airway resistance in the adult is approximately 15 cm H_2O/L/second at FRC. In disease states, several mechanisms may result in an increase in resistance. For example, contraction of bronchial smooth muscle produces airway narrowing and an increase in Raw in asthma (see Chap. 5). Edema of the bronchial mucosa and excessive airway secretions increase Raw in patients with chronic bronchitis. In emphysema, loss of tissue elasticity and a reduction in the tethering effect of the lung parenchyma on airways results in a decrease in airway caliber and an increase in Raw (see Chap. 6). Finally, intraluminal masses occluding an airway (e.g., bronchogenic carcinoma) increase Raw.

An important point that may not be readily apparent is that the magnitudes of many of the physical factors determining airway resistance and flow rates are different during the inspiratory and expiratory phases of the respiratory cycle. Furthermore, limitations to maximal expiratory flow rates exist, even in healthy lungs. Understanding the physiologic basis of expiratory flow limitation is important and requires analysis of several topics: the flow–volume loop, the isovolume pressure–flow curve, the maximal flow–static recoil curve, and the equal pressure point theory.

EXPIRATORY FLOW LIMITATION

An analysis of expiratory flow limitation in the lung begins with consideration of the *flow–volume loop.* A flow–volume loop is a plot of airflow rate versus lung volume (Fig. 2-15). The loop consists of two halves—an expiratory half, representing a maximal expiratory effort from TLC to RV (*expiratory vital capacity*), and an inspiratory half, representing a maximal inspiratory effort from the previously attained RV back to TLC (*inspiratory vital capacity*). A family of curves can be generated by having the subject exert different expiratory and inspiratory efforts, as shown in Figure 2-16.

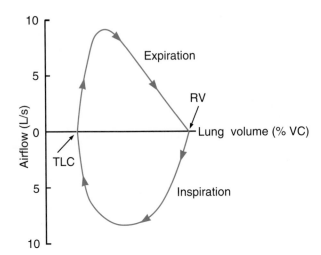

Figure 2-15. Schematic flow–volume loop. The loop is a plot of maximal expiratory and inspiratory airflow rates versus lung volume. See text for details.

Several features of the family of flow–volume plots are worth emphasizing:

1. The contours of the inspiratory and expiratory curves are different.
2. Peak expiratory flow occurs early in the expiratory phase of the loop.
3. The relationship between flow and volume is linear over the lower three quarters of the expiratory vital capacity.
4. During inspiration, greater inspiratory effort results in greater flow at all levels of the vital capacity.
5. During expiration, decreased effort results in decreased flow, but once a minimum "threshold" effort is exerted, further increases in effort produce increases in flow only during the initial quarter of the expiratory vital capacity. At low and moderate lung volumes, increased effort above the threshold does not result in increased flow. Flow is maximal (for the given lung volume) and is *effort independent.*

In trying to account for these observations, it is useful to consider a model of the respiratory system in which the lung is represented by an elastic sphere

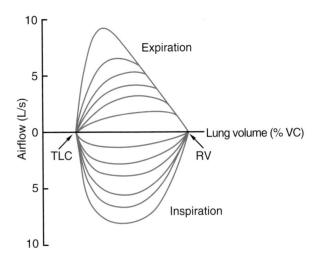

Figure 2-16. Family of flow–volume loops generated by a subject making inspiratory and expiratory maneuvers of varying effort between RV and TLC. See text for discussion.

Figure 2-17. Simplified model for analysis of pressure, flow, and volume relationships in the lung. The lung parenchyma is represented by a sphere connected to a rigid tube—the tracheobronchial tree—which opens to the atmosphere. The sphere and proximal three quarters of the tube are enclosed within an expansile "jacket" (the chest wall). **(A)** System at end-inspiration. Elastic recoil pressure is counterbalanced by pleural pressure (Ppl) of -20 cm H_2O; hence, alveolar pressure (Palv) is 0. Because Palv is equal to atmospheric pressure (or pressure at the airway opening, Pao) under these conditions, there is no pressure gradient for airflow. **(B)** System during quiet expiration. Relaxation of inspiratory muscles allows elastic recoil pressure to overcome Ppl. The net result is a Palv of $+15$ cm H_2O (Palv = Pel + Ppl = $(+20)$ + (-5) = $+15$) and a gradient of $+15$ cm H_2O for expiratory airflow. **(C)** System during forced expiration. Active contraction of expiratory muscles creates a positive Ppl $(+25$ cm $H_2O)$ that sums with the elastic recoil pressure $(+20$ cm $H_2O)$ to create a large Palv $(+45$ cm $H_2O)$. The pressure gradient for expiratory airflow is $+45$ cm H_2O. See text for additional details.

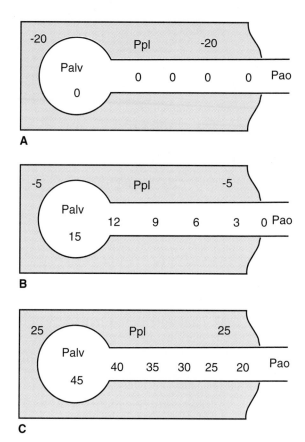

and the tracheobronchial tree by a rigid tube. The airway opens to the atmosphere. An expansile "jacket"—the chest wall—encloses the sphere and proximal three quarters of the tube (Fig. 2-17).

The driving pressure for airflow through the entire system (from alveoli to atmosphere) is the difference between alveolar pressure and pressure at the airway opening (atmospheric pressure). Alveolar pressure consists of two components, the elastic recoil pressure and the pleural pressure (Palv = Pel + Ppl). Furthermore, elastic recoil pressure is determined by the intrinsic elastic properties of the alveoli and the degree of stretch imposed on the lung (i.e., lung volume). The pleural pressure is generated by the elastic recoils of the lung and chest wall. At FRC, pleural pressure is approximately -5 cm H_2O. It becomes more negative with deeper inspiration and more positive with forced expiration. The pressure generated within the alveoli is dissipated in overcoming the resistances to airflow, including frictional resistance.

During relaxed expiration, airway pressure (intraluminal pressure) exceeds pleural pressure at all points along the airway (see Fig. 2-17B). During forced expiration, however, a point may be reached along the airway where pleural pressure exceeds intraluminal pressure (see Fig. 2-17C). The structural characteristics of the airway at this point assume critical importance in determining the airflow rate throughout the entire system. This is discussed more fully below.

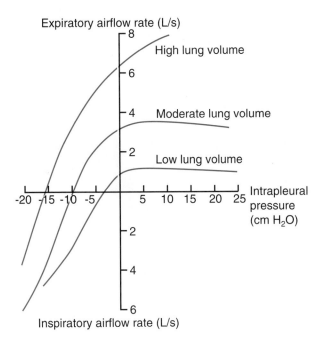

Figure 2-18. Isovolume pressure–flow curves for low, moderate, and high lung volumes. See text for details. (From West JB. Respiratory Physiology: The Essentials. 4th ed. Baltimore: Williams & Wilkins, 1990:108; based on Fry DL, Hyatt RE. Pulmonary mechanics: A unified analysis of the relationship between pressure, volume and gas flow in the lungs of normal and diseased human subjects. Am J Med 29:672–689, 1960.)

ISOVOLUME PRESSURE–FLOW CURVE

The next essential element in understanding the effect of lung volume on flow rate is the relationship between flow and pressure at constant lung volume, the *isovolume pressure–flow curve* (Fig. 2-18). A family of isovolume pressure–flow curves can be generated as follows. Flow is measured using a device called a pneumotachograph, and lung volume is measured using a plethysmograph or "body box" (see Chap. 4). Intrapleural pressure, as an index of respiratory effort, is measured using an intraesophageal balloon catheter. All three variables are plotted as a function of time during a series of respiratory maneuvers between TLC and RV; each maneuver is performed with different effort. The pressure points corresponding to a given lung volume are then plotted against the flow points at the same lung volume. The resultant curve is an isovolume pressure–flow curve, which expresses the rate of flow achieved as a function of effort (intraesophageal or intrapleural pressure) at a specified lung volume.

In examining these curves, several points are worth emphasizing. First, during inspiration, greater inspiratory effort produces greater inspiratory flow—that is, there are no flow maxima during inspiration. Second, at a given intrapleural pressure, expiratory flow is greater at higher lung volumes. Third, at high lung volumes, expiratory flow rises with increasing intrapleural pressure (increasing effort). Finally, at low and moderate lung volumes, flow rises with increased intrapleural pressure only to a point. Subsequently, flow remains constant despite further increases in effort; in other words, flow becomes effort independent once a critical pressure is reached. Indeed, these points of maximal flow on the isovolume pressure–flow curve correspond to the flows delineated on flow–volume loops at specified lung volumes.

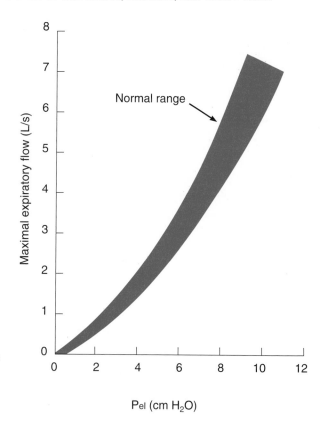

Figure 2-19. Maximal flow–static recoil (MFSR) curve. The normal range of maximal flow is shown. See text for details. (From Macklem PT. New tests to assess lung function. N Engl J Med 293:342, 1975.)

MAXIMAL FLOW–STATIC RECOIL CURVE

The final element to be considered in analyzing flow–volume loops stems from the previous discussion of static forces in the lung and the relationship between flow and static elastic recoil pressure—the *maximal flow–static recoil curve* (Fig. 2-19).

Maximal flow decreases almost linearly as elastic recoil pressure decreases. As noted, the elastic recoil pressure depends on lung volume; hence, maximal expiratory flow decreases as lung volume decreases, a relationship equally obvious from examination of the flow–volume curve.

Some authorities advocate use of the maximal flow–static recoil curve to determine whether the cause of reduced maximal expiratory flow is loss of elasticity (as in emphysema) or increased airway resistance (as in asthma). In the case of decreased flow due to loss of elasticity, the maximal flow–static recoil curve lies within the range of normal; however, maximal flow is limited because the static elastic recoil pressure reaches a limit. When maximal flow is decreased because of increased airway resistance, flow is reduced for a given static elastic recoil pressure. In other words, to achieve predicted maximal flow, more recoil pressure is required to overcome increased airway resistance.

EQUAL PRESSURE POINT THEORY

The groundwork has now been established for consideration of the theoretical "heart" of expiratory flow limitation, *equal pressure point theory.* Consider the

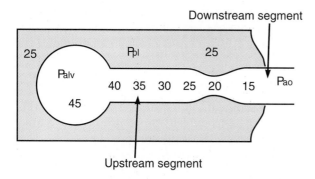

Downstream segment

Upstream segment

Figure 2-20. Model used for analysis of expiratory flow limitation, similar to that depicted in Figure 2-17. In this new model, the tube contains a collapsible region, dividing it into upstream and downstream segments. During forced expiration, creation of a negative transmural pressure results in narrowing of the tube and formation of a Starling resistor. Airflow rate becomes limited. See text for details.

model in Figure 2-20, one similar to that in Figure 2-17. In the new model, however, the tube is not entirely rigid; instead, it contains a collapsible segment.

The pertinent pressures are as noted previously. The collapsible segment divides the tube into "upstream" and "downstream" portions. Once again, pleural pressure is exerted equally against the elastic sphere and along the length of the tube.

During expiration, the pressure within the elastic sphere, Palv, exceeds the surrounding pressure, Ppl, by the amount Pel (i.e., Palv = Pel + Ppl). As Ppl changes, for example, with changes in respiratory effort, Palv changes by the same amount, so that the difference, Palv − Ppl, remains constant and equal to Pel (at constant sphere volume). Furthermore, there is a point somewhere along the tube where a pressure drop equivalent in magnitude to Pel occurs. The *transmural pressure* at this point, that is, the pressure across the tube wall, is zero. Further decrements in driving pressure as flow continues downstream (toward the airway opening) result in a negative transmural pressure. If the segment beyond the point where the intraluminal and pleural pressures are equal—the *equal pressure point*—is collapsible, the negative transmural pressure promotes narrowing of the segment. Airflow rate becomes limited. Complete collapse of the tube does not occur, however, because total occlusion results in a rise in the intraluminal pressure back to alveolar levels at a point just proximal to the collapsed segment. The segment immediately reopens because Palv always exceeds Ppl on expiration, and transmural pressure again becomes positive (intraluminal pressure greater than extraluminal).

The net result of these interacting forces is a *Starling resistor,* a system in which a collapsible segment produces a critical narrowing that limits flow. Under the circumstances prevailing in a Starling resistor, the critical pressure gradient determining flow is Palv − Ppl, not Palv − Pao (as in the example in Fig. 2-17). Furthermore, as Palv increases with increasing Ppl (Pel is constant at fixed lung volume), the driving pressure for flow, Palv − Ppl, remains constant, despite an increase in Palv − Pao. Hence, with constant resistance, expiratory flow remains constant, despite an increasing Ppl (increasing effort).

As might be predicted, with decreases in lung volume, the effective driving pressure, Pel, also decreases (decreased lung stretch); hence, the equal pressure point moves further upstream, toward alveoli. At high lung volumes, the equal pressure point lies in large, rigid airways like the trachea and main and lobar bronchi. Because these airways are not collapsible, expiratory flow is not limited, accounting for the effort-dependent part of the flow–volume loop. On the other hand, at low lung volumes, where the equal pressure point lies upstream, in collapsible (noncartilaginous) airways, a Starling resistor develops and expiratory flow no longer increases with increasing effort. Flow is effort independent.

DYNAMIC COMPLIANCE

The previous descriptions of the static and flow-resistive properties of the respiratory system may now be integrated to explain the concept of dynamic compliance, the measurement of which has clinical significance.

The lung, chest wall, and respiratory system compliances described earlier are measured under static, no-flow conditions. *Dynamic compliance* (Cdyn) refers to the change in volume relative to a change in pressure, measured under conditions of airflow. In practice, Cdyn is measured as the slope of the line drawn between the end-inspiratory and end-expiratory points of a dynamic pressure–volume curve (Fig. 2-21).

With normal airway resistance, Cdyn approximates Cstat and does not vary significantly with respiratory rate. With increased airway resistance, even when the increase is small and limited to the small, peripheral airways, Cdyn may decline, particularly at high respiratory rates, before routine measurements of airway function become abnormal. This variation in Cdyn with respiratory rate is called *frequency dependence of compliance*. Its physiologic basis is described below.

Consider a two-compartment lung model in which the compliances of the two compartments and the resistances of the two airways are equal (Fig. 2-22A). At a constant tidal volume, the amount of gas ventilating each unit is equal at all breathing frequencies. If one of the airways is narrowed, resistance to airflow to the affected unit increases (see Fig. 2-22B). At low breathing frequencies, there may be sufficient time for filling and emptying of this unit, so that overall ventilation to the two-compartment structure may not be affected. At higher breathing frequencies, however, less time is available for filling and emptying of the obstructed unit and, as a result, a smaller change in volume is achieved for a given change in pressure for the system as a whole. Therefore, Cdyn is reduced. Similarly, if one of the alveolar compartments is more distensible, (i.e.,

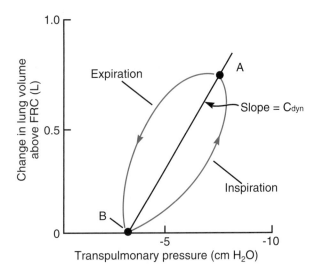

Figure 2-21. Dynamic pressure–volume curve obtained by measuring transpulmonary pressure (on the abscissa) and change in lung volume (on the ordinate) during a single breath. Inspiratory and expiratory portions of the curve are shown. Cdyn is the slope of the line drawn between end-inspiratory (**A**) and end-expiratory (**B**) points of the loop.

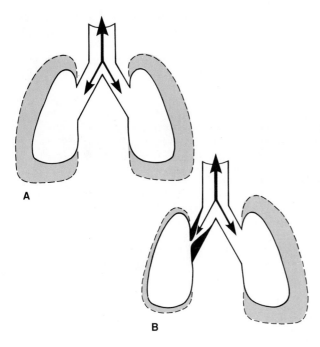

Figure 2-22. Dynamic compliance (Cdyn) in a two-compartment lung model. **(A)** Airway resistances and compliances of the two units are the same; the ventilation to each unit is the same at all breathing frequencies. **(B)** Airway resistance to one unit is increased. As a result, at high breathing frequencies, insufficient time for emptying and filling of the obstructed unit results in a smaller change in volume for a given change in pressure for the system as a whole. Therefore, Cdyn is reduced. The same result is noted when the compliance of one unit is increased. See text for details.

more compliant) than the other, it may be incompletely filled at the time expiration begins. Consequently, the overall volume change is less for the same filling pressure; Cdyn is reduced. The product of airway resistance (R) and lung compliance (C) is known as the *mechanical time constant* (RC).

Figure 2-23 shows a plot of the ratio, Cdyn/Cstat, versus breathing frequency. Normally, Cdyn/Cstat remains greater than 0.8 at all breathing frequencies; however, in patients with obstructive lung diseases, including those with so-called "small airways disease" due to smoking, the ratio falls as breathing frequency increases.

The foregoing sections have addressed the static and dynamic mechanical factors that dictate that work is necessary to move air into and out of the lungs.

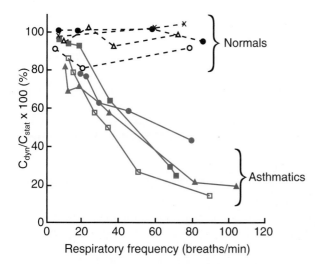

Figure 2-23. Frequency dependence of compliance in obstructive lung disease. Cdyn is expressed as a percentage of Cstat at different respiratory frequencies in healthy subjects (broken lines) and in patients with asthma (solid lines). Unlike healthy subjects, asthmatics demonstrate a fall in Cdyn/Cstat with increasing respiratory rate; that is, they show frequency dependence of compliance. (From Woolcock AJ, Vincent NJ, Macklem PT. Frequency dependence of compliance as a test for obstruction in the small airways. J Clin Invest 48:1100, 1969.)

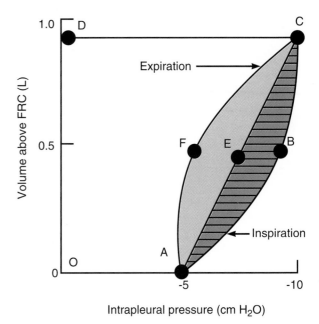

Figure 2-24. Work of breathing. The pressure–volume curve of the lung can be analyzed to determine the work necessary to overcome elastic forces (area OAECDO) and resistive forces (area ABCEA) during each breath. See text for discussion. (From West JB. Work of breathing. In: Respiratory Physiology: The Essentials. 4th ed. Baltimore: Williams & Wilkins, 1990:112.)

As a way of integrating these factors, the final section of this chapter deals briefly with the concept of *work of breathing*.

WORK OF BREATHING

When the respiratory muscles generate force to move the lung and chest wall, work is performed. This work may be expressed as a function of pressure and volume:

$$W = \int P\Delta V \qquad\qquad [2\text{-}15]$$

where

W = work
P = pressure
ΔV = change in lung volume

During inspiration, intrapleural pressure falls and lung volume rises above FRC. Recalling that work is the product of pressure and volume, consideration of Figure 2-24 indicates that work done on the lung during inflation is given by the area of trapezoid OABCDO. This work consists of two components: one required to overcome elastic forces, designated by area OAECDO, and another to overcome airway resistance (and tissue viscosity), designated by area ABCEA. The work for expiration is represented by the area AECFA. Because the latter falls within area OAECDO, the work is accomplished by the energy stored in the stretched elastic lung parenchyma during inspiration.

The work of breathing is increased with decreased distensibility of the lungs, as in pulmonary fibrosis (area OAECDO increased), or with increased airway resistance, as in asthma (area ABCEA increased). Clinically, the work of breathing can be measured during mechanical ventilation of a patient who is paralyzed pharmacologically.

SELECTED READING

Grippi MA, Metzger LF, Krupinski AV, Fishman AP. Pulmonary function testing. In: Fishman AP, ed. Pulmonary Diseases and Disorders. 2nd ed. New York: McGraw-Hill, 1988:2469–2521.

Hyatt RE, Schilder DP, Fry DL. Relationship between maximal expiratory flow and degree of lung inflation. J Appl Physiol 13:331–336, 1958.

Mead J, Turner JM, Macklem PT, Little JB. Significance of the relationship between lung recoil and maximum expiratory flow. J Appl Physiol 22:95–108, 1967.

Pride NB, Permutt S, Riley RL, Bromberger-Barnea B. Determinants of maximal expiratory flow from the lungs. J Appl Physiol 23:646–662, 1967.

Roussos C, Macklem PT. The respiratory muscles. N Engl J Med 307:786–797, 1982.

Woolcock AJ, Vincent NJ, Macklem PT. Frequency dependence of compliance as a test for obstruction in the small airways. J Clin Invest 48:1097–1106, 1969.

Lippincott's Pathophysiology Series: Pulmonary Pathophysiology, edited by Michael A. Grippi. J. B. Lippincott Company, Philadelphia © 1995.

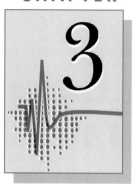

Distribution of Ventilation

Michael A. Grippi

As described in Chapters 1 and 2, the structural and mechanical properties of the lung and chest wall determine how gas moves into and out of the thorax. Before coming in contact with the alveolar–capillary membrane, inspired gas must flow along numerous airways interposed between the airway opening (nose or mouth) and alveoli. From a functional standpoint, the airways can be divided into *conducting* and *gas-exchanging* types (see Chap. 1). The conducting airways include the nose, mouth, pharynx, trachea, and bronchi to the level of the terminal bronchioles. The conducting airways do not participate in oxygen and carbon dioxide exchange. Rather, they provide a conduit to the gas-exchanging regions, which include the respiratory bronchioles, alveolar ducts, alveolar sacs, and alveoli. The distribution of inspired gas to the conducting airways and gas-exchanging regions has a profound effect on respiratory function.

DISTRIBUTION OF TIDAL VOLUME

As inspired air enters the lungs, a portion is distributed to the conducting airways and the remainder to the gas-exchanging areas (Fig. 3-1). The distribution depends, in part, on the relative volumes of these two regions. In the example shown in Figure 3-1, three units of gas are inspired. Two units enter the gas-exchanging region, along with one unit that previously resided in the conducting airways; one inspired unit remains in the conducting airways. The composition of the expired gas reflects the fact that two of the three inspired units participated in gas exchange and one did not.

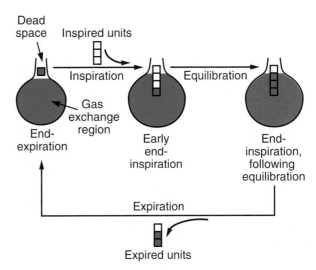

Figure 3-1. Distribution of tidal volume. Three units of ambient gas are inspired; two are distributed to the gas exchange region, along with the unit that previously resided in anatomic dead space. One of the freshly inspired units is distributed to dead space. The composition of alveolar gas at end-inspiration reflects equilibration between the freshly inspired gas (two units) and resident alveolar gas, whereas the composition of expired gas reflects a mixture of alveolar and dead space gas. (Modified from Forster RE II, Dubois AB, Briscoe WA, Fisher AB. Volume of pulmonary ventilation. In: The Lung: Physiologic Basis of Pulmonary Function Tests. 3rd ed. Chicago: Year Book Medical Publishers, 1986:40.)

The amount of gas inspired with each breath is the *tidal volume* (VT). The volume of gas entering or leaving the respiratory system per minute is the *minute ventilation* ($\dot{V}E$), calculated as the product of VT and *respiratory frequency* (f). Usually, *expired* ventilation is measured, as denoted by the "E" in the symbol for minute ventilation. For an adult of average size, VT is 0.5 to 0.7 L; f is 10 to 12 breaths/minute. Therefore, normal $\dot{V}E$ is approximately 5 to 8 L/minute.

DEAD SPACE

As described previously, gas delivered to the conducting airways does not participate in gas exchange. In effect, such airways are "dead" as far as carbon dioxide elimination is concerned; accordingly, this "dead space" is termed *anatomic dead space*. In pathologic states, diseased areas of the lung also contribute to dead space (see Chap. 13). Hence, dead space can be designated as *physiologic dead space*, which includes anatomic dead space (Fig. 3-2). As a rule, anatomic dead space, expressed in milliliters, is approximately equal to ideal body weight, expressed in pounds. The remainder of the tidal volume can be considered as "alveolar volume," because it is distributed to alveoli and related gas-exchanging structures.

Recall that

$$\dot{V}E = VT \cdot f \qquad [3\text{-}1]$$

where

$\dot{V}E$ = minute ventilation
VT = tidal volume
f = respiratory frequency

Substitution of the sum of alveolar volume (VA) and dead space volume (VD) for VT yields the following expression:

$$\dot{V}E = (VA + VD) \cdot f \qquad [3\text{-}2]$$

or

$$\dot{V}E = (VA \cdot f) + (VD \cdot f) \qquad [3\text{-}3]$$

The term, (VA · f), represents *minute alveolar ventilation* ($\dot{V}A$); the term, (VD · f), represents *minute dead space ventilation* ($\dot{V}D$).

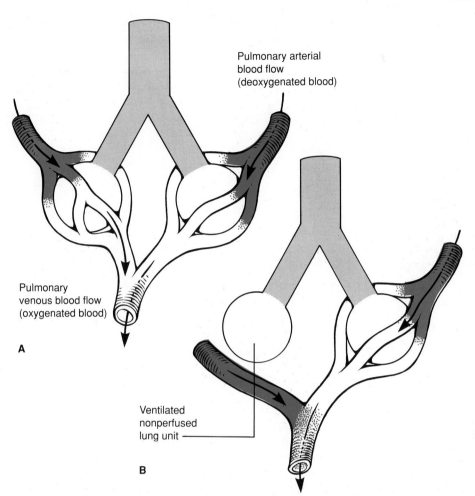

Figure 3-2. Types of dead space. **(A)** Anatomic. Blood flow is coupled ("matched") to gas distribution in both units. The only areas where gas exchange does not take place are the conducting airways (shaded); hence, all the dead space in this model is anatomic. Pulmonary venous blood is fully oxygenated. **(B)** Physiologic. Although in one unit ventilation is coupled to pulmonary blood flow (unit on the right), in the other it is not. In this model, physiologic dead space includes anatomic dead space and the nonperfused lung region (unit on the left). Pulmonary venous blood is partially oxygenated.

CALCULATION OF PHYSIOLOGIC DEAD SPACE

Inspired air contains a negligible amount of carbon dioxide. Therefore, all of the carbon dioxide in expired gas comes from the alveoli after the pulmonary circulation unloads it there. During expiration, carbon dioxide–laden alveolar gas is, in effect, "diluted" in the dead space, producing a drop in carbon dioxide concentration in expired gas relative to its alveolar concentration ("dead space" refers to physiologic dead space, not just anatomic). Using a simple mass-balance equation, the *ratio of physiologic dead space to tidal volume*, V_D/V_T, can be calculated.

The total amount of carbon dioxide (CO_2) in the respiratory system at any instant in time is the product of the initial volume in which the CO_2 is contained—the alveolar volume—and the concentration of CO_2 in the alveoli.

Alveoli contain a mixture of gases, including O_2, CO_2, N_2, and water vapor, each of which exerts a kinetic energy and, hence, a pressure (*partial pressure*). Alveolar CO_2 concentration is calculated as the partial pressure of alveolar CO_2 divided by the sum of the partial pressures of the gases and water vapor in the alveoli (see Chap. 9). Because the sum of partial pressures in the alveoli equals barometric pressure, alveolar *CO_2 content* can be written as:

$$\text{Alveolar } CO_2 \text{ content} = V_A \cdot \frac{P_{ACO_2}}{P_B} \qquad [3\text{-}4]$$

where

$$
\begin{aligned}
V_A &= \text{alveolar volume} \\
P_{ACO_2} &= \text{partial pressure of } CO_2 \text{ in alveoli} \\
P_B &= \text{barometric pressure}
\end{aligned}
$$

The total amount of CO_2 remains the same when the alveolar CO_2 is mixed with dead space volume. Therefore, the amount of CO_2 excreted with each tidal volume breath can be expressed as:

$$V_T \cdot \frac{P_{\bar{E}CO_2}}{P_B} = V_A \cdot \frac{P_{ACO_2}}{P_B} \qquad [3\text{-}5]$$

where

$$P_{\bar{E}CO_2} = \text{mean partial pressure of } CO_2 \text{ in expired gas}$$

Equation [3-5] can be written more simply as:

$$V_T \cdot P_{\bar{E}CO_2} = V_A \cdot P_{ACO_2} \qquad [3\text{-}6]$$

Equation [3-6] indicates that the amount of CO_2 exhaled with each breath, determined as the product of breath volume and partial pressure of CO_2 in exhaled gas, is equal to the amount of CO_2 in the alveoli. CO_2 is neither lost nor added to the gas evolved into the alveoli from the pulmonary circulation; the CO_2 is simply diluted to a new partial pressure ($P_{\bar{E}CO_2}$) by the addition of physiologic dead space. Substituting ($V_D + V_A$) for V_T in equation [3-6] yields:

$$(V_D + V_A) \cdot P_{\bar{E}CO_2} = V_A \cdot P_{ACO_2} \qquad [3\text{-}7]$$

Rearrangement of equation [3-7] and substitution of ($V_T - V_D$) for V_A yields:

$$V_D = V_T \cdot \frac{P_{ACO_2} - P_{\bar{E}CO_2}}{P_{ACO_2}} \qquad [3\text{-}8]$$

Equation [3-8] is more commonly expressed as:

$$\frac{V_D}{V_T} = \frac{P_{ACO_2} - P_{\bar{E}CO_2}}{P_{ACO_2}} \qquad [3\text{-}9]$$

Equation [3-9], known as the *Bohr equation,* indicates that the ratio of dead space to tidal volume can be calculated as the difference between the P_{CO_2} of alveolar gas and expired gas, divided by the alveolar P_{CO_2}. Because alveolar P_{CO_2} closely approximates arterial P_{CO_2} (Pa_{CO_2}), V_D/V_T can be calculated by concurrently measuring the P_{CO_2} in an arterial blood gas specimen and in a sample of expired gas.

As a sample calculation, consider a normal subject whose minute ventilation is 6 L/minute, achieved by breathing with a tidal volume of 0.6 L and a respiratory rate of 10 breaths/minute. An arterial blood gas specimen reveals a Pa_{CO_2} of 40 mmHg, and measurement of a mixed expired gas sample shows a $P\bar{E}_{CO_2}$ of 28 mmHg. Substitution of these measurements into equation [3-9] yields:

$$\frac{V_D}{V_T} = \frac{40 - 28}{40} = 0.30$$

Hence, V_D is $(0.30 \cdot 600 \text{ ml})$ or 180 ml. V_A is $(600 \text{ ml} - 180 \text{ ml})$ or 420 ml. In an otherwise healthy adult, V_D/V_T is approximately 0.30 to 0.35.

EFFECT OF VENTILATORY PATTERN ON V_D/V_T

In the previous sample calculation, the tidal volume and respiratory rate were specified, enabling calculation of V_D and V_A once V_D/V_T was determined. Consider what happens when a healthy, 70-kg subject uses three different breathing patterns to maintain the same minute ventilation (Fig. 3-3).

In Figure 3-3A, $\dot{V}_E$ is 6 L/minute, V_T is 600 ml, and f is 10 breaths/minute. A 70-kg subject has a dead space volume of approximately 150 ml. (As noted

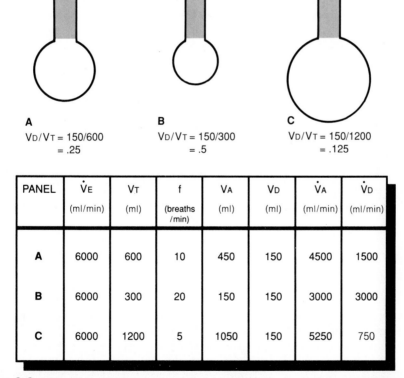

PANEL	$\dot{V}_E$ (ml/min)	V_T (ml)	f (breaths /min)	V_A (ml)	V_D (ml)	$\dot{V}_A$ (ml/min)	$\dot{V}_D$ (ml/min)
A	6000	600	10	450	150	4500	1500
B	6000	300	20	150	150	3000	3000
C	6000	1200	5	1050	150	5250	750

Figure 3-3. Effect of breathing pattern on dead space, alveolar ventilation, and V_D/V_T. Dead space is denoted by the shaded area. In each panel minute ventilation is 6 L/minute, and the respiratory system is shown at end-inspiration. **(A)** Tidal volume is 600 ml and respiratory rate is 10 breaths/minute. **(B)** Tidal volume is halved and respiratory rate is doubled. **(C)** Tidal volume is doubled and respiratory rate is halved. Despite a constant minute ventilation, the ratio of dead space to tidal volume varies markedly. See text for details.

previously, the "rule-of-thumb" is 1 ml of dead space per pound of body weight.) Therefore, $\dot{V}_D$ is 1500 ml (150 · 10) and $\dot{V}_A$ is 4500 ml (450 · 10). V_D/V_T is 150/600 or 0.25.

In Figure 3-3B, the subject has increased his respiratory rate to 20 breaths/minute. If the $\dot{V}_E$ of 6 L/minute is maintained, V_T is 300 ml. With a V_D of 150 ml, $\dot{V}_D$ is now 3000 ml/minute and $\dot{V}_A$ is 3000 ml/minute. V_D/V_T is increased to 150/300 or 0.5. This rapid, shallow breathing pattern is inefficient with respect to CO_2 elimination, because one half of every breath ventilates dead space.

Finally, in Figure 3-3C, the subject has increased his V_T to 1200 ml and decreased his respiratory rate to 5 breaths/minute. $\dot{V}_E$ is still 6 L/minute, but $\dot{V}_D$ is 750 ml/minute and $\dot{V}_A$ is 5250 ml/minute. V_D/V_T is decreased to 150/1200 or 0.125. In all three circumstances total ventilation is the same; however, alveolar ventilation is markedly different. As discussed later, alveolar ventilation is a critical determinant of the rate of CO_2 elimination.

RELATIONSHIP BETWEEN ALVEOLAR VENTILATION AND RATE OF CO_2 PRODUCTION

The rate of CO_2 production ($\dot{V}CO_2$) for a healthy, resting 70-kg subject is about 200 ml per minute. The respiratory control system is "set" to maintain a $Paco_2$ of 40 mmHg (see Chap. 16). Under steady-state conditions, the rate at which CO_2 is eliminated from the body equals the rate at which it is produced. The relationship among $Paco_2$, $\dot{V}CO_2$, and $\dot{V}_A$ is:

$$\dot{V}_A = K \cdot \frac{\dot{V}CO_2}{Paco_2} \qquad [3\text{-}10]$$

where K, a constant, equals 0.863 when $\dot{V}_A$ is expressed at BTPS and $\dot{V}CO_2$ at STPD.

Equation [3-10] indicates that at a constant rate of CO_2 production, $Paco_2$ varies inversely with alveolar ventilation (Fig. 3-4). Although the change in $Paco_2$ and, hence, in $Paco_2$ (which approximates $Paco_2$, as discussed in Chaps. 9 and 13) can be determined using Figure 3-4, the relative magnitude of change in Pco_2 (alveolar or arterial) produced by a change in $\dot{V}_E$ depends on the relationship between $\dot{V}_A$ and $\dot{V}_E$, that is, V_D/V_T (see section on Calculation of Physiologic Dead Space, earlier). The higher V_D/V_T is, the greater is the change in $\dot{V}_E$ necessary to produce alterations in $\dot{V}_A$ and $Paco_2$.

RELATIONSHIP AMONG ALVEOLAR VENTILATION, ALVEOLAR Po_2, AND ALVEOLAR Pco_2

Just as $Paco_2$ is determined by the balance between CO_2 production and alveolar ventilation, alveolar Po_2 (Pao_2) is a function of the rate of oxygen uptake across the alveolar–capillary membrane (see Chap. 9) and alveolar ventilation. Furthermore, because the partial pressure of the other gas in the alveoli (i.e., nitrogen) and the partial pressure of water vapor are constant, Pao_2 and $Paco_2$ vary reciprocally as alveolar ventilation is altered. Figure 3-5 shows the increase in Pao_2 as $\dot{V}_A$ is increased.

As noted, the sum of the partial pressures of O_2, CO_2, N_2, and water vapor in the alveolus equals barometric pressure. Because the partial pressures of nitrogen and water vapor are constant, the partial pressure of either O_2 or CO_2

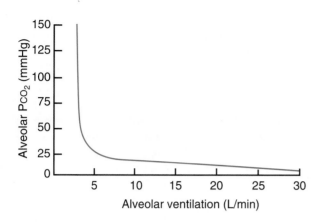

Figure 3-4. Relationship between alveolar ventilation and alveolar P_{CO_2}. Alveolar P_{CO_2} varies inversely with alveolar ventilation. The magnitude of the effect of a change in minute ventilation on alveolar P_{CO_2} depends on the relationship between dead space ventilation and total ventilation. The relationship is plotted for a person of average size who has a normal, stable rate of CO_2 production (about 200 ml/minute).

can be calculated if the partial pressure of the other is known. The calculation is based on the *alveolar gas equation:*

$$P_{AO_2} = P_{IO_2} - P_{ACO_2}\left(F_{IO_2} + \frac{1 - F_{IO_2}}{R}\right)$$ [3-11]

where

P_{IO_2} = P_{O_2} in inspired gas
F_{IO_2} = fractional concentration of O_2 in inspired gas
R   = respiratory exchange ratio

R, the *respiratory exchange ratio,* expresses the rate of CO_2 production relative to the rate of O_2 consumption ($\dot{V}_{O_2}$); i.e., R = $\dot{V}_{CO_2}/\dot{V}_{O_2}$. Under steady-state conditions, the respiratory exchange ratio equals the *respiratory quotient* (RQ), which describes the ratio of carbon dioxide production to oxygen consumption at the cellular level. This relationship depends on the relative contributions of carbohydrates and fats as fuel sources, with the former generating more CO_2 per gram metabolized.

According to the alveolar gas equation, P_{AO_2} can be calculated as the partial pressure of O_2 in the inspired gas (P_{IO_2}) minus a term that includes P_{ACO_2} and a factor that takes into account the change in total gas volume if oxygen uptake differs from carbon dioxide output: [F_{IO_2} + (1 − F_{IO_2})/R]. In a healthy, resting adult of average size, $\dot{V}_{O_2}$ is about 250 ml/minute; $\dot{V}_{CO_2}$ is approximately 200

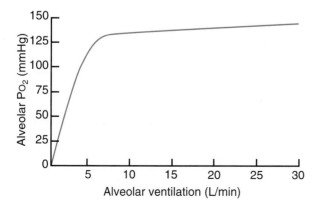

Figure 3-5. Relationship between alveolar ventilation and alveolar P_{O_2}. Alveolar P_{O_2} rises with increases in alveolar ventilation up to a point and then reaches a plateau.

ml/minute. R is, therefore, 200/250 or 0.8. Note that the term, $[F_{IO_2} + (1 - F_{IO_2})/R]$, reduces to 1.2 when $F_{IO_2} = 0.21$, and to 1.0 when $F_{IO_2} = 1.0$ (assuming $R = 0.8$ in each case).

As a sample calculation of P_{AO_2}, consider a healthy subject who is breathing room air and has a measured P_{aCO_2} of 40 mmHg (which closely approximates P_{ACO_2}). Assuming a barometric pressure of 760 mmHg and a water vapor pressure of 47 mmHg (inspired ambient air becomes fully saturated with water at normal body temperature), P_{IO_2} is calculated as the product of the total partial pressure of the "dry" gases in the alveoli and the fractional concentration of oxygen; that is, $P_{IO_2} = (760 - 47) \cdot 0.21$. Hence, $P_{AO_2} = [(760 - 47) \cdot 0.21] - 40 [0.21 + (1 - 0.21)/0.8] = 149 - 48 = 101$ mmHg.

REGIONAL DISTRIBUTION OF TIDAL VOLUME

Thus far, the discussion has focused on the relative distribution of each inspired breath between conducting airways and gas-exchanging regions of the lung. At first glance, it might appear that the lung is functionally homogeneous, and that the portion of each breath reaching the gas-exchanging regions is uniformly distributed. The lung, however, is quite heterogeneous with regard to regional mechanical properties of the airways and parenchyma. This heterogeneity accounts for differences in the distribution of each breath.

Normally, in an upright subject, a pleural pressure gradient exists between the top and bottom of the lung (Fig. 3-6). The pleural pressure is greatest (i.e., most negative) at the top; it is least (i.e., least negative) at the bottom. The gradient is about 0.25 cm H_2O for each centimeter of vertical height. Recalling that transpulmonary pressure, Pl, equals Palv − Ppl (see Chap. 2), it follows that transpulmonary pressure is greater at the lung apex than at the base. The larger apical transpulmonary pressure results in greater alveolar distention at the top of the lung (Fig. 3-7).

The larger transpulmonary pressure and alveolar size at the apex mean that this region functions along a different portion of the lung's pressure–volume curve than does the basilar area (Fig. 3-8). Application of an inflation pressure produces a greater change in lung volume at the base than at the apex. In Figure 3-8, the change in distending pressure, ΔP, produces more inflation

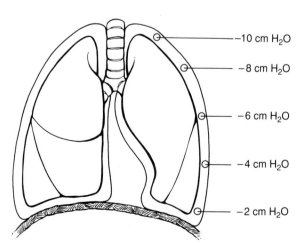

Figure 3-6. Pleural pressure gradient in the upright chest. Pressures are measured at end-expiration. See text for details.

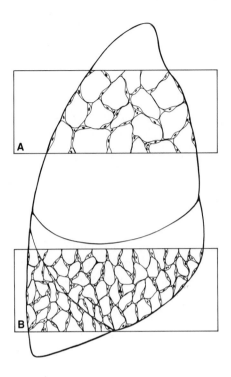

Figure 3-7. Schematic of apical and basal alveolar size. The lung is depicted at FRC. Apical alveoli **(A)** are larger than basilar **(B)**.

at the bottom of the lung (ΔV_1) than at the top (ΔV_2). This is easily seen, because the slope of the pressure–volume curve is greater at the base than at the apex. In other words, static lung compliance is higher in the base (see Chap. 2), and, consequently, more of each tidal volume breath is distributed to the base.

Although it is true that the lung base is larger, and, therefore, might be expected to receive more of the inspired breath, regardless of mechanical differences between regions, the preferential basilar distribution holds even when ventilation is adjusted ("normalized") for regional lung volume (Fig. 3-9). This actually enhances the efficiency of gas exchange, because pulmonary blood flow also predominates at the base (see Chap. 13).

If transpulmonary pressure at the base becomes negative, that is, if pleural pressure exceeds alveolar pressure (as may occur with loss of lung elasticity due

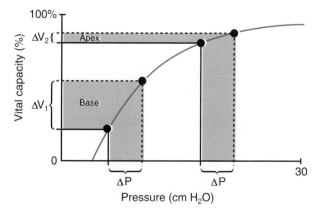

Figure 3-8. Pressure–volume plot of the lung. Changes in volume from two regions of the same lung are shown during application of inflation pressure, ΔP. The change in lung volume at the base, ΔV_1, is greater than the change at the apex, ΔV_2. Even when allowance is made for the fact that there are more alveoli at the base than at the apex, the greater change in lung volume at the base still holds. See text and Figure 3-9. (Modified from Murray JF. Ventilation. In: Murray JF, ed. The Normal Lung. 2nd ed. Philadelphia: WB Saunders, 1986:92.)

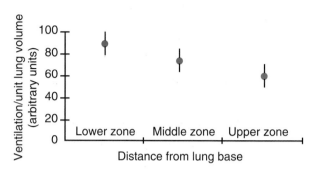

Figure 3-9. Measurement of regional lung ventilation by inhalation of radioactive xenon gas. The subject inhales a bolus of xenon-133. A camera then scans upper, middle, and lower lung zones to quantitate regional ventilation. Each regional measurement is divided by lung volume ("normalized"). Because the lung is larger at the base (where there are more alveoli), more xenon is expected to go there. Even when the apical–basal difference in lung volume is taken into account, however, ventilation to the base is greater. (Modified from West JB. Ventilation. In: Respiratory Physiology: The Essentials. 4th ed. Baltimore: Williams & Wilkins, 1990:19.)

to aging or emphysema), airways may become compressed at the end of expiration, as discussed later. If blood flow in the base persists under these circumstances, gas exchange is impaired as a result of ventilation-perfusion mismatch (see Chap. 13).

The factors responsible for the pleural pressure gradient include the weight of the suspended, upright lung "pulling" on the lung apex and the tethering of the lung centrally at the hilum.

CAUSES OF UNEVEN DISTRIBUTION OF VENTILATION IN DISEASE STATES

Despite the tremendously wide range of diseases that affect the lung by altering the distribution of ventilation, the underlying pathophysiologic mechanisms can be distilled to a basic few (Fig. 3-10).

Many common clinical disorders, such as asthma and chronic bronchitis, are characterized by increases in airway resistance (see Chaps. 2, 4, 5, and 6). Although the increase in airway resistance may be seen throughout the lung, it is usually not uniform. Figure 3-10A depicts two idealized lung units, one of which is supplied by an airway with normal resistance and the other by one with increased resistance. With each breath, a greater proportion of the inspired volume is distributed to the nonobstructed unit. The net effect on gas exchange depends on the extent to which blood flow is redistributed from the obstructed to the normally ventilated unit.

In Figure 3-10B, localized changes in lung elasticity (the reciprocal of compliance, as described in Chap. 2) result in an uneven distribution of ventilation. Diseases like emphysema (decreased elasticity) and pulmonary fibrosis (increased elasticity) produce this pattern of abnormality. Over the course of repeated breaths, lung units with increased elasticity receive a greater proportion of inspired volume. In some disorders (e.g., emphysema), a combination of altered regional compliance and airway resistance may prevail (see Fig. 3-10C). The increased airway resistance is "dynamic," occurring with expiration (see Chap. 2, Fig. 2-20). The result is marked nonuniformity of ventilation; most inspired gas goes to nonobstructed regions with normal compliance.

Finally, in some pulmonary disorders, airway resistance and lung elasticity may be normal, but a regional limitation to lung expansion results in maldistribution of ventilation (see Fig. 3-10D). Clinical examples include lung compression by a pleural effusion and limited expansion of one hemithorax due to unilateral diaphragm paralysis.

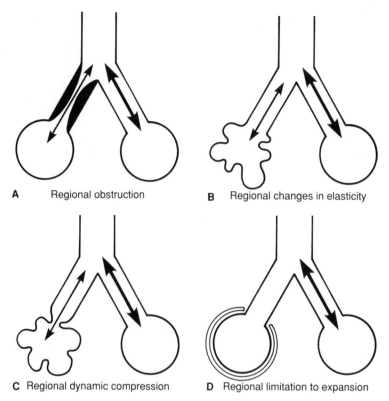

A Regional obstruction

B Regional changes in elasticity

C Regional dynamic compression

D Regional limitation to expansion

Figure 3-10. Models of non-uniform lung ventilation. **(A)** Partial obstruction of the airway to one lung unit. **(B)** Altered elasticity of one lung unit. **(C)** Localized dynamic compression of the airway to one lung unit. **(D)** Limited expansion of one lung unit during inflation. In each model, over time the normal unit receives a greater fraction of the total inspired volume. See text for details. (Modified from Forster RE II, Dubois AB, Briscoe WA, Fisher AB. Pulmonary ventilation. In: The Lung: Physiologic Basis of Pulmonary Function Tests. 3rd ed. Chicago: Year Book Medical Publishers, 1986:61.)

TESTS OF NONUNIFORM LUNG VENTILATION

Although a number of tests have been used to assess nonuniformity of ventilation, only one is described here—the *single-breath nitrogen test*. Another method, determination of frequency dependence of compliance, was described in Chapter 2. Regional distribution of ventilation has also been measured using inhaled radioactive gases (e.g., xenon).

During the single-breath nitrogen test, the subject makes a maximal inspiration of pure oxygen after first emptying his lungs to residual volume; that is, he makes a vital capacity inspiration of oxygen. The subject then exhales slowly back to residual volume, and the volume of exhaled gas is quantitated using a spirometer. The concentration of nitrogen in the expirate is monitored using a nitrogen meter. Figure 3-11 shows the four phases of the so-called "nitrogen washout curve" obtained in this manner.

During early expiration, gas from the upper airways is exhaled. Because this region contains pure oxygen from the prior inspiration, the nitrogen concentration is zero (phase I). Next, nitrogen-containing gas from anatomic dead space is washed out as alveoli deflate; the nitrogen concentration rises abruptly (phase II). Subsequently, alveolar gas is exhaled. In healthy people with minimal inhomogeneity of ventilation, this phase of the curve (phase III) is flat and is known as the *alveolar plateau*.

In patients with a variety of parenchymal and airway diseases, phase III is not flat. In fact, the slope of phase III (% N_2 concentration/L exhaled volume) provides a measure of the inhomogeneity of ventilation. Presumably, some poorly ventilated lung regions receive little of the inspired oxygen. Consequently, these regions have a high alveolar nitrogen concentration relative to

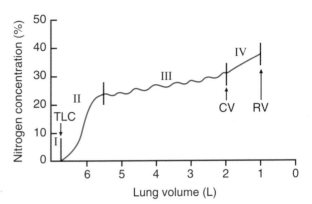

Figure 3-11. Single-breath nitrogen washout curve, demonstrating four phases. TLC, total lung capacity; CV, closing volume; RV, residual volume. See text for details.

normally ventilated areas; there is less dilution of the nitrogen by the inspired oxygen. The poorly ventilated areas tend to empty last, contributing to the rise in nitrogen concentration during phase III.

Examination of Figure 3-11 also shows that after the alveolar plateau, there is another abrupt rise in the nitrogen concentration of expired gas (phase IV). The proposed mechanism underlying phase IV is closure of small airways at the lung bases at low lung volumes.

During the early part of the inspiration of pure oxygen, small airways (respiratory bronchioles) in the lung bases may be compressed to closure by the weight of the lung itself. As a consequence, these regions may receive little of the early inspirate (oxygen). By the time inspiration to total lung capacity is complete, however, much more of the gas has been distributed to the lung bases, which have a larger volume than the apices, and which operate on a steeper portion of the pressure–volume curve (see earlier section on Regional Distribution of Tidal Volume). Consequently, there is more dilution of endogenous alveolar nitrogen in the bases than in the apices. During expiration, apical and basilar lung zones empty, constituting phase III of the curve. When small airway closure at the bases occurs toward the end of expiration, however, the nitrogen-rich apical lung zones contribute proportionately more gas, creating phase IV.

The lung volume representing that portion of the vital capacity remaining at the onset of phase IV of the nitrogen washout curve is known as the *closing volume*. The sum of closing volume and residual volume is called the *closing capacity*. In healthy, young people, airway closure occurs at about 10% of the vital capacity above residual volume. By the seventh decade, airway closure may occur at up to 40% of the vital capacity above residual volume. Patients with even minor degrees of airway obstruction may show significant elevations in closing volume.

SELECTED READING

Forster RE II, Dubois AB, Briscoe WA, Fisher AB. Pulmonary ventilation. In: The Lung: Physiologic Basis of Pulmonary Function Tests. 3rd ed. Chicago: Year Book Medical Publishers, 1986:25–64.

Hlastala M. Ventilation. In: Crystal RG, West JB, eds. The Lung: Scientific Foundations. New York: Raven Press, 1991:1209–1214.

Murray JF. Ventilation. In: Murray JF, ed. The Normal Lung. 2nd ed. Philadelphia: WB Saunders, 1986:77–113.

West JB. Ventilation. In: Respiratory Physiology: The Essentials. 4th ed. Baltimore: Williams & Wilkins, 1990:11–20.

Lippincott's Pathophysiology Series: Pulmonary Pathophysiology, edited by Michael A. Grippi. J. B. Lippincott Company, Philadelphia © 1995.

CHAPTER

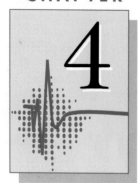

4

The Physiologic Basis of Pulmonary Function Testing

Mark A. Kelley

The concepts presented in earlier chapters constitute the framework for tests used in the quantitative evaluation of lung function. Pulmonary function testing is an important part of clinical medicine and serves a number of roles: (1) to establish the diagnosis of pulmonary disease and to assess its severity; (2) to document the effectiveness of therapy for various pulmonary disorders (e.g., the response to bronchodilators in patients with asthma; see Chap. 5); (3) to chart the course of a disease through serial testing; and (4) to educate patients and, perhaps, facilitate alterations in lifestyle (e.g., convincing smokers to stop smoking if lung dysfunction is demonstrated).

This chapter focuses on pulmonary function testing and its physiologic basis. Emphasis is placed on frequently used tests that illustrate fundamental differences among prevalent pulmonary disorders. Other, less commonly used tests are also outlined to illustrate additional physiologic principles. Finally, several clinical scenarios are presented to highlight how diagnostic problems can be solved using routine pulmonary function testing.

PRINCIPLES OF PULMONARY FUNCTION TESTING

The respiratory system accommodates gas exchange under a wide variety of circumstances, including rest and vigorous exercise. With exercise, the requirements for increased O_2 consumption and CO_2 elimination necessitate even greater efficiency of gas exchange and ventilation.

As noted in Chapters 1 through 3, lung structure is designed to maximize ventilatory efficiency. Functionally, the respiratory system may be divided into three components: (1) the airways, (2) the lung parenchyma, and (3) the chest bellows.

The airways range from the semirigid, central airways (trachea and lobar bronchi) to the more flexible, smaller airways that extend to the lung periphery. As discussed in Chapter 2, airflow patterns vary from very turbulent, in the central airways, to laminar, in the smaller airways. These smaller airways may be compressed during forced expiration. Consequently, airflow, in both healthy and pathologic states, is limited during expiration. This is an important concept in pulmonary function testing, because analysis of the *expiratory* portion of ventilation uncovers most lung disorders.

As presented in detail in Chapter 2, the second functional component, the elastic lung parenchyma, behaves like a balloon. Energy is required for inflation; without continued energy investment to maintain inflation, the lung deflates. Disorders that make the lung stiff (e.g., pulmonary fibrosis) inhibit full inflation, whereas disorders that destroy the lung's elasticity (e.g., emphysema) reduce the force with which the lung deflates.

The third functional component—the chest bellows—consists of the thoracic cage, intercostal muscles, and diaphragm (see Chap. 1). Because the lung itself has no intrinsic means of initiating respiration, the thoracic cage and respiratory musculature must create the forces necessary for ventilation. Respiratory muscles are active during inspiration; muscles of expiration usually are operative only in certain disease states and during exercise. Disorders of the thoracic cage or respiratory muscles may influence respiratory "pump" function, resulting in respiratory failure (see Chap. 18).

Alteration in any of these three functional components may cause dyspnea and measurable abnormalities in pulmonary function. In fact, pulmonary function testing can be used to assess each of these components, individually.

Major groups of clinically important pulmonary function tests include spirometry, tests of respiratory muscle strength, measurement of lung volume, and diffusing capacity. A discussion of diffusing capacity is provided in Chapter 9. Each of the other groups of tests is described in the following sections.

SPIROMETRY

Spirometry is the single most important test of pulmonary function. During spirometry, the patient inhales and exhales with full effort. Measurements are made of airflow rate and change in volume of the respiratory system. Most clinical information is provided from analysis of the expiratory maneuver.

WATER-SEALED SPIROMETER

For decades, a simple system for spirometry was employed that measured lung volume using a sealed chamber (Fig. 4-1). While seated, the patient breathes into the chamber, which consists of a movable cylinder inverted over a water bath. Changes in lung volume are measured as changes in the volume of the cylinder, determined by connecting the cylinder to a calibrated, rotating drum. In the example shown in Figure 4-1, inspiration results in an upward deflection, and expiration in a downward deflection, on the drum.

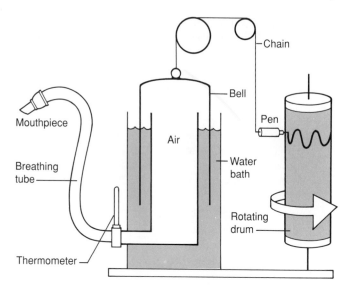

Figure 4-1. Conventional water-sealed spirometer. The air-filled bell, inverted over a water bath, is connected to a rotating drum on which the spirometry tracing is inscribed. The drum rotates at a fixed, known speed, and the paper on the drum is calibrated, allowing measurement of changes in lung volume and airflow rate. See text for details.

The fundamental measurement of spirometry is the *vital capacity* (VC), which is the maximal volume of air that can be inhaled (inspiratory VC) or exhaled (expiratory VC). To measure the expiratory VC, the patient inhales to his or her greatest lung volume and then exhales until air can no longer be expelled.

As discussed later, some air remains in the lungs even after a maximal expiratory maneuver. This volume is termed the *residual volume* (RV). The sum of the vital capacity and residual volume is the *total lung capacity* (TLC). The residual volume cannot be determined by spirometry alone; it requires additional measurements of lung volume (see section on Measurement of Lung Volumes, later).

As noted, rate of airflow is a major determinant of ventilatory capacity. Airflow rate can be measured as a timed expiratory vital capacity maneuver. Using a spirometer like that described in Figure 4-1, the vital capacity is timed by having the cylinder rotate at a known speed. With the vertical axis constituting volume (VC), and the horizontal axis providing a measurement of time, airflow rate (volume/time) is calculated.

A typical spirometric tracing using this technique is shown in Figure 4-2. The lung volume at the top of the spirogram is TLC. As the patient exhales, a curvilinear pattern is inscribed, which then flattens out at the end of exhalation as the patient's lung volume approaches RV. Several key measurements are derived from this expiratory maneuver.

The *forced expiratory volume in 1 second* (FEV_1) is the amount of air exhaled in the first second. Commonly, the FEV_1 is expressed as a percentage of the *forced vital capacity* (FVC). In a healthy subject, at least 70% of the FVC is exhaled within the first second. In patients with severe obstructive airway disease, as little as 20% to 30% may be exhaled in the first second. This ratio, the $FEV_1/FVC\%$, is an extremely useful and reproducible measurement.

Another useful measurement from spirometry is the airflow rate during the middle portion of the expiratory maneuver: the *forced expiratory flow between 25% and 75% of forced vital capacity*, or $FEF_{25\%-75\%}$. With this measurement, the average airflow rate between 25% and 75% of the exhaled volume is calculated.

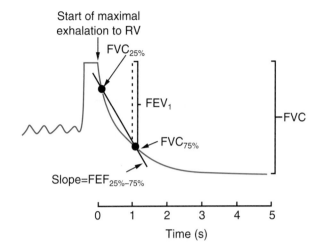

Figure 4-2. Spirometric measurements obtained during a forced expiration from TLC to RV. See text for definitions and discussion.

FLOW–VOLUME LOOP

Simple mechanical equipment like the water-sealed spirometer shown in Figure 4-1 has largely been supplanted by electronic devices that make possible accurate measurements of inspiratory and expiratory airflow. These devices also permit measurement of flow rate as a function of lung volume. To understand the relationship between airflow rate and lung volume, it is useful to analyze the *flow–volume loop* (Fig. 4-3).

After a period of tidal volume breathing, the subject makes a maximal inspiration, inscribing a flow tracing with an elliptical shape (curve AEB). The volume at maximal inspiration (point B) is TLC. Subsequently, the patient exhales forcefully, inscribing the FVC portion of the tracing (curve BCDA). Maximal expiratory airflow rate is seen early in the tracing (point C); the airflow rate then trails off (point D) before the curve returns to its original position (point A). Hence, the flow–volume loop describes the relationship between airflow rate and volume throughout inspiration and expiration and contains the same

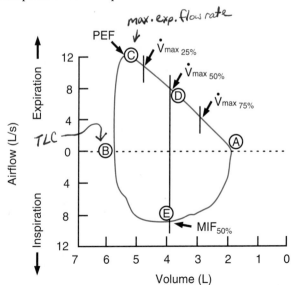

Figure 4-3. Normal maximal flow–volume loop. Inspiration begins at point A; exhalation commences at point B. Peak expiratory flow (PEF) occurs at point C. Maximal expiratory flow at mid-vital capacity ($\dot{V}max_{50\%}$) is at point D, whereas maximal inspiratory flow (MIF$_{50\%}$) is at point E.

information found in the simple spirogram; however, additional useful measurements are easily made.

Obviously, the characteristics of airflow during inspiration and expiration are markedly different. Airflow is fairly symmetric during inspiration; the highest airflow rate is achieved at approximately the halfway point. This point is termed the *maximal mid-inspiratory flow rate at 50% of vital capacity* ($MIF_{50\%}$).

In contrast, the maximal expiratory airflow rate occurs very early in expiration; airflow rate then decreases linearly throughout the rest of exhalation. The highest expiratory airflow rate is the *peak expiratory flow* (PEF). As described for the simple spirogram, the airflow rate between 25% and 75% of the forced vital capacity can be determined from the flow–volume curve. A more convenient frame of reference, however, is the airflow rate at the middle of forced exhalation, the $\dot{V}max_{50\%}$. In general, the $MIF_{50\%}$ is 1.5 times the $\dot{V}max_{50\%}$ because increased airway resistance during expiration limits expiratory airflow (see Chap. 2).

Although the flow–volume loop contains much of the same information provided by the simple spirogram, the visual relationship between flow and volume provides insight into the functional characteristics of both upper and lower airways. Analysis of the flow–volume loop may be useful in difficult diagnostic cases, as described later in this chapter (see section on Clinical Examples).

EXAMPLES OF COMMON CLINICAL APPLICATIONS OF SPIROMETRY

Spirometry may be used to define two major physiologic patterns of abnormalities: *obstructive* and *restrictive* (Fig. 4-4).

In obstructive disorders, the primary physiologic abnormality is increased airway resistance (see Chaps. 5 and 6). In the simplest case (e.g., asthma), the lung parenchyma is normal, but the airways are narrowed. Therefore, although the FVC may be preserved, airflow rate is reduced, and the $FEV_1/FVC\%$ is decreased. As seen in Figure 4-4B, the slope of the expiratory tracing is markedly reduced compared to normal; the FEV_1 and $FEV_1/FVC\%$ are decreased. The $FEF_{25\%-75\%}$, not shown in the figure, is also reduced.

Restrictive disorders are characterized by limited inflation of the thorax. In many restrictive disorders, the lung parenchyma is altered so that the lung is stiff and difficult to inflate (see Chap. 7). Airway function usually remains normal, and, therefore, airflow rate is preserved. Although the FVC and FEV_1 are reduced, the $FEV_1/FVC\%$ is normal (see Fig. 4-4C). Not shown in the figure is the decreased $FEF_{25\%-75\%}$. In restrictive lung disorders, reduced lung volume reduces elastic recoil (see Chap. 2). Hence, the $FEF_{25\%-75\%}$ may be decreased in the absence of airway obstruction.

The same functional abnormalities for restrictive and obstructive disorders are described by the expiratory limb of the flow–volume loop (Fig. 4-5), the physiologic basis of which is described in Chapter 2. For the patient with restrictive disease, the flow–volume loop appears as a smaller version of the normal loop. The expiratory tracing has a normal shape. All values, including airflow rates, are reduced because lung volume is decreased. In contrast, in obstructive airway diseases, the shape of the flow–volume loop is markedly abnormal. The expiratory limb includes a reduced peak airflow rate and a markedly distorted contour; airflow rate is reduced throughout expiration.

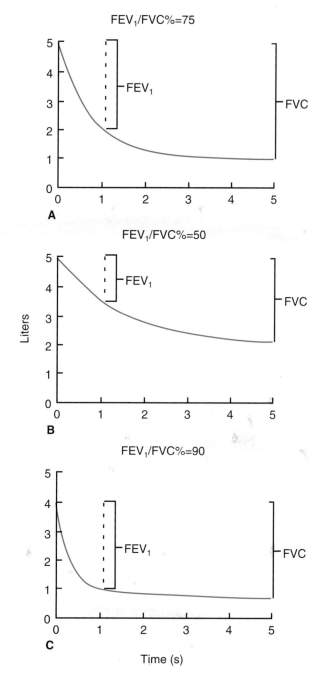

Figure 4-4. Representative spirometric tracings. **(A)** Healthy subject. **(B)** Patient with obstructive airway disease. **(C)** Patient with restrictive lung disease. The FEV$_1$/FVC% is reduced in obstruction and preserved in restriction.

TESTS OF RESPIRATORY MUSCLE STRENGTH

Occasionally, neuromuscular disorders mimic parenchymal lung disease. Just as parenchymal lung disease may result in limited expansion of the thorax, loss of respiratory muscle power may produce similar abnormalities in pulmonary function tests. If the underlying lung is healthy, the physiologic problem is essentially one of "power failure," in which inspiration is impaired and the VC reduced. The resultant pulmonary function test pattern resembles restrictive

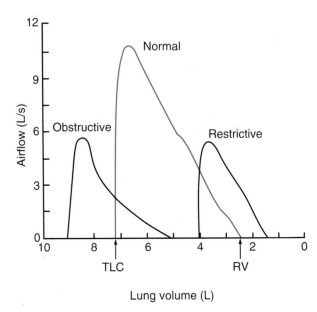

Figure 4-5. Representative expiratory flow–volume loops from a healthy subject and patients with obstructive or restrictive lung diseases. With obstruction, lung volume is increased, and the curve is shifted to the left. Expiratory airflow rates are diminished at all lung volumes. With restriction, lung volume is reduced, and the curve is shifted to the right. Although peak flow is reduced, expiratory airflow rates are actually *increased* compared with normal airflow rates *at the same lung volume.*

parenchymal lung disease. This pattern may also be seen with lack of patient cooperation or motivation. From a practical standpoint, the clinical problem is whether the restrictive pattern represents restrictive lung disease, neuromuscular disease, or poor patient effort.

To evaluate these possibilities, the force of inspiratory and expiratory muscle contraction can be measured. The patient is asked to make a maximal inspiratory or expiratory effort against a pressure gauge, and the resultant pressure, generated isometrically, is measured.

The forces developed by the respiratory muscles are directly related to lung volume. Maximal inspiratory pressure (MIP) is achieved at the smallest lung volume (RV) when the length–tension relationship of the diaphragm is optimized (see Chap. 2). Conversely, maximal expiratory pressure (MEP) is achieved at TLC. Patients with neuromuscular disease often cannot achieve normal maximal pressures, which suggests the underlying cause of the restrictive pulmonary abnormality. In contrast, patients who are poorly cooperative often do attain these pressures quite easily, helping to make the distinction between poor cooperation and neuromuscular weakness. Importantly, maximal inspiratory and expiratory pressures are specific tests of respiratory muscle function, and they are, for the most part, unaffected by underlying lung disease.

A useful test of the patient's overall pulmonary function, including muscle strength, is the *maximal voluntary ventilation* (MVV). In this maneuver, the patient breathes as rapidly and as deeply as possible over a 12-second interval. The resultant exhaled volume is measured and extrapolated over a minute (i.e., the measurement is expressed in liters per minute). Empirically, it has been observed that the MVV is 35 to 40 times the FEV_1.

MEASUREMENT OF LUNG VOLUMES

Thus far, spirometry has been emphasized as the major tool in the diagnosis and quantification of a variety of lung disorders. In some patients, however, direct measurement of lung volumes may provide additional insight into abnormalities initially detected on spirometry. For example, restrictive lung diseases reduce VC. The VC also may be reduced due to airway obstruction, however, and an important clinical question arises in this context: Is the problem pure airway obstruction, or is it a combination of obstructive and restrictive disorders?

As an example, consider a heavy smoker who is being evaluated for occupational lung disease. Although smoking is commonly associated with airway obstruction (see Chap. 6), many occupational lung diseases produce a restrictive pattern. In the presence of airway obstruction, the finding of a reduced VC does not allow the distinction to be made. In this case, measurement of lung volumes is particularly useful in facilitating interpretation of the spirometry.

DEFINITIONS

Several lung volume measurements have become standard in clinical pulmonary function testing (Fig. 4-6). The volume of air in the patient's lungs in the resting, end-expiratory position, measured with the subject's glottis open to atmosphere, is the *functional residual capacity* (FRC). During quiet breathing, the inspiratory volume is the *tidal volume* (VT). *Total lung capacity* (TLC) is the volume of air in the lungs after a maximal inspiration from FRC. The volume difference between FRC and TLC is the *inspiratory capacity* (IC). The volume exhaled during a maximal expiratory maneuver from TLC is the (expiratory) *vital capacity* (VC). The volume remaining in the lung after an expiratory vital capacity maneuver is the *residual volume* (RV). The difference between FRC and RV is the *expiratory reserve volume* (ERV). All lung volumes can be calculated from measurements of the VC and FRC. FRC can be measured using one of two techniques: *helium dilution* or *body plethysmography*.

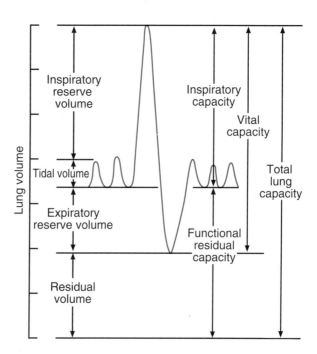

Figure 4-6. Subdivisions of lung volume as defined in the spirogram. See text for definitions and discussion.

HELIUM DILUTION TECHNIQUE

The helium dilution technique (Fig. 4-7) is based on the simple principle of conservation of mass. An inert tracer gas, helium, contained within a breathing circuit of known volume, is diluted by the addition of an unknown volume— the lung at FRC. After an appropriate time for equilibration of gases throughout the system, measurement of the new, decreased helium concentration re-

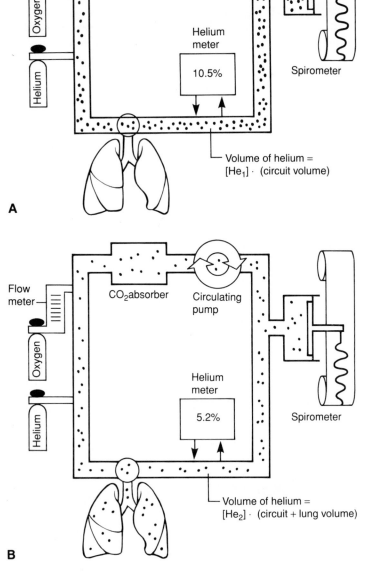

Figure 4-7. Closed-circuit helium dilution method for measurement of FRC. **(A)** System before patient is connected. **(B)** System after patient is connected and equilibrium is achieved. The initial helium concentration in the circuit (He_1) is compared with the final concentration after rebreathing (He_2). If the spirometer circuit volume (V_s) and its dead space volume (V_d) are known, FRC can be calculated as:

$$FRC = V_s \cdot \left(\frac{He_1 - He_2}{He_2}\right) - V_d$$

See text for details. (From Grippi MA, Metzger LF, Krupinski AV, Fishman AP. Pulmonary function testing. In: Fishman AP, ed. Pulmonary Diseases and Disorders. 2nd ed. New York: McGraw-Hill, 1988:2474.)

flects the total volume into which this gas is distributed throughout the lung and breathing circuit. Because the latter volume is known, the former can be calculated.

As depicted in Figure 4-7, the subject breathes on a circuit, which includes a sealed spirometer and CO_2 absorber. A supply of oxygen is connected to the system. Ongoing removal of CO_2 by the CO_2 absorber and repletion of oxygen from the external source allow the patient to ventilate continuously while connected to the circuit (see Fig. 4-7A). Before the patient is connected, the circuit is filled with a gas mixture which contains a known concentration of helium. As the patient breathes on the system, the helium is diluted throughout the lung and the circuit (see Fig. 4-7B). After equilibration, the new helium concentration is a measure of the new volume of distribution of the gas.

The volume of the spirometer circuit (V_s) is known; the initial helium concentration in the circuit (He_1) and final concentration after rebreathing (He_2) are measured. The total amount of helium present initially (the product of initial helium concentration and initial circuit volume) equals the total amount of helium after equilibration (the product of final helium concentration and final system volume; final system volume is initial volume plus FRC):

$$V_s \cdot He_1 = (V_s + FRC) \cdot He_2 \qquad [4\text{-}1]$$

Solving equation [4-1] for FRC yields the following expression:

$$FRC = V_s \cdot (He_1 - He_2) / He_2 \qquad [4\text{-}2]$$

The value for FRC calculated in this way actually includes a small volume of dead space in the spirometer circuit that must be subtracted to give the patient's true FRC.

Although the helium dilution method is simple in principle, its accuracy depends on complete gas mixing within the lung. In healthy subjects, complete mixing (equilibration) may take only several minutes. In patients with poorly ventilated lung regions (see Chap. 3), such as those with obstructive airway disease, equilibration may take much longer, however. Therefore, the helium dilution method may be inaccurate and require long testing times in patients with nonuniform lung ventilation.

BODY PLETHYSMOGRAPHY

Body plethysmography is a faster and usually more reliable method of measuring lung volume than the helium dilution method; however, it requires more sophisticated technology. The principle of body plethysmography is based on *Boyle's law*, which describes the constant relationship between the pressure (P) and volume (V) of a gas at a constant temperature:

$$P_1 V_1 = P_2 V_2 \qquad [4\text{-}3]$$

where

P_1 = initial gas pressure
V_1 = initial gas volume
P_2 = pressure after change in gas volume
V_2 = volume after change in gas pressure

The subject, seated in an airtight plethysmograph ("body box"), breathes through a mouthpiece connected through a shutter to the outside atmosphere (Fig. 4-8). The shutter can be opened and closed electronically. At FRC, the subject pants against the closed shutter. The gas contained within the lungs is alternately compressed (during expiration) and decompressed (during inspiration). Changes in pressure measured at the subject's mouth (equivalent to alveolar pressure) and changes in thoracic gas volume (as reflected by changes in pressure within the airtight body box) during the panting maneuver are displayed continuously on an oscilloscope.

Thoracic gas volume (VTG), equivalent to FRC, is measured according to Boyle's law:

$$P_I \cdot V_{TG} = (P_I + \Delta P_A) \cdot (V_{TG} + \Delta V) \qquad [4\text{-}4]$$

where

$$\begin{aligned}
P_I \quad &= \text{initial mouth pressure at FRC} \\
&\quad \text{(i.e., atmospheric or barometric pressure)} \\
\Delta P_A &= \text{change in mouth pressure during panting} \\
\Delta V &= \text{change in lung volume during panting}
\end{aligned}$$

Solving equation [4-4] for VTG yields:

$$V_{TG} = \frac{\Delta V}{\Delta P_A} \cdot (P_I + \Delta P_A) \qquad [4\text{-}5]$$

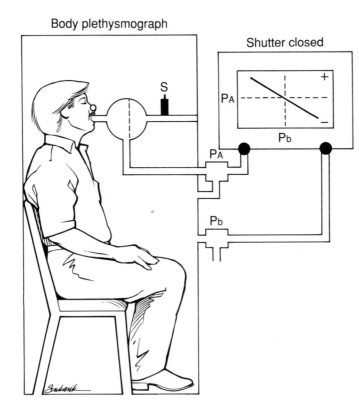

Body plethysmograph

Shutter closed

Figure 4-8. Body box method for measurement of thoracic gas volume (VTG). When the shutter (S) is closed at FRC, the subject makes panting inspiratory and expiratory efforts. As lung volume increases with intrathoracic gas decompression during inspiration, *box pressure (Pb) increases;* the opposite occurs during expiration. The relationship between mouth pressure (PA) and change in lung volume (ΔV)—or box pressure—is displayed on a screen. VTG is calculated as:

$$V_{TG} = \left(\frac{\Delta V}{\Delta P_A}\right) \cdot P_1$$

where PI is initial mouth pressure at FRC (i.e., atmospheric or barometric pressure). See text for details.

Since ΔP_A is negligible relative to P_I, equation [4-5] can be rewritten as:

$$V_{TG} = \frac{\Delta V}{\Delta P_A} \cdot P_I \qquad\qquad [4\text{-}6]$$

V_{TG} is expressed in liters. P_I, barometric pressure, is measured directly. The fractional term in equation [4-6], $\Delta V/\Delta P_A$, is the slope of the line drawn through the volume–pressure loop recorded on the oscilloscope of the body box (see Fig. 4-8). The tracing on the oscilloscope is actually alveolar pressure (P_A) versus body box pressure (P_b). The latter term, however, is directly related to changes in lung volume within the box, because the box is calibrated so that known changes in volume correspond to consistently measurable changes in pressure. Hence, for practical purposes, the term, ΔV, can be substituted for ΔP_b.

Body plethysmography provides a very rapid measure of lung volume and can be applied multiple times over a short interval. Some subjects, however, do not tolerate the body box because of claustrophobia. In addition, subjects may have a body habitus that precludes its use (e.g., extreme obesity).

COMMON PATTERNS OF ABNORMAL PULMONARY FUNCTION TESTS

Based on measurements of airflow rate and lung volume, several common *patterns* of pulmonary function test abnormalities may be described (Table 4-1).

In the *restrictive pattern,* the pathophysiologic hallmark is limited lung expansion, resulting in reduced lung volumes and a decrease in the driving force for expiratory airflow. The airways and airway resistance are normal, however. Spirometry demonstrates reductions in FVC and FEV_1, but preservation of $FEV_1/FVC\%$. Because of the loss of lung volume, the absolute airflow rate is reduced, as indicated by a low $FEF_{25\%-75\%}$. Lung volumes, including FRC, are decreased, giving a "shrunken lung" pattern.

In contrast, the *obstructive pattern* is characterized by reductions in expiratory airflow rates. The $FEV_1/FVC\%$ and $FEF_{25\%-75\%}$ are reduced. The FVC is usually normal or reduced, depending on whether the disease process affects other lung volumes. In the case of mild obstruction, such as mild asthma, the

TABLE 4-1. *COMMON PATTERNS OF PULMONARY FUNCTION ABNORMALTIES*

MEASUREMENT	RESTRICTIVE DISORDERS	OBSTRUCTIVE DISORDERS Mild	Severe
FVC	↓↓	Normal	↓
FEV_1	↓↓	↓	↓↓
$FEV_1/FVC\%$	Normal	↓	↓↓
$FEF_{25\%-75\%}$	↓↓	↓	↓↓
FRC	↓	Normal	↑
RV	↓	Normal	↑
TLC	↓	Normal	↑

FVC may be preserved, although spirometry demonstrates evidence of airway obstruction (reduced $FEV_1/FVC\%$). In more severe airway obstruction, such as severe emphysema, air trapping and loss of lung elastic recoil result in increases in RV and FRC. Consequently, FVC is diminished. FRC also may be increased, and TLC is normal or increased. The ratio of RV to TLC exceeds the normal value of 0.3.

With an obstructive pattern, it is clinically useful to document whether the obstruction is influenced by administration of a bronchodilator (see Chap. 5). Improvement in airflow rates after inhalation of an aerosol of a β-agonist suggests that the obstruction is caused, at least in part, by bronchospasm. Obstructive airway disease is considered reversible or "bronchodilator responsive" when the FEV_1 improves by at least 15% after administration of an inhaled bronchodilator.

Spirometry can also be used to document alterations in pulmonary function during an "inhalation challenge." For example, some patients with suspected asthma have normal results on spirometry. For diagnostic purposes, it may be useful in such patients to document whether bronchospasm can be induced pharmacologically. In the *methacholine challenge test,* a parasympathomimetic drug, methacholine, is inhaled in increasing doses administered sequentially. Spirometry is performed after each dose to assess the effect of the agent on expiratory airflow rate. In asthmatic patients, bronchospasm develops after a relatively low cumulative dose of methacholine.

EVALUATION OF UPPER AIRWAY OBSTRUCTION

As noted, the flow–volume loop may give information beyond that provided by simple spirometry. One important use of the flow–volume loop is the clinical assessment of suspected upper airway obstruction. Two important physiologic principles are worth underscoring in this regard.

The first principle is that breathing through a "fixed obstruction" (i.e., an obstruction whose geometry does not vary with the phase of respiration) limits airflow *in both inspiration and expiration.* The contours of the flow–volume loop generated by a healthy subject performing vital capacity maneuvers through narrow, rigid tubes are altered (Fig. 4-9). If the fixed obstruction occurs anywhere in the central airways, the flow–volume loop shows reduced airflow rates in both inspiration and expiration.

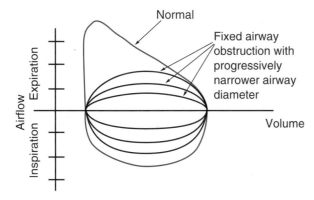

Figure 4-9. Flow–volume loops obtained with normal airways and with fixed airway obstruction. As the subject breathes through increasingly narrow fixed obstructions, both inspiratory and expiratory flow rates are progressively reduced.

The second physiologic principle is that dynamic factors affecting airways exert differing effects on airflow rate, depending on whether the airway is intrathoracic or extrathoracic (Fig. 4-10). Within the thorax, the airway is held open during inspiration by negative pleural pressure. During forced expiration, however, positive pleural pressure surrounding the airway compresses it, reducing airway diameter. Consequently, airway resistance is selectively increased during expiration.

In contrast, for extrathoracic airways, creation of negative intraluminal pressure during inspiration results in airway narrowing. During expiration, the intraluminal pressure becomes positive, making the airway diameter larger. Normally, large airways behave as semirigid tubes and are only modestly compressible. If the airways become narrowed or unusually pliable, however, airway resistance may vary markedly during respiration.

FUNCTIONAL CATEGORIES OF UPPER AIRWAY OBSTRUCTION

Based on the physiologic principles just described, three functional categories of upper airway obstruction may be defined on the basis of the flow–volume loop: (1) *fixed obstruction,* (2) *variable intrathoracic obstruction,* and (3) *variable extrathoracic obstruction* (Fig. 4-11).

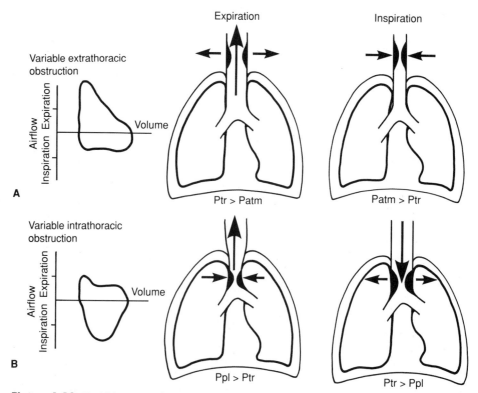

Figure 4-10. Variable upper airway obstruction. **(A)** Variable extrathoracic obstruction. Forced expiration increases intratracheal pressure (Ptr) above atmospheric pressure (Patm); airway diameter is nearly normal. During inspiration, Ptr is less than Patm; inspiratory airflow is reduced. **(B)** Variable intrathoracic obstruction. Forced expiration increases intrapleural pressure (Ppl) which exceeds Ptr; the intrathoracic airway is narrowed and expiratory airflow obstruction develops. During inspiration, Ptr exceeds Ppl and airway narrowing is minimized.

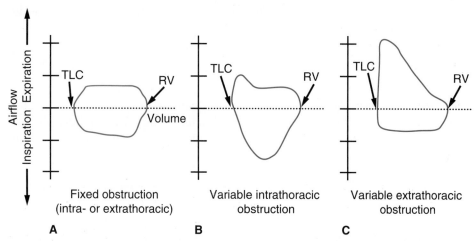

Figure 4-11. Flow–volume loop in fixed and variable upper airway obstructions. **(A)** Fixed obstruction. **(B)** Variable intrathoracic obstruction. **(C)** Variable extrathoracic obstruction. See text for discussion.

For both fixed and variable intrathoracic obstructions, spirometry reveals decreases in $FEV_1/FVC\%$ and $FEF_{25\%-75\%}$, indicating a limitation to expiratory airflow. The shape of the flow–volume curve is markedly different in the two disorders, however.

Fixed Obstruction

With a fixed obstruction (see Fig. 4-11A), such as tracheal stenosis due to a prior tracheostomy, the curve is flattened or truncated, and the normally easily discernible flow peak is absent. The expiratory flow pattern resembles that during inspiration; the mid-inspiratory and mid-expiratory airflow rates are approximately equal. This is in contrast to the usual relationship, where inspiratory airflow rate is approximately 1.5 times expiratory airflow rate.

Variable Intrathoracic Obstruction

With a variable intrathoracic obstruction (see Fig. 4-11B), such as a tracheal tumor above the carina, airway dynamics potentiate airway compression selectively during expiration. Expiratory airflow rate is reduced, and the contour of the expiratory flow–volume loop is flattened. During inspiration, however, the airflow rate and shape of the loop are normal.

Variable Extrathoracic Obstruction

Variable extrathoracic obstructions, such as vocal cord paralysis or vocal cord tumors, cause airflow limitation selectively during inspiration (see Fig. 4-11C). The presence of such an obstruction might also be predicted by an alteration in the relationship between the mid-inspiratory and mid-expiratory airflow rates: The mid-inspiratory airflow rate is markedly decreased compared to the mid-expiratory airflow rate, suggesting impairment of inspiratory flow.

ADDITIONAL PULMONARY FUNCTION TESTS OF CLINICAL OR PHYSIOLOGIC IMPORTANCE

Compared with the tests described previously, the following tests are used less commonly in clinical practice; however, they illustrate important pathophysiologic principles. For each test described, technical aspects are covered only briefly. Emphasis is placed on the underlying physiology.

MEASUREMENT OF AIRWAY RESISTANCE AND SPECIFIC CONDUCTANCE

Airway resistance (Raw) depends on lung volume (see Chap. 2). As lung volume increases, the lung parenchyma exerts a tethering action on intrapulmonary airways, increasing their diameter and reducing airway resistance. The relationship between Raw and its reciprocal, *airway conductance* (Gaw), is illustrated in Figure 4-12.

Variation in Raw with lung volume can be accurately determined using the body box (Fig. 4-13), the application of which in measurement of lung volume was described previously.

While seated in the body box, the subject pants through the open shutter connected to a flow-measuring device called a pneumotachograph. This maneuver produces, on the screen of the body box instrumentation, a closed loop that represents the relationship between airflow ($\dot{V}$) and box pressure (P_b), that is, $\dot{V}/P_b$. The shutter is then closed, and a loop representing alveolar pressure and box pressure (P_A/P_b) is generated. From these two measurements, airway resistance can be calculated as:

$$Raw = \frac{P_A/P_b}{\dot{V}/P_b} = \frac{P_A}{\dot{V}} \qquad [4\text{-}7]$$

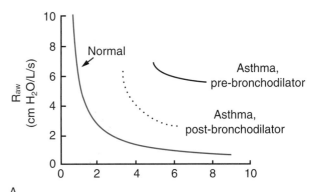

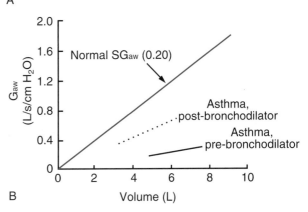

Figure 4-12. Changes in airway resistance and conductance with lung volume. **(A)** Airway resistance (Raw) in a healthy subject and in a patient with asthma before and after administration of an inhaled bronchodilator. **(B)** Airway conductance (Gaw) in a healthy subject and in an asthmatic patient before and after administration of an inhaled bronchodilator. Gaw is linearly related to lung volume; the slope represents *specific airway conductance* (SGaw). In asthma, Raw decreases and Gaw and SGaw increase after bronchodilator administration.

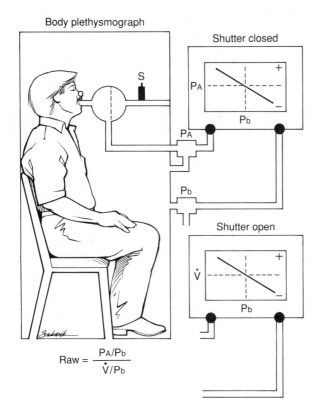

Body plethysmograph

Shutter closed

Shutter open

$$Raw = \frac{P_A/P_b}{\dot{V}/P_b}$$

Figure 4-13. Body box method for measurement of Raw. The relationship between pressure at the airway opening, equivalent to alveolar pressure (P$_A$), and box pressure (P$_b$), is obtained when the shutter (S) is closed. The relationship between flow ($\dot{V}$) and P$_b$ is obtained when the shutter is open. See text for details.

If this determination is made at several different lung volumes, the relationship between airway resistance and lung volume may be plotted.

PULMONARY COMPLIANCE

Occasionally, measurement of lung distensibility provides clinically useful information. As described in Chapter 2, lung inflation requires generation of a pressure across the lung's surface. In turn, inflation creates an elastic recoil pressure that promotes deflation. The magnitude of the pressure favoring deflation depends on the inflation volume (Fig. 4-14).

In an isolated lung, the inflation pressure is the pressure exerted across the wall of the alveolus, that is, the difference between alveolar pressure and surrounding pleural pressure. Alveolar pressure at any lung volume can be measured in the body box, as described previously. Pleural pressure can be measured directly using a catheter placed in the pleural space, or indirectly, by measuring intraesophageal pressure, which provides a relatively noninvasive and reliable estimate of pleural pressure.

The normal pressure–volume relationship of the lung is curvilinear. In the mid-portion of the vital capacity the curve is steep, but as the lung nears full inflation, progressively higher pressures are observed. Pulmonary fibrosis, a restrictive disease, is characterized by stiff lungs and a flat pressure–volume curve (see Chap. 7). Relatively small changes in volume are associated with large changes in pressure (Fig. 4-15). In contrast, emphysema, an obstructive disorder in which there is loss of lung elasticity, is characterized by a steep pressure–

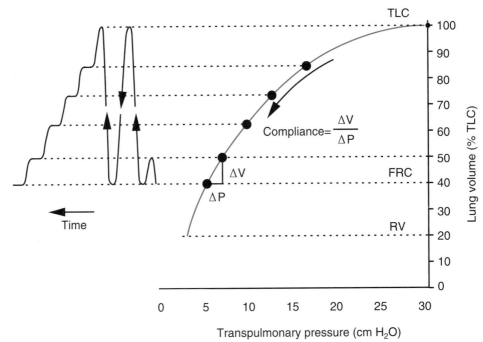

Figure 4-14. Static lung compliance. During deflation from TLC (lefthand side of figure), step decreases in lung volume (ΔV) are related to corresponding decreases in transpulmonary pressure (estimated using an intraesophageal balloon). The pressure–volume function is curvilinear, and the compliance at any point along the curve is $\Delta V/\Delta P$.

volume curve (see Chap. 6). Large changes in lung volume are accompanied by small changes in inflation pressure.

The balloon model of the lung, initially described in Chapter 2, is a useful construct for remembering these concepts. With restrictive lung diseases, the balloon-like lung becomes stiffer; it is less compliant and harder to inflate. Although the stiffer balloon is harder to inflate, once inflated, it exerts a high pressure. In emphysema, the lung loses its elasticity, becomes overly compliant and, during inflation, behaves more like a cellophane bag than a balloon. The cellophane bag is easy to inflate; however, it does not deflate very readily.

Figure 4-15. Pressure–volume curves in a healthy subject and in patients with emphysema or restrictive lung disease. The pressure–volume curve in emphysema is steeper (increased compliance), and the maximal elastic recoil pressure at TLC is reduced. The pressure–volume curve in restrictive lung disease (e.g., pulmonary fibrosis) is flatter (decreased compliance), and the maximal elastic recoil pressure at TLC is increased.

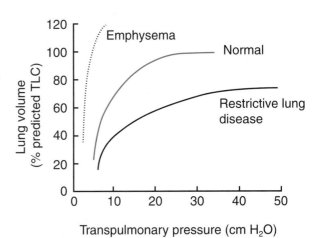

TESTS FOR SMALL AIRWAY DISEASE

When first developed, tests for detecting obstruction confined to the small airways (those <2 mm in diameter) were popular, based on the hypothesis that obstructive airway disease might still be reversible when confined to the small airways. Because of an uncertain correlation between the results of these tests and the natural history of obstructive airway disease, however, tests of small airway function have not been widely used. Nonetheless, two such tests illustrate several physiologic principles regarding airflow: (1) the *helium-oxygen flow–volume curve* and (2) measurement of *closing volume*, described initially in Chapter 3.

Helium–Oxygen Flow–Volume Curve

The helium-oxygen flow–volume curve takes advantage of the fact that the density of the inert gas, helium, is lower than that of air. When helium is breathed, its lower density results in a reduction of turbulent flow in large, central airways and enhancement of airflow rates where turbulent flow exists. Because airway resistance is higher in a turbulent-flow system (see Chap. 2), a reduction in turbulence is associated with a reduction in resistance. In contrast to the large airways, airflow in small airways is laminar; laminar flow is not density dependent. Therefore, breathing a gas of lower density has little influence on flow and resistance in small airways.

In performing the helium–oxygen flow–volume maneuver, the subject breathes a helium–oxygen gas mixture after first generating a flow–volume loop while breathing room air. As a result of reduced turbulence and resistance, in a healthy subject the flow–volume loop shows an increase in the expiratory airflow rate measured at 50% of the expiratory vital capacity—the $\Delta\dot{V}max_{50\%}$ (Fig. 4-16). In a patient with obstruction limited to the small airways, however,

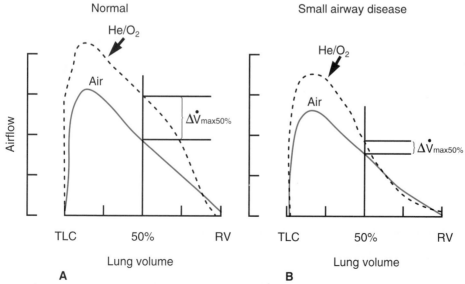

Figure 4-16. Helium–oxygen flow–volume curves. **(A)** Healthy subject. **(B)** Patient with small airway disease. $\Delta\dot{V}max_{50\%}$ is increased to a greater extent in the healthy subject breathing helium–oxygen than in the patient with small airway disease. See text for discussion.

where airflow is primarily laminar, breathing the helium–oxygen mixture fails to improve the airflow rate. Therefore, $\Delta\dot{V}max_{50\%}$ is much smaller in patients whose airway obstruction is caused by small airway disease (see Fig. 4-16B).

Closing Volume

Another test of small airway function, which highlights a different set of physiologic principles, is measurement of *closing volume* (see Chap. 3).

Smaller, peripheral airways are compressed during expiration, becoming progressively narrowed as residual volume is approached. This results in lower airflow rates at low lung volumes and, eventually, closure of small airways. In pathologic disorders of small airways, this effect is exaggerated. Consequently, small airways are narrowed and close earlier in expiration. The closing volume measurement is designed to measure the lung volume at which flow in small airways ceases.

CLINICAL EXAMPLES

To illustrate the usefulness of the previously described pulmonary function tests in clinical problem solving, several prototypic cases are described below.

CASE 1

A 65-year-old man complains of shortness of breath for the past year. He is a heavy cigarette smoker and has a chronic cough, producing several tablespoons of white sputum each morning. He has no known cardiac disease, but he is worried that he may have emphysema. His physical examination reveals diffusely diminished breath sounds. A chest radiograph shows hyperinflation, but it is otherwise negative. Results of spirometry are shown in Table 4-2. Test results are shown before and after the administration of an inhaled bronchodilator.

TABLE 4-2. *CASE 1: PULMONARY FUNCTION TESTS*

PULMONARY FUNCTION TEST	BEFORE BRONCHODILATOR		AFTER BRONCHODILATOR	
	Actual Value	Percent Predicted	Actual Value	Percent Change
FVC (L)	4.0	103	4.2	5
FEV_1 (L)	2.4	80	2.9	20
$FEV_1/FVC\%$	60		68	
$FEF_{25\%-75\%}$ (L/s)	2.0	51	2.4	20
$FIF_{25\%-75\%}$ (L/s)	4.0	68	4.4	10
MVV (L/min)	110	79	115	5

Initial spirometry shows moderate airway obstruction, as indicated by the reduced $FEV_1/FVC\%$ (60%). The FVC is preserved. Therefore, the patient has pure obstructive disease. The etiology may be a reversible process, such as asthma, or an irreversible disorder, such as emphysema. An endobronchial lesion (e.g., an intrathoracic malignancy) is also a possibility. In this case, an inhaled bronchodilator was administered to help differentiate among the considerations. Repeat spirometry demonstrates that the airway obstruction is largely reversible, as indicated by an increase in FEV_1 by 20%. This strongly suggests that the patient has a component of asthma. Reversibility of obstruction on spirometry is associated with a more favorable prognosis and suggests that bronchodilator therapy will be useful.

CASE 2

A 25-year-old woman who had been hospitalized for several months with the adult respiratory distress syndrome (see Chap. 14), has made a complete recovery after prolonged endotracheal intubation. Three months after discharge, she notes progressive shortness of breath. On physical examination, her chest is clear. Chest radiograph shows only mild interstitial changes. Results of spirometry are shown in Table 4-3.

TABLE 4-3. *CASE 2: PULMONARY FUNCTION TESTS*

PULMONARY FUNCTION TEST	ACTUAL VALUE	PERCENT PREDICTED
FVC (L)	4.0	108
FEV_1 (L)	2.0	65
$FEV_1/FVC\%$	50	
$FEF_{25\%-75\%}$ (L/s)	2.0	50
$FIF_{25\%-75\%}$ (L/s)	2.0	50
MVV (L/min)	50	41

Spirometry reveals a normal FVC, but reduced FEV_1 and $FEV_1/FVC\%$. A subtle clue in the spirometry is that the mid-inspiratory airflow rate matches the mid-expiratory airflow rate. Normally, the inspiratory airflow rate is at least 50% greater than the expiratory airflow rate. These findings suggest that obstruction is present during both inspiration and expiration.

A flow–volume loop shows a contour similar to that in Figure 4-11A, suggesting that the patient has a fixed upper airway obstruction. In this case, the obstruction was the result of tracheal stenosis from the prior endotracheal intubation. Examination of the inspiratory spirogram may be essential in correctly diagnosing the cause of obstructive airway disease.

CASE 3

A 50-year-old woman with no significant past medical history is referred for unexplained shortness of breath. An extensive cardiovascular evaluation is negative. She has no smoking history; her physical examination and chest radiograph are normal. Spirometry is shown in Table 4-4.

TABLE 4-4.   *CASE 3: PULMONARY FUNCTION TESTS*

PULMONARY FUNCTION TEST	ACTUAL VALUE	PERCENT PREDICTED
FVC (L)	2.0	64
FEV_1 (L)	1.8	70
$FEV_1/FVC\%$	90	
$FEF_{25\%-75\%}$ (L/s)	2.0	59
$FIF_{25\%-75\%}$ (L/s)	4.0	78
MVV (L/min)	90	93
MIP (cm H_2O)	32	88
MEP (cm H_2O)	63	90

The patient has a reduced FVC and a normal $FEV_1/FVC\%$, suggesting restrictive lung disease or a neuromuscular disorder. The normal MIP, MEP, and MVV rule against the latter diagnosis, however. Because the patient's degree of respiratory impairment does not seem to match the rest of her clinical picture, a flow–volume loop is obtained (Fig. 4-17). As can be seen, the patient did not complete the FVC maneuver. There was an abrupt, premature termination of expiration; the patient's tracing did not return to the starting point on the curve. Such a finding may be the result of technical problems, or may represent poor patient cooperation. In either case, without an analysis of the flow–volume loop, spirometry would have given the mistaken impression of significant pulmonary disease.

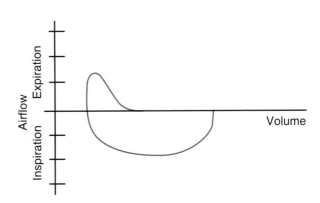

Figure 4-17. Flow–volume loop generated with poor patient effort or coordination.

CASE 4

A 60-year-old male shipyard worker is referred for disability evaluation. He has had significant exposure to asbestos and has been a heavy cigarette smoker. Examination of the chest reveals decreased breath sounds and a few fine rales scattered throughout both lung fields. The chest radiograph shows hyperinflation and mild accentuation of the interstitial markings. Spirometry, before and after administration of an inhaled bronchodilator, and lung volumes are shown in Table 4-5.

TABLE 4-5. *CASE 4: PULMONARY FUNCTION TESTS*				
PULMONARY FUNCTION TEST	**BEFORE BRONCHODILATOR**		**AFTER BRONCHODILATOR**	
	Actual Value	**Percent Predicted**	**Actual Value**	**Percent Change**
FVC (L)	2.4	60	2.4	0
FEV_1 (L)	1.4	44	1.5	7
$FEV_1/FVC\%$	58		63	
$FEF_{25\%-75\%}$ (L/s)	1.3	33	1.2	0
$FIF_{25\%-75\%}$ (L/s)	4.0	67	4.0	0
MVV (L/min)	49	34	50	2
RV (L)	4.6	205		
TLC (L)	7.0	112		
FRC (L)	5.2	142		

The patient's initial spirometry shows a reduced FVC and a moderate degree of airflow obstruction that is not bronchodilator responsive. These findings are compatible with emphysema. The pattern of obstruction, however, including the reduced FVC, could also be caused by a combination of obstructive airway disease and restrictive lung disease related to asbestos exposure. Measurement of lung volumes is an important test in determining which process predominates.

The patient's RV, FRC, and TLC are markedly elevated. Hence, restrictive lung disease is excluded as a cause of the reduced FVC. Instead, the elevated lung volumes strongly suggest that the patient has loss of lung elastic recoil and that the major pathophysiologic process is airway obstruction secondary to emphysema.

SELECTED READING

Briscoe WA, Dubois AB. The relationship between airway resistance, airway conductance, and lung volume in subjects of different age and body size. J Clin Invest 37:1279–1285, 1958.

Cosio M, Ghezzo H, Hogg JC, et al. The relations between structural changes in small airways and pulmonary-function tests. N Engl J Med 298:1277–1281, 1977.

Despas PJ, Leroux M, Macklem PT. Site of airway obstruction in asthma as determined by measuring maximal expiratory flow breathing air and a helium–oxygen mixture. J Clin Invest 51:3235–3243, 1972.

Dosman J, Bode F, Urbanetti J, et al. The use of a helium–oxygen mixture during maximum expiratory flow to demonstrate obstruction in small airways in smokers. J Clin Invest 55:1090–1099, 1975.

DuBois AB, Botelho SY, Bedell GN, Marshall R, Comroe JH Jr. A rapid plethysmographic method for measuring thoracic gas volume: A comparison with a nitrogen washout method for measuring functional residual capacity in normal subjects. J Clin Invest 35:322–326, 1956.

DuBois AB, Botelho SY, Comroe JH Jr. A new method for measuring airway resistance in man using a body plethysmograph: Values in normal subjects and in patients with respiratory disease. J Clin Invest 35:327–335, 1956.

Kryger M, Bode F, Antic R, Anthonisen N. Diagnosis of obstruction of the central and upper airways. Am J Med 61:85–93, 1976.

Lippincott's Pathophysiology Series: Pulmonary
Pathophysiology, edited by Michael A. Grippi.
J. B. Lippincott Company, Philadelphia © 1995.

CHAPTER

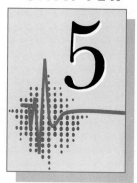

5

Mechanisms of Bronchoconstriction and Asthma

Richard K. Murray

In the preceding chapter on pulmonary function testing, the physiologic characterization of respiratory disorders as "obstructive" or "restrictive" (or both) was highlighted. Obstructive pulmonary disorders are very common. Asthma is the prototype of the *reversible* disorders in this category, affecting approximately 5% of the population of the United States.

This chapter focuses on our current understanding of the pathophysiology of bronchoconstriction and asthma. The pathology, role of airway inflammation, and mechanisms of airway smooth muscle contraction are considered. Subsequently, the effects of airway narrowing on pulmonary function tests are reviewed. Finally, an overview of management, based on underlying pathophysiology, is presented.

OVERVIEW OF MECHANISMS OF AIRWAY NARROWING IN ASTHMA

Airway narrowing arises through several mechanisms (Fig. 5-1). One important mechanism is contraction of airway smooth muscle (ASM), which is found throughout the trachea and bronchi. ASM contracts in response to a variety of stimuli, including neurotransmitters and inflammatory mediators. ASM contraction narrows the airway lumen and markedly increases airway resistance (see Chaps. 2 and 4).

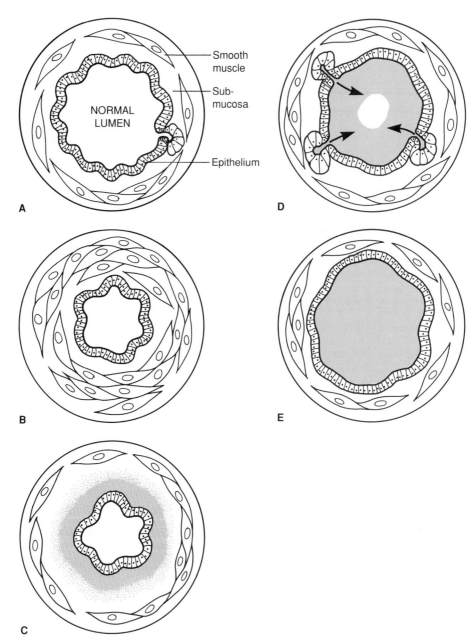

Figure 5-1. Mechanisms of airway narrowing in asthma. **(A)** The normal airway is lined by an intact epithelium, below which is the submucosa containing blood vessels. Glands secrete mucus into the airway lumen. Layers of smooth muscle and discontinuous areas of cartilage are present. **(B)** In an asthma exacerbation, narrowing of the lumen occurs as a consequence of smooth muscle contraction and possible hyperplasia or hypertrophy. **(C)** Thickening of the submucosal space by edema and cellular infiltration. **(D)** Inspissated secretions. **(E)** Accumulation of cellular debris resulting from epithelial damage and airway inflammation.

Another mechanism of airway narrowing is based on airway wall thickening. The acute effects of asthma, such as airway wall cellular infiltration and edema, as well as the chronic effects of airway inflammation, such as smooth muscle hyperplasia and hypertrophy, lead to narrowing of the airway lumen or amplification of the effects of ASM contraction.

Finally, accumulation of airway secretions, mucus casts, and cellular debris may partially occlude the airway lumen, leading to increased resistance.

Although contraction of ASM can be reversed rapidly with administration of bronchodilator drugs, the other two mechanisms of airway narrowing are not immediately reversible. Recent insights into the pathology of asthma, which includes airway wall thickening and excess secretions, have provided direction in the investigation of basic pathophysiologic mechanisms.

PATHOLOGY OF ASTHMA

Historically, most information on the pathology of asthma was derived from autopsy studies. The usual findings include airway inflammation with the presence of neutrophils, eosinophils, and mononuclear cells, and epithelial cell damage. More recently, lung biopsies performed through the flexible fiberoptic bronchoscope have confirmed the presence of these inflammatory changes, even in patients with mild asthma. Other common findings include mucus hypersecretion and an increase in ASM mass due to hypertrophy or hyperplasia. In patients with chronic asthma, the numbers of airway eosinophils, mast cells, macrophages, and T-helper lymphocytes are increased. Figure 5-2 shows examples of epithelial destruction and increased muscle mass in bronchial biopsy specimens from an asthmatic patient.

Before considering the relationship between the pathologic findings and pathophysiology of asthma, it is useful to consider in some detail the normal regulation of airway caliber.

REGULATION OF AIRWAY CALIBER

Airway diameter is under active regulation by a number of control mechanisms, including the autonomic nervous system (Fig. 5-3).

Cholinergic (parasympathetic) motoneurons innervate the airways via the vagus nerve, synapsing near ASM cells. These neurons release the neurotransmitter, *acetylcholine,* which is a potent stimulator of ASM contraction.

Although *sympathetic neurons* might be predicted to relax ASM, in humans there is little direct effect of the sympathetic nervous system in determining airway caliber. Indirect effects of the sympathetic nervous system by way of the adrenal gland may play a minor role in the normal regulation of airway diameter.

The *nonadrenergic noncholinergic (NANC) nervous system* exerts powerful excitatory and inhibitory influences over ASM tone. NANC system neurons in the vagus nerve release the peptides, *substance P* and *vasoactive intestinal peptide (VIP)*, which contract and relax ASM cells, respectively. Substance P-releasing neurons also participate in local reflex arcs in which local irritation of nerve endings (e.g., because of epithelial cell damage or release of inflammatory mediators) leads to reflex contraction of ASM. VIP-releasing neurons relax ASM by increasing

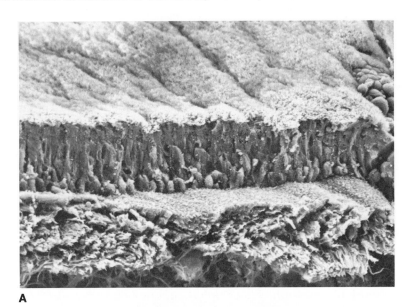

A

Figure 5-2. Scanning electron micrographs of normal and asthmatic airway walls. **(A)** Normal airway. Surface epithelium (top of figure) is attached to a thin basement membrane with underlying collagen (magnification, ×400). **(B)** Asthmatic airway. Epithelial destruction, as a consequence of mechanical and inflammatory effects, is seen. The exposed basement membrane may permit enhanced access of luminal mediators to underlying smooth muscle which, in the figure, is increased dramatically in size (rounded masses) as a result of hypertrophy or hyperplasia (magnification, ×250). (From Jeffrey P. Morphology of the airway wall in asthma and COPD. Am Rev Respir Dis 143: 1156, 1991.)

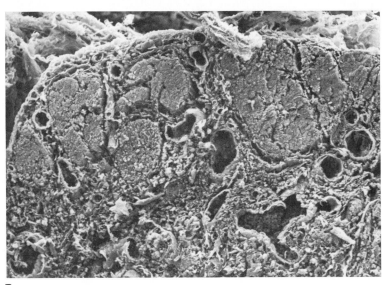

B

intracellular *cyclic adenosine monophosphate (cAMP)* levels. The neurons of the NANC system appear to be the most potent relaxant component of the nervous system that are involved in regulation of airway caliber.

Finally, there is little evidence that physiologic changes in circulating levels of cortisol or other hormones play an important role in the regulation of airway diameter in humans.

AIRWAY INFLAMMATION AND INFLAMMATORY MEDIATORS IN ASTHMA

Studies performed in asthmatics using bronchoalveolar lavage, in which saline is repeatedly instilled and aspirated from a local lung region through a

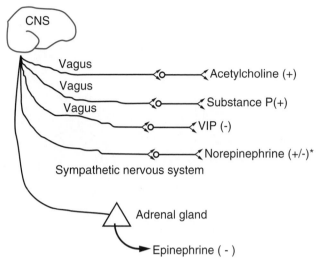

Figure 5-3. The autonomic nervous system and control of airway diameter. Parasympathetic neurons travel in the vagus nerve and synapse close to airway smooth muscle. These neurons release acetylcholine, which causes contraction (+). Nonadrenergic, noncholinergic (NANC) excitatory neurons also travel in the vagus and release the potent neuropeptide, substance P, which causes ASM contraction. NANC inhibitory neurons release the neuropeptide, vasoactive intestinal peptide (VIP), which causes ASM relaxation (−). Sympathetic neurons, acting through the adrenal gland, may cause minor changes in airway tone due to changes in circulating levels of catecholamines.

fiberoptic bronchoscope, have demonstrated a large number of biologically active molecules in alveoli, collectively referred to as *mediators*. These mediators play an important role in airway inflammation, and a variety of cells are active in their elaboration (Fig. 5-4).

ROLE OF LYMPHOCYTES

T lymphocytes appear to be important in local immunologic regulation of the airways. In particular, release of the cytokine, interleukin-2 (IL-2), by T lymphocytes plays an autocrine (self-stimulatory) role. T lymphocytes, in concert with antigen-presenting macrophages, release a number of other cytokines as well, including IL-3, IL-4, IL-5, and IL-6. Cytokines have important effects on B lymphocytes (e.g., stimulation of production of specific antibody), mast cells, and eosinophils (e.g., cell priming and activation). The mast cells and eosinophils may bind specific IgE molecules, and cross-linking of IgE by antigen may be an important initiating event in exacerbations of asthma.

ROLE OF MAST CELLS

When mast cells are activated, a number of preformed and newly formed mediators are released. Examples include histamine, leukotrienes, bradykinin, and various prostaglandins. Among the biologic effects of these mediators are chemotaxis of white cells, contraction of airway and vascular smooth muscle, cytotoxicity for airway epithelium, and activation of other effector cells. Mast cell mediators and their biologic effects are summarized in Table 5-1.

ROLE OF EOSINOPHILS

Eosinophils that are recruited into the lung and activated also release previously formed and newly synthesized mediators (Table 5-2). The pathologic ef-

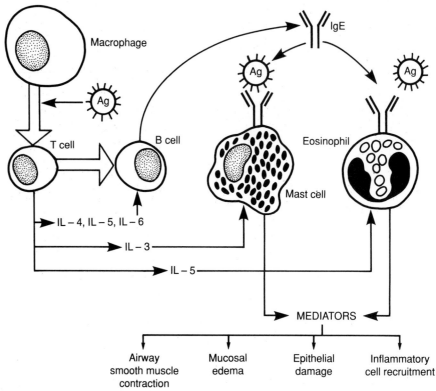

Figure 5-4. Interactions between immune effector cells and the airways. Macrophages participate in antigen (Ag) presentation to T cells, which stimulate B cells to produce specific IgE antibodies. Interleukins -4, -5, and -6 (IL-4, IL-5, IL-6), elaborated from the T cell, participate in the B-cell stimulation. IL-3 and IL-5 help "prime" mast cells and eosinophils, respectively. Both mast cells and eosinophils may be coated with IgE and interact with antigen, resulting in activation of either effector cell. The resultant release of mediators leads to airway inflammation, mucosal thickening, epithelial damage, and airway narrowing. (From Murray RK, Panettieri RA Jr. Management of asthma: The changing approach. In: Fishman AP, ed. Update: Pulmonary Diseases and Disorders. New York: McGraw-Hill, 1992:74.)

fects of these mediators include airway inflammation, epithelial cell damage, mucosal edema, and ASM contraction.

ROLE OF AIRWAY EPITHELIUM

Cytotoxic effects of mediators on epithelium further complicate the pathologic picture of asthma. Loss of the epithelial "barrier" function and a decrease in production of *epithelial-derived relaxant factor*—a substance that promotes ASM relaxation—may exacerbate airway hyperreactivity. The interplay among mediators, epithelium, smooth muscle, and local neural reflexes is shown schematically in Figure 5-5.

THE MEDIATOR "SOUP"

The mediator "soup" that emerges from the interplay between lymphocytes and effector cells includes a huge number of biologically active molecules.

TABLE 5-1. *MAST CELL MEDIATORS*

MEDIATOR	EFFECTS IN ASTHMA
Preformed Mediators	
Histamine	Airway smooth muscle contraction, mucus secretion
Chemotactic factors	Chemotaxis of eosinophils and neutrophils
Tryptase	Generation of bradykinin; degradation of vasoactive intestinal peptide
Newly Formed Mediators	
Superoxide	Cytotoxicity
Leukotrienes C4, D4, E4	Airway smooth muscle contraction, mucosal edema, and mucus secretion
Prostaglandin D_2	Airway smooth muscle contraction
Prostaglandin E_2	Mucosal edema
Thromboxane	Airway smooth muscle contraction
Bradykinin	Mucosal edema, airway smooth muscle contraction
Platelet activating factor	Bronchoconstriction (?)
Cytokines	
Granulocyte–monocyte colony-stimulating factor	Stimulation, maturation, and priming of eosinophils
Interleukin-3 Interleukin-5	Stimulation, maturation, and priming of eosinophils

TABLE 5-2. *EOSINOPHIL MEDIATORS*

MEDIATOR	EFFECTS IN ASTHMA
Preformed Mediators	
Major basic protein	Cytotoxicity, epithelial cell damage
Eosinophil cationic protein	Cytotoxicity, neurotoxicity
Eosinophil-derived neurotoxin	Unknown
Eosinophil peroxidase	Unknown
Newly Formed Mediators	
Platelet activating factor	Bronchoconstriction (?)
Leukotriene B4	Mucosal inflammation, chemotaxis
Leukotriene C4	Airway smooth muscle contraction, edema, mucus secretion
15-hydroxyeicosatetraenoic acid	Activation of mast cells

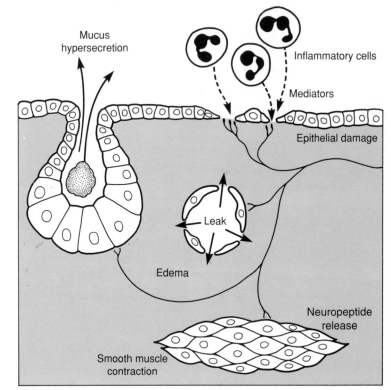

Figure 5-5. Interaction of airway epithelium, autonomic nervous system, and cellular mediators in asthma. Inflammatory cells in the airway lumen exert a cytotoxic effect on the epithelium, enhancing mediator access to exposed neurons and underlying smooth muscle. Activation of local neural reflexes (involving antidromic conduction) leads to airway smooth muscle contraction and vasogenic edema, the latter from effects on vascular smooth muscle. In addition, direct effects of inflammatory mediators and neural reflexes contribute to mucus hypersecretion, potentiating airway obstruction.

Some important mediators have been identified (e.g., leukotriene D_4, LTD4) and have been specifically targeted for possible therapeutic intervention (e.g., development of competitive antagonists or inhibitors of their production). Unfortunately, no single mediator dominates the pathogenesis of asthma, and the approach to treatment of airway inflammation remains based on the use of corticosteroids. Although corticosteroids are very effective antiinflammatory drugs, they exert a number of undesirable side effects. As more is learned about specific adhesion factors responsible for cell trafficking and the cytokines responsible for activation of specific effector cells, a more focused approach using antiinflammatory agents should emerge.

AIRWAY SMOOTH MUSCLE CONTRACTION

As noted, a number of neurohumoral substances and inflammatory mediators exert potent effects on ASM. In a sense, ASM forms the common final pathway for the transduction of these biologic compounds' effects into airway narrowing. To understand the ways in which the biology of the system might be modified pharmacologically, it is necessary to explore the basics of intracellular signaling and the roles of membrane ion channels and β-receptors in regulating ASM tone.

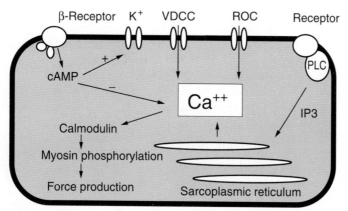

Figure 5-6. Signal transduction in airway smooth muscle. Pathways related to activation of contractile agonists of airway smooth muscle are highlighted. An agonist that binds with its specific surface receptor, coupled through a G protein, activates phospholipase C (PLC). As a result, phosphatidylinositol bis-phosphate is cleaved to diacylglycerol and inositol tris-phosphate (IP3); the concentration of IP3 rises, and calcium is released from the sarcoplasmic reticulum. The rise in intracellular calcium results in activation of calmodulin, an increase in myosin light chain kinase activity, phosphorylation of myosin, cross-bridge cycling, and contractile force production. Extracellular calcium may stimulate contraction through voltage-dependent calcium channels (VDCC) or receptor-operated channels (ROC). Stimulation of cell surface β-receptors by β-adrenergic agents results in G protein interaction with adenylate cyclase, leading to a rise in cAMP. cAMP activates protein kinase A, initiates phosphorylation of intracellular proteins, and has functional effects on airway smooth muscle contraction. Inhibition of phosphodiesterase increases the intracellular effects of cAMP.

INTRACELLULAR SIGNALING IN AIRWAY SMOOTH MUSCLE

Most agents that exert an effect on ASM act through specific *surface receptors.* A contractile substance or *agonist,* such as acetylcholine, histamine, or LTD4, binds to a specific surface receptor to initiate a cascade of biochemical events that, ultimately, leads to an increase in smooth muscle cell contraction. The agonist's effect may be negated by blocking the receptor with an *antagonist* (e.g., an anticholinergic agent or antihistamine) or by manipulating subsequent biochemical events within the cell. The latter approach is sometimes referred to as *functional antagonism.*

Figure 5-6 highlights the biochemical events that follow agonist–receptor binding. With binding, membrane-bound *phospholipase C* is activated (by a guanosine triphosphate-binding protein, G_q). The membrane lipid, phosphatidylinositol bis-phosphate is cleaved into *inositol tris-phosphate* (IP3) and diacylglycerol. IP3 is a soluble, intracellular "second messenger" that releases calcium from intracellular stores (sarcoplasmic reticulum). The increase in cytosolic calcium, which may also arise from calcium influx through cell membrane calcium channels, initiates a series of calcium-dependent biochemical events.

As a result of these events, *myosin light chain kinase* is activated and actin–myosin cross-bridge cycling occurs, in a manner analogous to that in skeletal muscle. Hence, factors that modulate calcium mobilization in response to stimulation by a contractile agonist alter ASM contractile force. In addition, they present a target for development of functional antagonists of a variety of contractile substances.

ION CHANNELS IN AIRWAY SMOOTH MUSCLE

In addition to agonist–receptor interactions, a number of ion channels participate in the regulation of ASM tone (see Fig. 5-6).

Voltage-dependent calcium channels (VDCC) are a membrane-depolarization mechanism by which intracellular calcium concentration and ASM contraction are augmented. Inhibition of calcium channels by organic calcium channel blockers (e.g., dihydropyridines), in turn, inhibits ASM contraction. Inhibition of VDCC, however, does not fully block ASM contraction, in part because of the major contribution of intracellular calcium release to the production of contractile force. In addition, other pathways for calcium influx, such as receptor-operated channels, appear to be present in this tissue.

Finally, potassium channels regulate the steady-state flux of potassium across the membrane and set the cell's resting membrane potential. These channels may be "opened" by potassium channel agonists, which hyperpolarize the cell. Hyperpolarization decreases the contribution of VDCC and results in decreased ASM contraction.

THE β-ADRENERGIC SYSTEM

Another important regulatory pathway in ASM is the *β-adrenergic system* (see Fig. 5-6). This system transduces the effect of β-adrenergic agents, such as isoproterenol, by activation of the GTP-binding protein, G_s, which stimulates adenyl cyclase. Increased adenyl cyclase activity increases cAMP production and activation of protein kinase A. Protein kinase A phosphorylates a variety of intracellular targets, leading to important biochemical alterations. This effect may be mimicked by agents that prevent the breakdown of cAMP, such as phosphodiesterase inhibitors (e.g., theophylline).

Previously, all β-adrenergic effects were thought to be exerted through an increase in cAMP and activation of protein kinase A. It has been shown, however, that specific subunits of the G_s protein that couple the β-receptor to adenyl cyclase can act as soluble second messengers, exerting potentially important effects on the potassium channel.

Little evidence exists to support the notion that an intrinsic abnormality of ASM causes the development of asthma. Although this possibility has not been completely excluded, subtle abnormalities in immune regulation, changes in the pattern or degree of mediator production, or release of neurohumoral substances seem more likely explanations.

PHYSIOLOGIC CONSEQUENCES OF AIRWAY OBSTRUCTION

Physiologic derangements produced by the cellular and biochemical events described previously may be profound. They are associated with predictable clinical findings and results on pulmonary function testing.

ALTERATIONS IN RESPIRATORY MECHANICS

During an asthma attack, increased resistance to airflow, which is accentuated during expiration, causes air trapping and an increase in FRC—

"hyperinflation." Hyperinflation, noted on the chest radiograph as flattening of the diaphragm, results in an increase in the work of breathing, because the muscle fibers of the flattened diaphragm are no longer operating at the optimal point on their length–tension curve (see Chap. 2). In addition, the hyperinflated lung occupies a new position on the pressure–volume curve. A larger change in intrathoracic pressure is required to effect a change in lung volume. Hence, in addition to overcoming increased airway resistance, the asthmatic must use less efficient respiratory muscles to inflate stiffer lungs. Furthermore, these pathophysiologic effects increase oxygen consumption and carbon dioxide production by the diaphragm.

ALTERATIONS IN GAS EXCHANGE

In addition to the adverse mechanical effects observed in asthma, deleterious changes in gas exchange also occur. The most important is the mismatching of ventilation and pulmonary blood flow, so-called "ventilation–perfusion mismatching," described in Chapter 13.

Normally, ventilation and perfusion are closely coupled or "matched" within regions of the lung. When ventilation–perfusion relationships are altered, areas that are relatively underventilated are responsible for a drop in arterial oxygenation. On the other hand, regions that are relatively underperfused contribute to inefficient ventilation and impairment of CO_2 elimination.

ALTERATIONS IN SPIROMETRY AND LUNG VOLUMES

In asthmatic patients experiencing an acute exacerbation of their disease, pulmonary function tests characteristically demonstrate an obstructive pattern (see Chap. 4). Between attacks, patients have normal or near-normal pulmonary function, although airway hyperreactivity to nonspecific stimuli still may be demonstrated. In addition to having a normal FVC, FEV_1, and $FEV_1/FVC\%$, well-controlled patients have a normal maximal voluntary ventilation (MVV) and $FEF_{25\%-75\%}$.

During an asthma attack, airway obstruction leads to reductions in $FEF_{25\%-75\%}$, FEV_1, FVC, and $FEV_1/FVC\%$. The MVV is also decreased due to prolongation of the expiratory phase. Patients inspire more forcefully to shorten the inspiratory time. Because of the resultant prolongation in the expiratory phase, a decrease in the inspiratory-to-expiratory time ratio is common. In addition, lung volumes (TLC, RV, and FRC) increase because of air trapping.

As the patient responds to treatment, many of the pulmonary function test abnormalities resolve, although some derived measures may actually worsen. For example, as the FEV_1 and FVC improve with treatment, the $FEV_1/FVC\%$ may worsen. Ultimately, most spirometric tests and lung volume measurements normalize, although subtle abnormalities, such as the decrease in $FEF_{25\%-75\%}$, may persist for several weeks. Typical changes in pulmonary function tests during an exacerbation of asthma are summarized in Figure 5-7.

BRONCHOPROVOCATION

Bronchoprovocational challenge is a test of potential value in patients in whom the diagnosis of asthma is suspected, but not definitively established.

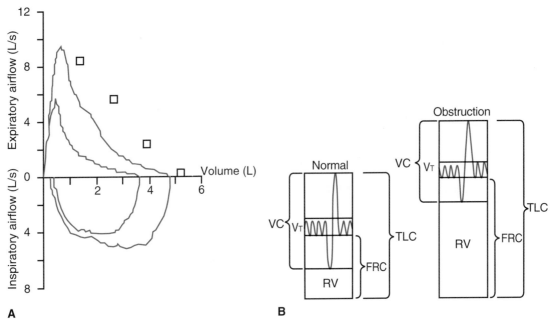

Figure 5-7. Pulmonary function tests in an exacerbation of asthma. **(A)** Flow–volume loop. The inner loop, obtained before administration of an inhaled bronchodilator, demonstrates severe obstruction and reduced expiratory and inspiratory flows. After treatment, marked improvement in flow is noted (outer loop); however, the expiratory curve has not returned to predicted normal (boxes). **(B)** Routine spirometry and lung volumes. TLC, FRC, and RV are increased; the patient is "hyperinflated." VC and VT are decreased.

The patient inhales progressively higher concentrations of nebulized methacholine or histamine, each of which is capable of stimulating airway obstruction in both healthy subjects and asthmatics. In asthmatics, however, the concentration required to lower the airflow rate by 20% (the PD_{20} or "provocative dose") is several orders of magnitude less than in healthy subjects. Hence, measurement of the PD_{20} can help establish the diagnosis of asthma in a patient with otherwise normal pulmonary function tests.

THERAPY OF ASTHMA

The pathophysiologic consequences of asthma that, in the extreme case, culminate in respiratory failure (see Chap. 18) are summarized in Figure 5-8. Physiologically targeted approaches to asthma management include use of drugs to relax ASM (bronchodilators) and to suppress airway inflammation (antiinflammatory agents).

BRONCHODILATORS

Bronchodilators act primarily by inhibiting ASM contraction; they include *specific antagonists* and *functional antagonists.*

Examples of specific antagonists of ASM contraction are anticholinergics (e.g., atropine and ipratropium bromide), antihistamines, and LTD4 blockers.

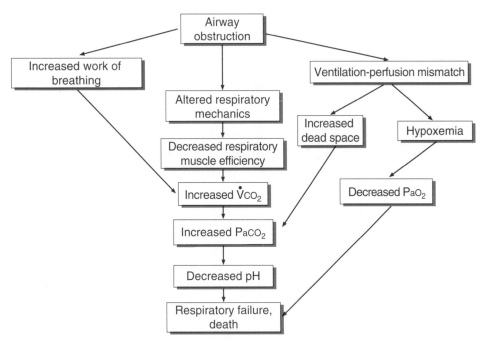

Figure 5-8. Pathophysiologic consequences of airway obstruction on work of breathing, respiratory mechanics, and ventilation–perfusion (V̇/Q̇) matching. Mechanical and gas-exchange abnormalities decrease respiratory muscle efficiency and interfere with CO_2 elimination. Ultimately, life-threatening respiratory and metabolic acidoses develop (see Chap. 10). Interventions include use of bronchodilators and antiinflammatory agents, supplemental oxygen, and mechanical ventilation. See text for discussion. (From Murray RK, Panettieri RA Jr. Management of asthma: The changing approach. In: Fishman AP, ed. Update: Pulmonary Diseases and Disorders. New York: McGraw-Hill, 1992:72.)

In addition, agents that inhibit lipoxygenase and reduce production of LTD4 by inflammatory cells constitute examples of specific antagonists.

Functional antagonists of ASM contraction, which oppose the effects of a variety of mediators and neurohumoral substances, include β-adrenergic agents, phosphodiesterase inhibitors, calcium channel blockers, and potassium channel agonists (see Fig. 5-6).

β-Adrenergic Agents

β-Adrenergic agents, such as isoproterenol, or β_2-selective compounds, such as albuterol, are very effective bronchodilators. These substances increase cAMP levels within ASM cells, oppose agonist-induced calcium mobilization, and oppose membrane depolarization through activation of potassium channels. Furthermore, β-adrenergic agents may be delivered locally in aerosols; aerosolized β_2-selective drugs are relatively free of systemic side effects.

Phosphodiesterase Inhibitors

Phosphodiesterase inhibitors (e.g., theophylline) may also increase cAMP levels within ASM cells. Whether this increase occurs with therapeutic drug levels is debated. Theophylline is a less effective bronchodilator than are the β-adrenergic agents. In addition, because theophylline is taken orally, its use is limited by systemic side effects.

Calcium Channel Blockers

To date, calcium channel blockers have been disappointing as bronchodilators. Because VDCC in ASM are modulated by dihydropyridines, the ineffectiveness of these agents most likely reflects the complexities of calcium homeostasis in ASM and the fact that inhibition of VDCC, alone, is insufficient to prevent agonist-induced calcium mobilization.

Potassium Channel Agonists

Potassium channel agonists have been used successfully as bronchodilators, but their use has been complicated by effects on vascular smooth muscle, resulting in systemic hypotension.

ANTIINFLAMMATORY AGENTS

Antiinflammatory agents used in asthma management include corticosteroids and cromolyn sodium.

Corticosteroids

Corticosteroids may be given orally, intramuscularly, or intravenously. Alternatively, corticosteroids can be administered in aerosols. The advantage of inhaled corticosteroids is the relative absence of corticosteroid side effects.

Corticosteroids have a number of effects on airways that are useful in management of asthma: (1) reduction in the number of inflammatory cells (eosinophils, neutrophils, and macrophages); (2) inhibition of secretion of prostaglandins and leukotrienes by effector cells; and (3) reduction in airway edema.

Corticosteroids interact with an intracellular steroid receptor that evokes nuclear responses, including the production of *lipocortin*. Although the details of the mechanism of action of corticosteroids remain incompletely understood, inhibitory effects on phospholipase A2 (which results in limitation of arachidonic acid availability for new mediator formation) and on IL-1 and IL-2 have been described. Corticosteroids have also been shown to have few direct effects on ASM.

The effects of corticosteroids on airway inflammation in asthma are depicted in Figure 5-9. In addition to inhibiting the release of mediators from effector cells, corticosteroids interrupt cytokine-mediated intercellular communication. Unlike bronchodilators, corticosteroids are effective during the "late phase" of asthma, that is, 4 to 6 hours after exposure to an inciting antigen. In the late phase, airway obstruction is heavily affected by inflammatory infiltration of the airways, mediator release, and resistance to β-adrenergic agents. Corticosteroids are also effective in treating airway hyperreactivity, suggesting that the cellular mechanisms underlying the late phase may be operative in chronic airway hyperreactivity.

Cromolyn Sodium

Cromolyn sodium, a drug that "stabilizes" mast cells, is also considered an antiinflammatory agent. Although cromolyn protects against allergen-induced bronchospasm, it has no bronchodilatory effects. The precise mechanism of action of cromolyn remains uncertain.

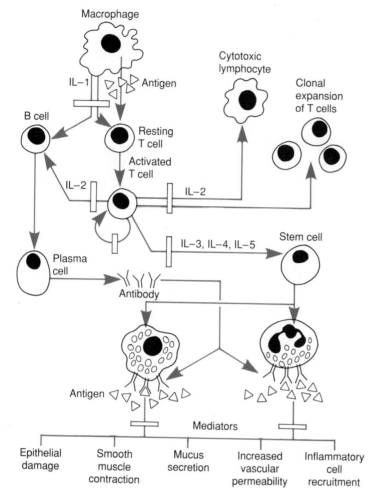

Figure 5-9. Mechanisms of airway inflammation and effects of corticosteroids. Macrophages present antigen to T cells and, via interleukin-1 (IL-1), activate T and B cells. Activated T cells are autostimulatory (via IL-2), leading to clonal expansion of T cells, development of cytotoxic lymphocytes, and activation of B cells. Activated T cells also release IL-3, IL-4, and IL-5, leading to maturation, priming, and activation of eosinophils and mast cells. Plasma cells secrete immunoglobulins, which are bound to mast cells and eosinophils. Cross-linking of the immunoglobulins leads to further activation of mast cells and eosinophils, and release of both preformed and newly formed mediators that affect the airway. As shown by the blocked pathways, corticosteroids inhibit mediator formation in mast cells and eosinophils and interrupt cell-to-cell communication through cytokines. Inhibition of eosinophil maturation and activation may be a particularly important effect of corticosteroids in asthma. (From Chang KF, Wiggins J, Collins J. Corticosteroids. In: Weiss EB, Stein M, eds. Bronchial Asthma: Mechanisms and Therapeutics. 3rd ed. Boston: Little, Brown & Co., 1993:803.)

Other Agents

Other antiinflammatory approaches that have been tried in very small numbers of patients include use of the potent immunosuppressive agents, methotrexate and cyclosporine. Although these drugs may be effective in controlling asthma or in allowing a reduction in corticosteroid dose, each is associated with severe side effects.

POTENTIAL NEW STRATEGIES IN THE THERAPY OF ASTHMA

Our current understanding of the pathophysiology of asthma suggests a number of potential treatment strategies. Delineation of specific molecular pathways important in generating ASM contractile force should lead to new targets for intervention. These targets might include specific inhibitors of phospholipase C, phosphodiesterase, the IP3 receptor, and receptor-operated calcium channels. As the role of cytokines is clarified, more specific inhibition of lymphocyte-mediated cell priming and activation may be possible. In addition, specific inhibitors of key adhesion molecules may prevent trafficking of effector cells (e.g., eosinophils) to the lung. Such approaches may allow more specific antiinflammatory agents to be delivered to the airways without risk of the systemic side effects of corticosteroids.

SELECTED READING

Barnes PJ. A new approach to the treatment of asthma. N Engl J Med 321:1517–1527, 1989.

Coburn RF, Baron CB. Coupling mechanisms in airway smooth muscle. Am J Physiol 258:119–133, 1990.

Kotlikoff MI. Ion channels in airway smooth muscle. In: Coburn RF, ed. Airway Smooth Muscle in Health and Disease. New York: Plenum Press, 1989: 169–182.

Leff AR. Endogenous regulation of bronchomotor tone. Am Rev Respir Dis 137: 1198–1216, 1988.

McFadden ER Jr, Gilbert IA. Medical progress: Asthma. N Engl J Med 327:1928–1937, 1992.

Lippincott's Pathophysiology Series: Pulmonary Pathophysiology, edited by Michael A. Grippi. J. B. Lippincott Company, Philadelphia © 1995.

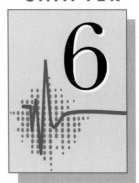

Chronic Obstructive Pulmonary Disease

Reynold A. Panettieri, Jr.

Although the term *chronic obstructive pulmonary disease (COPD)* encompasses a wide variety of disorders, including asthma, chronic bronchitis, emphysema, cystic fibrosis, bronchiectasis, and congenital bullous lung disease (Table 6-1), its use usually is restricted to two clinical entities: chronic bronchitis and emphysema. Asthma is the prototype of reversible airway diseases (see Chap. 5); the term COPD implies, in part, *irreversible* airway obstruction. Although there may be some overlap between asthma and the irreversible obstructive disorders, considerable overlap exists between the clinical manifestations of chronic bronchitis and emphysema (Fig. 6-1).

This chapter provides an overview of the pathology, pathogenesis, and pathophysiologic hallmarks of COPD, including alterations in respiratory mechanics, ventilation–perfusion relationships, work of breathing, and control of ventilation. Clinical considerations, including management based on the underlying pathophysiology, are highlighted. Finally, important pathophysiologic aspects of cystic fibrosis and bronchiectasis are summarized.

PATHOLOGY AND PATHOGENESIS

The morphologic findings in chronic bronchitis and emphysema provide insight into the underlying pathophysiology. Although both chronic bronchitis and emphysema are categorized as chronic obstructive pulmonary diseases, their pathology and pathophysiology are notably different.

TABLE 6-1. *THE OBSTRUCTIVE PULMONARY DISEASES*
Asthma
Chronic bronchitis
Emphysema
Bronchiectasis
Cystic fibrosis
Congenital bullous lung disease

CHRONIC BRONCHITIS

The diagnosis of chronic bronchitis is established on clinical grounds; however, a number of important morphologic changes in the airways characterize the disorder (Fig. 6-2).

As described in Chapter 1, the normal bronchus is lined by *pseudostratified columnar epithelium,* which consists predominantly of ciliated cells (see Fig. 6-2A). The airway epithelium rests on a thin basement membrane that overlies the loose connective tissue of the *lamina propria.* Below the lamina propria lies a layer of smooth muscle that is adjacent to another layer of loose connective tissue—the *submucosa. Mucus glands* are present within the submucosal layer.

In chronic bronchitis, the submucosal glands are enlarged due to hypertrophy and hyperplasia (see Fig. 6-2B). The *Reid index* provides a measure of the proportion of bronchial glands relative to bronchial wall thickness. Normally, mucous glands make up less than 40% of total wall thickness, constituting a normal Reid index of less than 0.4; in chronic bronchitis, the Reid index may exceed 0.7. These changes may be accompanied by goblet cell hyperplasia and bronchial wall edema secondary to inflammation—factors that further narrow airway diameter and increase resistance (see later section on Pathophysiologic Hallmarks).

The underlying mechanisms for the changes seen in chronic bronchitis remain unknown. Cigarette smoking, however, appears to be causally related. In addition, acute or chronic exposures to dusts, toxic fumes, air pollution, and respiratory viruses have been implicated.

Figure 6-1. The spectrum of obstructive airway diseases. A variety of pathologic processes result in airflow limitation, and considerable overlap exists among the pathophysiologic mechanisms operative in asthma, chronic bronchitis, and emphysema. (Modified from Woolcock A, Morgan MDL. Bronchitis, emphysema and bullae. In: Turner-Warwick M, Hodson ME, Corrin B, Kerr IH, eds. Slide Atlas of Respiratory Diseases, Vol. IV. London: Gower Medical Publishing, 1990:9.2.)

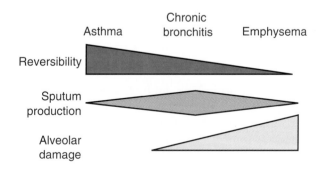

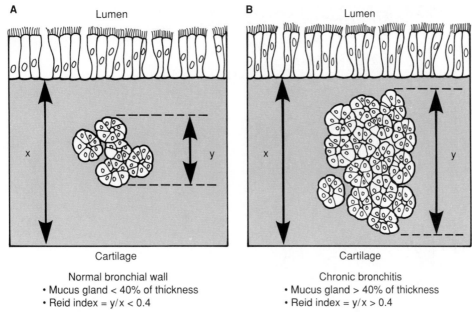

Figure 6-2. Histopathology of chronic bronchitis and the Reid index. **(A)** Normal bronchus. **(B)** Chronic bronchitis. Marked hyperplasia of mucus glands. The Reid index is > 0.4. See text for details. (Modified from Woolcock A, Morgan MDL. Bronchitis, emphysema and bullae. In: Turner-Warwick M, Hodson ME, Corrin B, Kerr IH, eds. Slide Atlas of Respiratory Diseases, Vol. IV. London: Gower Medical Publishing, 1990:p 9.5.)

EMPHYSEMA

Emphysema is defined anatomically as an irreversible increase in the size of air spaces distal to the terminal bronchioles. Two major subtypes have been recognized: centrilobular and panacinar (Fig. 6-3).

Centrilobular emphysema occurs most commonly as a result of, or in association with, cigarette smoking; the proximal portion of the terminal bronchiole is affected (see Fig. 6-3B).

Panacinar emphysema occurs in elderly patients and patients with α_1-antiprotease deficiency (see below); the entire respiratory bronchiole is affected (see Fig. 6-3C). Although these pathologic subtypes are distinctive, the degree of functional impairment, rather than the histologic status, determines the clinical course of emphysema.

Substantial alveolar–capillary wall destruction in emphysema results in enlargement of the acini or air spaces. Elastic recoil is reduced, and profound alterations in the coupling of ventilation and perfusion occur (see Chap. 13). Furthermore, airway collapse during expiration may arise because of reduced radial traction on the airways due to loss of alveoli, and reduced intraluminal pressure from lower lung elastic recoil (see Chap. 2). Increases in mucous secretion and airway smooth muscle contraction further decrease expiratory airflow rates. An increase in lung volume due to increased lung compliance and air trapping is also observed (see section on Pathophysiologic Hallmarks, later).

Although the pathogenesis of emphysema remains a matter of speculation, two important observations in the 1960s influenced contemporary thinking about the role of proteases and antiproteases in this disease. First, development

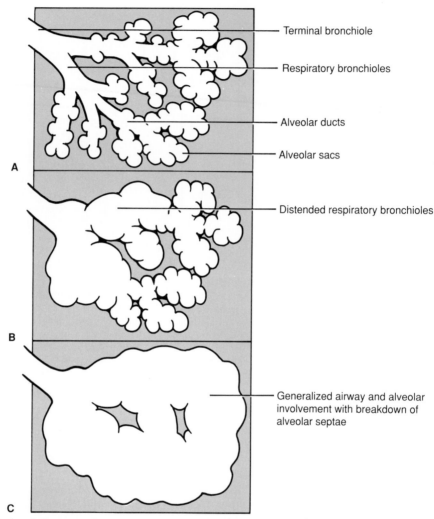

Figure 6-3. Types of emphysema. **(A)** Normal lung acinus. **(B)** Centrilobular emphysema. **(C)** Panacinar emphysema. See text for descriptions. (Modified from Netter FH. Chronic obstructive pulmonary disease. In: Divertie MB, ed. CIBA Collection of Medical Illustrations, Vol. 7: Respiratory System. Summit, NJ: CIBA, 1979:138.)

of emphysema in patients with an inherited deficiency of α_1-antitrypsin, a plasma protein that inhibits neutrophil elastase, suggested that α_1-antitrypsin may play an etiologic role. Second, recognition that, in experimental animals, intratracheal instillation of proteases induced emphysema suggested that enzymes may destroy the extracellular matrix of the lung and result in COPD. These observations are the basis for the *protease–antiprotease theory,* according to which a decrease in antiprotease activity or an increase in protease activity (or both) destroys the lung elastic fiber network (Fig. 6-4).

Alveolar macrophages and neutrophils are the major sources of proteases and elastases in the lung. When activated, these cells secrete enzymes that are important in modulating immune responses. With a deficiency of antiprotease activity, such as from decreased liver synthesis of α_1-antiprotease (as seen in α_1-antitrypsin deficiency) or inactivation of the protein by oxidation, the elastic

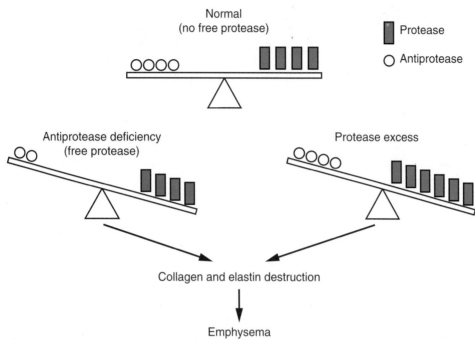

Figure 6-4. Protease–antiprotease model of emphysema. Normally, proteolytic enzyme activity is inactivated by antiproteases (e.g., α_1-antitrypsin). In emphysema, excess proteolytic activity destroys elastin and collagen—the major extracellular matrix proteins responsible for maintaining integrity of the alveolar–capillary membrane. Excess proteolytic activity may arise through an increase in protease levels, a decrease in antiprotease activity, or a combination of the two. The end result is destruction of the alveolar–capillary membrane and an increase in lung compliance, two hallmarks of emphysema.

architecture of the alveolar walls may be destroyed. Cigarette smoke may induce a relative increase in elastase activity by increasing the elastase burden in the lung (i.e., by recruiting neutrophils into the lung) and by oxidizing endogenous antiproteases. Although most patients with emphysema are either current or former cigarette smokers, COPD develops in only about 15% of smokers.

PATHOPHYSIOLOGIC HALLMARKS

The chief pathophysiologic hallmark of chronic bronchitis and emphysema is a limitation in airflow rates, particularly expiratory airflow. Major disturbances in respiratory mechanics, ventilation–perfusion matching, work of breathing, and control of ventilation are also observed. In chronic bronchitis, the integrity of the alveolar–capillary surface is maintained; however, airway resistance is increased due to mucus hypersecretion and bronchial wall inflammation, as described previously. In emphysema, many of the physiologic alterations represent a chronic adaptive response to loss of alveolar–capillary surface area and elastic recoil.

ALTERATIONS IN RESPIRATORY MECHANICS

Abnormalities in respiratory mechanics constitute a primary finding in obstructive airway diseases and are fundamentally related to the clinical findings.

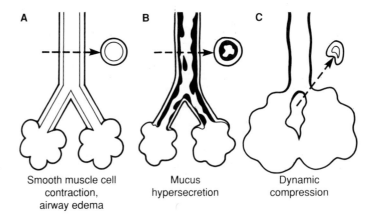

Figure 6-5. Mechanisms of airflow limitation in emphysema. **(A)** Airway smooth muscle contraction and airway edema. **(B)** Mucus hypersecretion. **(C)** Dynamic airway compression. See text for discussion.

Analysis of respiratory mechanics in these disorders is conveniently divided into four areas: expiratory airflow rates, lung volumes, lung compliance, and airway resistance.

Expiratory Airflow Rates

In COPD, the reduction in airflow rates arises through several mechanisms (Fig. 6-5): (1) partial airway occlusion by excess secretions (especially in chronic bronchitis); (2) airway narrowing secondary to smooth muscle contraction, bronchial wall edema, and airway inflammation; and (3) reduction in lung elasticity and loss of tethering forces exerted on the airway lumen (see Chap. 2). The last factor is particularly noteworthy in emphysema, in which noncartilaginous, moderate-sized airways are floppy and narrowed, especially during forced expiration (Fig. 6-6).

Figure 6-7 shows the forced expiratory spirogram of a patient with COPD. Both the FEV_1 and $FEF_{25\%-75\%}$ are diminished. In addition, expiratory time is profoundly increased, in part because of increased airway resistance. Prolonga-

Figure 6-6. Dynamic airway compression. Expiratory flow depends on intraluminal pressure, radial traction on the airways, and pleural pressure. **(A)** Normal airway. Radial traction created by lung elastic recoil tethers open the airway during forced expiration. Alveolar pressure drives airflow along the airway. **(B)** Emphysema. During expiration, the airway collapses due to the loss of radial traction associated with a reduction in lung elastic recoil. Alveolar pressure is also reduced. (Modified from Woolcock A, Morgan MDL. Bronchitis, emphysema and bullae. In: Turner-Warwick M, Hodson ME, Corrin B, Kerr IH, eds. Slide Atlas of Respiratory Diseases, Vol. IV. London: Gower Medical Publishing, 1990:9.6.)

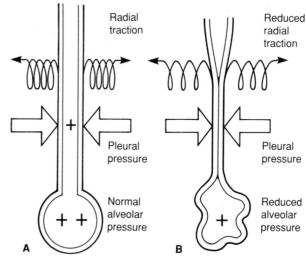

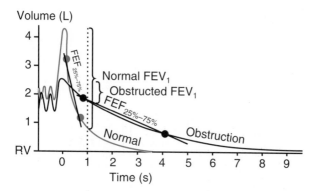

Figure 6-7. Spirometry in obstructive airway diseases. In COPD, expiratory airflow rates (FEV_1, FVC, and $FEF_{25\%-75\%}$) are diminished. Forced expiratory time is invariably prolonged as a result of increased airway resistance.

tion of expiration prevents adequate emptying of alveoli, contributing to air trapping and an increase in TLC (see Chap. 4).

The relationship between airflow and lung volume is described by the flow–volume curve (Fig. 6-8). Peak expiratory and mid-expiratory airflow rates are reduced. The curve is shifted to a higher lung volume range because of hyperinflation.

Lung Volumes

Most patients with COPD have increased static lung volumes (Fig. 6-9); a number of mechanisms account for this finding.

Airway obstruction from bronchial wall edema, smooth muscle contraction, and inflammatory cell infiltration slows alveolar emptying and increases RV. This mechanism is responsible for the hyperinflation in patients with chronic bronchitis. In addition, loss of lung elastic recoil decreases the driving pressure for expiratory airflow from alveoli to mouth. The tethering forces surrounding the airways are reduced, potentiating airway collapse. These effects predominate in patients with emphysema. The increase in airway resistance and loss in driving pressure promote movement of the equal pressure point "upstream," toward the distal bronchi, which do not contain cartilage. Consequently, dynamic air-

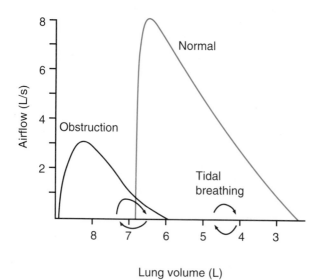

Figure 6-8. Maximal expiratory flow–volume curve in obstructive airway disease. Diminished expiratory flow occurs over the entire flow–volume curve as a result of increased resistance in large and small airways. In severe COPD, even tidal volume breaths may become flow limited, as demonstrated by overlap between the tidal breathing and maximal expiratory curves. (Modified from Netter FH. Chronic obstructive pulmonary disease. In: Divertie MB, ed. CIBA Collection of Medical Illustrations, Vol. 7: Respiratory System. Summit, NJ: CIBA, 1979:141.)

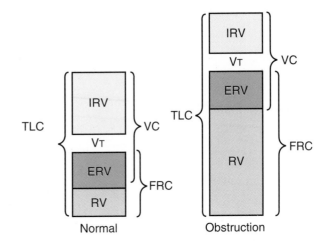

Figure 6-9. Lung volumes in COPD. TLC, FRC, and RV are increased; VC and IRV are decreased. See text for discussion.

way compression develops, resulting in gas trapping and hyperinflation (see Chap. 2).

As demonstrated in Figure 6-9, an increase in RV due to loss of elastic recoil "encroaches" on the VC; FRC is increased, as is TLC. In general, the effects of airway obstruction on lung volumes are comparable whether the obstruction is the result of loss of lung elastic recoil or airway narrowing. Loss of elastic recoil is irreversible, however, whereas bronchial wall edema and airway smooth muscle contraction may improve with treatment.

Lung Compliance

Although measurements of lung compliance are not made routinely in the clinical evaluation of patients with COPD, the findings are those expected on the basis of the underlying pathophysiology.

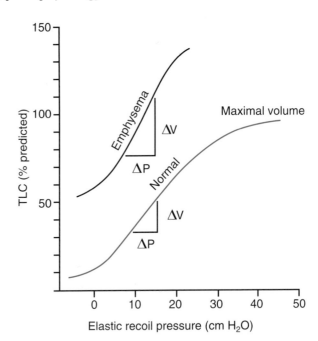

Figure 6-10. Static lung compliance in emphysema. The pressure–volume curve is shifted upward and to the left. Lung compliance is increased.

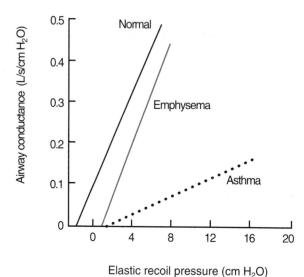

Figure 6-11. Airway conductance in obstructive lung diseases. Airway conductance, a measure of expiratory flow, depends on airway diameter. Because the measurement is performed during isovolumic breathing maneuvers (i.e., when lung volume remains constant), expiratory flow limitation due to loss of elastic recoil (as seen in emphysema) is minimized. In chronic bronchitis and asthma, airway obstruction is caused by intrinsic narrowing of the airways by smooth muscle contraction, bronchial wall edema, and mucus hypersecretion. Airway conductance is decreased. (Modified from Colebatch HJH, Finucane KE, Smith MM. Pulmonary conductance and elastic recoil relationships in asthma and emphysema. J Appl Physiol 34:143–153, 1973.)

Patients with chronic bronchitis and asthma have static compliances that closely approximate normal values, because the lung parenchyma is little affected in these diseases. In patients with emphysema, however, an alteration in lung elastic recoil is accompanied by an increase in lung compliance. The static compliance curve is shifted upward and to the left (Fig. 6-10).

Airway Resistance

As expected, airway resistance is increased in patients with COPD. Airway conductance, the reciprocal of resistance, is reduced. Measurement of airway resistance can help distinguish airway obstruction due to intrinsic narrowing of the airway (e.g., asthma) from that due to loss of lung elastic recoil (e.g., emphysema); although airway resistance is elevated in both disorders, the increase is usually more marked in asthma (Fig. 6-11).

VENTILATION–PERFUSION RELATIONSHIPS

Disruption of the close relationship between regional ventilation and blood flow (ventilation–perfusion matching) is common in patients with COPD. As a result, alterations in both oxygenation and alveolar ventilation arise, as discussed in Chapter 13. Perfusion of poorly ventilated areas (low ventilation–perfusion ratios) results in a reduction in arterial oxygenation. Conversely, overventilation of poorly perfused areas (high ventilation–perfusion ratios) results in an increase in dead space ventilation and impaired CO_2 excretion (see Chaps. 3 and 13).

These abnormalities may not be evident at rest. During exercise, however, oxygen demand increases. If the alveolar–capillary surface area is reduced (e.g., because of emphysema), additional gas-exchange units may not be "recruitable." The lack of alveolar–capillary reserve is manifested as exercise-induced hypoxemia (see Chap. 19).

As discussed in Chapter 9, the single-breath diffusing capacity for carbon monoxide (DLCO) is a useful clinical measurement of the lung's capacity to transfer oxygen across its surface. Many factors affect the DLCO, including ventilation–perfusion matching, area and thickness of the alveolar–capillary membrane, number of perfused pulmonary capillaries, and mean transit time of red blood cells through the capillaries. Because of loss of alveolar–capillary units, patients with emphysema have a reduced DLCO. Furthermore, the magnitude of the reduction correlates with disease severity. In patients with chronic bronchitis or asthma, gas-exchanging units are preserved, and the DLCO is normal or mildly reduced.

Several chronic adaptive responses are seen in patients with COPD who experience a prolonged reduction in arterial P_{O_2}, that is, prolonged *hypoxemia*. In emphysema, destruction of alveolar–capillary units results in a rise in pulmonary artery pressure; hypoxic pulmonary vasoconstriction contributes to the pulmonary hypertension (see Chap. 12). Because the right ventricle must generate a greater pressure to overcome the increased pulmonary artery pressure, right ventricular hypertrophy and dilation occur. Ultimately, increases in cardiac output due to febrile illnesses or worsening hypoxemia induce overt right ventricular failure. In addition, chronic hypoxemia may induce an increase in red blood cell production (*reactive erythrocytosis*) that further increases blood viscosity and exacerbates right ventricular failure.

WORK OF BREATHING AND OXYGEN COST OF BREATHING

The work of breathing is increased in patients with airflow limitation, regardless of the underlying cause. Several pathophysiologic mechanisms are responsible.

Inadequate expiratory time and increased airway resistance produce an increase in end-expiratory lung volume (FRC). The increase in FRC results in shortening of the diaphragm, placing the muscle at a mechanical disadvantage (see Chap. 2). Use of accessory muscles of respiration, such as the sternocleidomastoid and trapezius, and active recruitment of expiratory muscles increase oxygen demand. If the underlying mechanical and metabolic abnormalities are not corrected, the patient with severe airflow limitation may experience respiratory muscle failure. Alveolar ventilation declines, reducing the work of breathing; however, the reduced alveolar ventilation results in an increase in arterial P_{CO_2}, or *hypercapnia* (see Chap. 18).

CONTROL OF VENTILATION

Hypercapnia is a common finding in many patients with advanced COPD; it is uncommon in patients with asthma, except during a severe attack. Although patients with chronic bronchitis and emphysema may have comparable degrees of obstruction according to pulmonary function tests, some experience hypercapnia, whereas others do not. The precise pathophysiologic basis for the difference remains unknown (see Chaps. 16 and 18). Possible mechanisms of hypercapnia include a decrease in the central drive to breathe and increases in the work of breathing, dead-space ventilation, and the rate of CO_2 production.

CLINICAL MANIFESTATIONS

Patients with COPD usually come to a physician seeking relief from shortness of breath or cough. Typically, the patient is in the sixth or seventh decade

TABLE 6-2. *CHRONIC BRONCHITIS VERSUS EMPHYSEMA*		
CLINICAL FEATURE	**EMPHYSEMA (PINK PUFFER, TYPE A)**	**CHRONIC BRONCHITIS (BLUE BLOATER, TYPE B)**
Age	Older	Younger
Stature	Tall, thin	Stocky, obese
Cor pulmonale	Late in course	Early in course
Hypoxemia	Mild	Prominent
Hypercapnia	Late in course	Early in course
Lung compliance	Increased	Normal
D_{LCO}	Reduced	Normal
Airway obstruction	Severe	Moderate
Hematocrit	Normal	Increased

of life and gives a history of cigarette smoking. He or she complains of the insidious onset of shortness of breath with exertion. Similar symptoms occurring in the fourth or fifth decade should prompt consideration of alternative diagnoses, including asthma, α_1-antitrypsin deficiency, or congenital bullous lung disease (see Table 6-1).

Other manifestations that occur late in the course of the disease usually represent complications of COPD. For example, leg swelling suggests right-sided congestive heart failure and significant pulmonary hypertension. Morning headache, lethargy, and confusion are common symptoms of CO_2 retention. Frequently, dyspnea on exertion is a manifestation of severe expiratory flow limitation and limited breathing reserve.

The classic descriptions of the patient with pure chronic bronchitis (the "blue bloater") or pure emphysema (the "pink puffer") summarize many of the clinical manifestations of severe COPD (Table 6-2).

The pink puffer (type A COPD) is tachypneic. Respirations are labored and pursed-lip breathing (tensing of the upper and lower lips which are maintained in a rounded position during expiration) is seen. Arterial oxygenation is well preserved, however. The pink puffer suffers primarily from emphysema.

In contrast, the blue bloater (type B COPD) is cyanotic secondary to hypoxemia. In addition, hypercapnia, leg swelling, and right-sided congestive heart failure are present. The blue bloater suffers primarily from chronic bronchitis.

Physical examination suggests evidence of chronic severe airflow limitation and hypoxemia. Auscultation of the chest often reveals distant breath sounds, expiratory wheezing, and prolongation of the expiratory phase. If airway obstruction is moderate or severe, the increased lung volume may be evident as an increased anteroposterior diameter of the chest, hyperresonant lung fields, and limited respiratory excursion of the diaphragm. Signs of pulmonary hypertension and right-sided congestive heart failure, such as neck vein distention, hepatomegaly, and peripheral edema, usually occur in patients with longstanding hypoxemia due to ventilation–perfusion mismatching. Consequently, they are most apt to occur in patients with chronic bronchitis (the blue bloater).

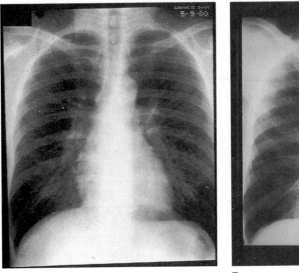
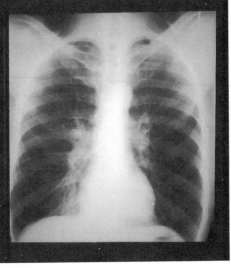

A   **B**

Figure 6-12. Posteroanterior chest radiographs in a healthy subject **(A)** and in severe emphysema **(B)**. Expiratory airflow limitation results in an increase in lung volume. The increased lung volume flattens the diaphragm and makes the lung fields appear more radiolucent.

COMMONLY PERFORMED DIAGNOSTIC TESTS

Although the diagnosis of COPD is established on clinical grounds, certain ancillary studies are used to confirm the diagnosis, exclude other considerations, and quantitate the severity of the disorder. The chest radiograph, pulmonary function tests, and arterial blood gases are especially useful.

CHEST RADIOGRAPH

The chest radiograph frequently shows hyperinflation, manifested as radiolucent lung fields, a flattened diaphragm, and a small, narrow cardiac silhouette (Fig. 6-12). Although the chest radiograph is useful in supporting a diagnosis of COPD, particularly emphysema, it is not specific, because patients experiencing an acute exacerbation of asthma or cystic fibrosis may have identical radiographic findings. Furthermore, the chest radiograph may not reflect the severity of COPD, as determined by pulmonary function tests.

PULMONARY FUNCTION TESTS

Pulmonary function tests are valuable in confirming the diagnosis of COPD, assessing its severity, evaluating reversibility, and determining prognosis.

Spirometry reveals decreases in FEV_1, FVC, and FEV_1/FVC%. Although most patients with COPD do not demonstrate an increase in FEV_1 in response to the administration of an inhaled bronchodilator, approximately 20% are bronchodilator-responsive—that is, the FEV_1 increases by at least 15% after drug administration (see Chap. 4).

As noted, lung volumes, determined by body plethysmography, are usually increased in emphysema, but they may be normal in chronic bronchitis. The increase in TLC is a consequence of expiratory airflow limitation and air trapping; FRC and RV are also increased (see Fig. 6-9).

The lung volumes measured by body plethysmography are often higher than those measured by the single-breath helium dilution technique (see Chap. 4). In the face of significant airflow obstruction, helium is incompletely distributed throughout the lung after a single breath, resulting in an underestimation of true lung volume.

As noted, in emphysema, the D_{LCO} is decreased because of loss of alveolar–capillary units. In contrast, the D_{LCO} is well preserved in patients with chronic bronchitis and asthma. Consequently, this test is of value in distinguishing patients with emphysema from those with chronic bronchitis or asthma.

ARTERIAL BLOOD GASES

Arterial blood gases are relatively insensitive measures of the severity of COPD. In the early stages of emphysema, a decline in arterial oxygenation during exercise is common. In the later stages of the disease, hypoxemia and hypercapnia may occur at rest. Reactive erythrocytosis, manifested by an increase in hematocrit, is a consequence of chronic hypoxemia that may be reinforced by high carboxyhemoglobin levels (see Chap. 10) caused by cigarette smoking.

MANAGEMENT OF COPD: PATHOPHYSIOLOGIC TARGETS

The treatment of COPD is aimed at altering the basic pathophysiologic mechanisms responsible for expiratory airflow limitation. Unfortunately, unlike asthma, chronic bronchitis and emphysema usually demonstrate irreversible airway narrowing.

IMPROVEMENT IN EXPIRATORY AIRFLOW LIMITATION

Because airflow limitation in COPD may be caused, in part, by bronchial smooth muscle contraction, bronchodilators are used frequently in treatment. Several categories of bronchodilators, including anticholinergics, β-agonists, and theophylline, as well as antiinflammatory agents (corticosteroids), have been used.

Anticholinergics and β-Agonists

Ipratropium bromide, an anticholinergic agent that blocks muscarinic receptors in airway smooth muscle, decreases vagal tone, inhibits smooth muscle contraction, and decreases mucus secretion. The bronchodilator potency of anticholinergic agents is not attenuated by continued administration, while prolonged use of β-agonists may result in a blunted bronchodilator response. β-agonists also may induce pulmonary vasodilation, which worsens ventilation–perfusion mismatching, occasionally resulting in a decrease in arterial P_{O_2}; ipratropium bromide does not have this effect.

Theophylline

Although theophylline has been used in the treatment of COPD for more than 100 years, the mechanisms by which this agent improves dyspnea and decreases airway obstruction remain unknown. Theophylline is a weak bronchodilator in comparison to β-agonists or ipratropium. In COPD, the therapeutic effect of theophylline may be a consequence of effects other than bronchodilation. Theophylline has been reported to increase the contractility of the "fatigued" diaphragm and to increase mucociliary action in healthy airways. Moreover, theophylline increases the hypoxic drive to breathe in hypercapnic patients with COPD; it also increases right and left ventricular function through vasodilation and direct myocardial stimulation.

Corticosteroids

As described, expiratory airflow limitation in COPD may be caused by bronchial wall edema and inflammation. Although the benefits of corticosteroids in the management of asthma are well documented (see Chap. 5), the efficacy of these agents in management of patients with stable COPD is less well established. Some patients with COPD who do not respond to bronchodilators improve with corticosteroid therapy.

COMPENSATION FOR VENTILATION–PERFUSION MISMATCH

Hypoxemia in COPD is the result of ventilation–perfusion mismatch (see Chap. 13). Administration of supplemental O_2 has been shown to reduce mortality in COPD. Supplemental O_2, however, may decrease the central drive to breathe, inducing modest increases in arterial PCO_2 (see Chap. 16). This phenomenon is most marked in patients experiencing an acute exacerbation of COPD.

REDUCTION IN THE WORK OF BREATHING

The work of breathing (see Chap. 2) is elevated in all patients with airflow limitation, and therapy is aimed at reducing the underlying increased airway resistance. Use of bronchodilators, antiinflammatory agents, and supplemental O_2 reduces airway resistance, decreases air trapping, improves O_2 delivery to respiratory muscles, and lessens the work of breathing.

Another therapeutic approach to decreasing the work of breathing focuses on respiratory muscle training and pulmonary rehabilitation. Rehabilitation programs may reduce dyspnea and improve exercise endurance time in patients with severe COPD.

SMOKING CESSATION

Smoking cessation represents an important intervention in management of patients with COPD. The benefits of smoking cessation are well established. Although destruction of alveolar–gas exchange units may be irreversible, smoking cessation profoundly slows further destruction. In young smokers (younger than 35 years old) who have mild airway obstruction ($FEV_1 > 60\%$ predicted), the FEV_1 returns to normal after the patient stops smoking. In older patients, cessation of smoking slows, but does not eliminate, further decrements in the FEV_1.

BRONCHIECTASIS AND CYSTIC FIBROSIS

Although the pathogenesis of bronchiectasis and cystic fibrosis differs from that of chronic bronchitis and emphysema, chronic airflow obstruction is a common clinical manifestation of these diseases as well.

BRONCHIECTASIS

Bronchiectasis is an abnormal dilation of medium-sized bronchi (diameter >2 mm) arising from destruction of the muscular and elastic components of airway walls. The dilation is commonly associated with chronic bacterial infection, and it may lead to irreversible airflow obstruction. Bronchiectasis often occurs in association with systemic diseases (e.g., cystic fibrosis and immunodeficiency states).

CYSTIC FIBROSIS

Cystic fibrosis, the most common genetic disease in caucasians (1 in 2500 live births), is transmitted as an autosomal recessive trait; 1 of every 20 caucasians is a carrier. Cystic fibrosis is a systemic disorder that affects exocrine glands, producing protean findings: sinusitis, nasal polyps, bronchiectasis, hyperglycemia, pancreatic insufficiency, and malnutrition.

The genetic defect of cystic fibrosis results in abnormalities of ion transport across epithelial cells. In particular, epithelial cells are impermeable to chloride ions. As a result, airway mucus is viscous and mucociliary clearance is impaired. Recurrent lower respiratory infections destroy airway architecture and induce irreversible airway obstruction.

The primary objectives in treatment of cystic fibrosis include control of infection, promotion of mucus clearance, and improved nutrition. Airflow obstruction is treated as described previously. Lung transplantation holds some therapeutic promise, as does gene therapy.

SELECTED READING

Campbell EJ, Senior RM. Emphysema. In: Fishman AP, ed. Update: Pulmonary Diseases and Disorders. New York: McGraw-Hill, 1992:37–51.

Reid LM. Chronic obstructive pulmonary diseases. In: Fishman AP, ed. Pulmonary Diseases and Disorders. New York: McGraw-Hill, 1988:1247–1272.

Snider GL. Chronic bronchitis and emphysema. In: Murray JF, Nadel JA, eds. Textbook of Respiratory Medicine. Philadelphia: WB Saunders, 1988: 1069–1107.

Snider GL. State of the art. Emphysema: The first two centuries—and beyond. Am Rev Respir Dis 146:1334–1344, 1992.

Lippincott's Pathophysiology Series: Pulmonary Pathophysiology, edited by Michael A. Grippi. J. B. Lippincott Company, Philadelphia © 1995.

CHAPTER

Lung Immunology and Interstitial Lung Diseases

Milton D. Rossman

Immunologically mediated diseases of the airways and lung parenchyma constitute a clinically important group of disorders that profoundly affect lung function. In many instances, immunologically mediated airway disorders behave like other obstructive diseases, especially asthma. Furthermore, although the number of causes of interstitial lung diseases, including those that are immunologically based, is large, there tends to be a common pathophysiologic denominator, characterized by a restrictive pattern on pulmonary function testing (see Chap. 4).

This chapter focuses on immune mechanisms affecting the lung and highlights associated pathologic processes. Important changes in lung volumes, airflow rates, gas exchange, and exercise testing are considered. In addition, a brief overview of the diagnostic approach and management, based on the underlying pathophysiology, is provided. Many of the concepts considered here are also covered in Chapters 2 through 6. Related pathophysiologic aspects of gas exchange are detailed in Chapters 9, 12, 13, and 19.

IMMUNE MECHANISMS OF THE LUNG RESULTING IN INTERSTITIAL LUNG DISEASE

A conceptually useful categorization of basic immune mechanisms of disease is the *Coombs and Gell classification,* according to which immune reactions in the lung can be divided into four types: (1) immediate hypersensitivity, (2) antibody-dependent cytotoxicity, (3) immune complex reactions, and (4) cell-mediated immune reactions (Table 7-1 and Fig. 7-1).

IMMEDIATE HYPERSENSITIVITY

The *immediate hypersensitivity* reactions, or *type I reactions,* are mediated by immunoglobulin E (IgE) (see Fig. 7-1A). Bound by its fragment of crystallization (Fc) to either mast cells or basophils, IgE causes degranulation of these cells on binding to antigen. The subsequent release of histamine, leukotrienes, and other soluble factors results in vasodilation, increased capillary permeability, and bronchoconstriction. Typically, type I reactions occur in the airways and result in an obstructive pattern on pulmonary function testing (see Chap. 4); pulmonary parenchymal (i.e., interstitial) involvement is uncommon. IgE-mediated reactions in the lung have been implicated in the pathogenesis of extrinsic asthma of childhood and certain forms of occupational asthma (e.g., that caused by exposure to trimetallic anhydride or toluene diisocyanate). These reactions are thought to be less important in intrinsic asthma of adulthood, however.

ANTIBODY-DEPENDENT CYTOTOXIC REACTIONS

In *antibody-dependent cytotoxic reactions,* or *type II reactions,* immunoglobulin G (IgG) molecules are produced that bind to "self" antigens (see Fig. 7-1B). This binding causes cell death, either by complement fixation or antibody-dependent, cell-mediated cytotoxicity. Macrophages or natural killer cells, which can bind to IgG by means of their Fc receptors, have been implicated in the pathogenesis. Goodpasture syndrome, clinically manifested as alveolar hemorrhage and renal failure, is characterized by the production of IgG antibodies directed against alveolar and glomerular basement membranes; it is the classic clinical example of a type II reaction.

TABLE 7-1. *BASIC IMMUNE MECHANISMS*

TYPE OF IMMUNE REACTION	MECHANISM	EXAMPLE OF RESULTANT PULMONARY DISEASE
I: Immediate hypersensitivity	IgE-mediated degranulation of mast cells and basophils; mediator release; IgG autoantibodies	Extrinsic asthma
II: Antibody-dependent cytotoxicity	IgG autoantibodies	Goodpasture syndrome
III: Immune complex reaction	Deposition of IgG immune complexes; mediator release	Hypersensitivity pneumonitis
IV: Cell-mediated immune reaction	T cell–mediated injury	Chronic beryllium disease; transplantation rejection

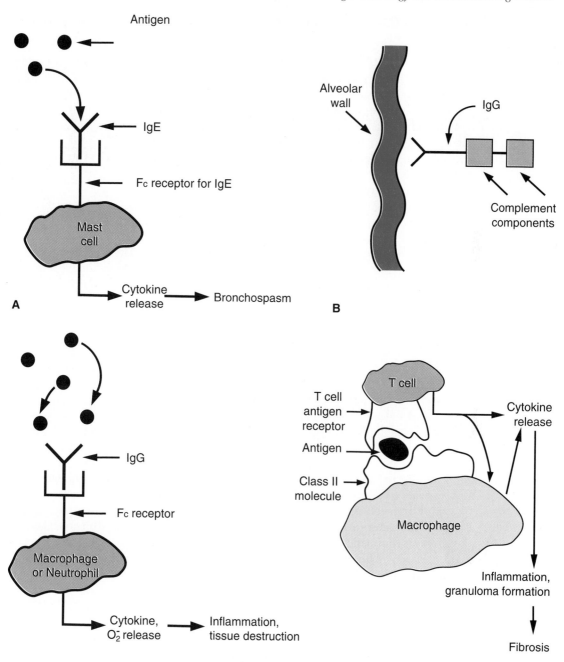

Figure 7-1. Four types of immunologic reactions in the lung. (**A**) Immediate hypersensitivity. (**B**) Antibody-dependent cytotoxicity. (**C**) Immune complex-mediated. (**D**) Cell-mediated. See text for details.

IMMUNE COMPLEX REACTIONS

Immune complexes, consisting of antigen and bound antibody, may be soluble or precipitated. The ratio of antibody to antigen and the size of the complex are important determinants of tissue localization and injury. Pulmonary disease secondary to immune complexes, or *type III reactions,* may be the result of local production and deposition of immune complexes, as likely occurs in hypersensitivity pneumonitis (see Fig. 7-1C). Alternatively, the underlying mechanism may entail transport of immune complexes to the lung through the circulation and precipitation or deposition of the complexes in the lung, such as in collagen vascular diseases.

Immune complexes activate complement, causing the release of histamine and leukotrienes, attracting and activating phagocytic cells. A persistent inflammatory reaction develops because of either continued deposition of immune complexes or failure to clear the complexes. Continued inflammation eventually leads to destruction of lung tissue and pulmonary fibrosis. Although the specific cause of idiopathic pulmonary fibrosis is unknown, the presence of high levels of immune complexes in the blood and lung suggests that the complexes play an important role in pathogenesis.

CELL-MEDIATED IMMUNE REACTIONS

Whereas the three types of immunologic reactions described previously are antibody mediated, *cell-mediated immune reactions,* or *type IV reactions,* are based on T-lymphocyte activity (see Fig. 7-1D). T lymphocytes identify foreign substances and initiate inflammation. If the antigen initiating a cell-mediated immune response is poorly "digestible," persistent inflammation develops, leading to granuloma formation and fibrosis. Chronic beryllium disease may be the best example of this process, in which cell-mediated immunity, alone, has been implicated in pathogenesis. In addition, sarcoidosis, a disease of unknown etiology, appears to be immunologically similar to chronic beryllium disease.

Although cell-mediated immune responses are important in the pathogenesis of mycobacterial and fungal diseases, humoral immunity appears also to play an important role. Similarly, both type III and type IV reactions play crucial roles in hypersensitivity pneumonitis. Finally, cell-mediated immune responses also are important in organ transplantation reactions.

PATHOLOGY OF INTERSTITIAL LUNG DISEASES

Pathologic changes induced by immunologic reactions may involve alveolar walls, alveolar air spaces, blood vessels, and small airways (Table 7-2). The predominant site and nature of the pathologic changes depend on the underlying etiology and immunologic mechanism. Anatomic sites of potential involvement are discussed in the following sections.

ALVEOLAR WALLS

As described in Chapter 1, the alveolar walls consist of a surface layer of surfactant, epithelial cells, and the interstitial space, which includes basement membranes, capillaries, and interstitial cells (Figs. 7-2 and 7-3). Interstitial lung

TABLE 7-2. *PATHOLOGIC CHANGES IN INTERSTITIAL LUNG DISEASES*

ANATOMIC SITE	PATHOLOGIC CHANGE	EXAMPLE OF PULMONARY DISEASE
Alveolar walls		
Inflammation	Accumulation of inflammatory cells and edema	Sarcoidosis, chronic beryllium disease
Fibrosis	Increased mesenchymal cells	Radiation fibrosis
	Increased extracellular matrix	
Destruction	Loss of alveoli	Honeycomb lung, emphysema
Air spaces		
Lymphocytic infiltration	Increased CD4 T cells	Sarcoidosis
	Increased CD8 T cells	Hypersensitivity pneumonitis
Neutrophilic infiltration	Increased neutrophils and eosinophils	Usual interstitial pneumonitis (UIP)
Blood vessels	Vasculitis	Wegener granulomatosis
Small airways	Bronchiolitis	Bronchiolitis obliterans with organizing pneumonia (BOOP)
	Granuloma formation	Sarcoidosis

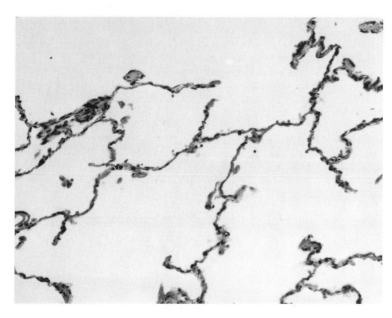

Figure 7-2. Light microscopic section of normal lung (hematoxylin and eosin, original magnification ×200). (Courtesy of Leslie A. Litzky, M.D.)

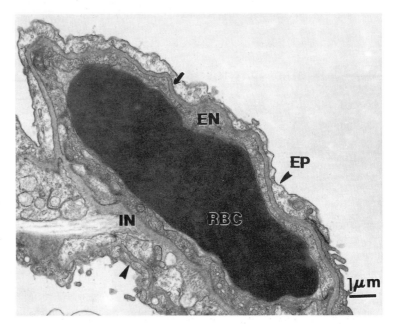

Figure 7-3. Electron micrograph of normal human alveolar wall (original magnification ×15,000). The thin side (arrow) is shown (see Chap. 14). The capillary endothelium (EN) is separated from the type I pneumocyte (EP, arrowheads). The interstitium (IN) is also shown. RBC, red blood cell. (Courtesy of Giuseppe G. Pietra, M.D.)

diseases from known or unknown causes are characterized by three distinct pathologic patterns in the alveolar walls.

The *inflammatory pattern* is thought to reflect an early and potentially reversible process. Alveolar walls are thickened due to accumulation of inflammatory cells (neutrophils, lymphocytes, and macrophages), edema fluid, and other extracellular substances (Fig. 7-4). The inflammatory pattern may be distinctive, such as well-formed granulomas in sarcoidosis and chronic beryllium disease, giant cell vasculitis in Wegener granulomatosis, or a nonspecific pattern in idiopathic pulmonary fibrosis.

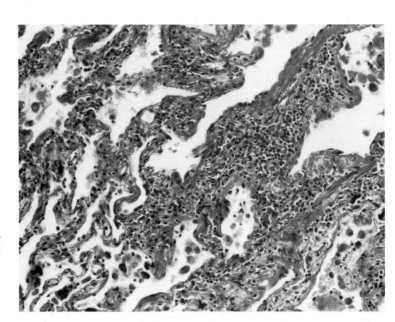

Figure 7-4. Cellular interstitial pneumonitis (hematoxylin and eosin, original magnification ×200). Diffuse interstitial widening is caused by a dense, chronic inflammatory infiltrate associated with hypersensitivity to tungsten carbide, an industrial grinding material. (Courtesy of Leslie A. Litzky, M.D.)

The *fibrotic pattern* may be seen in the alveolar walls of some patients with interstitial lung diseases (Fig. 7-5). The interstitium contains an increased number of mesenchymal cells, and the volume of extracellular matrix is greatly increased. Alveolar lining cells are cuboidal rather than flat, and type II cells predominate. Fibroblasts are present in the interstitial space, and the alveolar walls are thickened due to increased amounts of fibrous tissue. In general, this pattern responds poorly to therapy.

The third pathologic pattern is *lung destruction* (Fig. 7-6). Alveolar walls have "dropped out," and cystic or emphysematous areas in the lung are seen. Radiographically, this pattern represents a *honeycomb lung* and indicates end-stage disease. If the process is widespread, lung transplantation is the only therapeutic intervention.

These pathologic patterns of interstitial lung disease are not mutually exclusive. The extent of each process—inflammation, fibrosis, and destruction—depends on the etiology of the disease, its duration, and response to therapy.

ALVEOLAR AIR SPACES

Although the pathologic changes in interstitial lung disorders are localized predominantly in the alveolar walls, distinct changes in the air spaces also occur. Using the technique of *bronchoalveolar lavage,* in which the distal airways and alveolar spaces are filled with saline that is then aspirated for analysis, changes in cellular constituents and levels of soluble substances in these portions of the lung can be assessed.

In active inflammatory processes involving the alveolar walls, increased numbers of inflammatory cells are recovered in the bronchoalveolar lavage fluid. In reversible processes (e.g., hypersensitivity pneumonitis), the cells are predominantly lymphocytes. The quantity and type of lymphocyte in the lavage fluid reflect the primary pathologic process within the alveolar walls. The presence

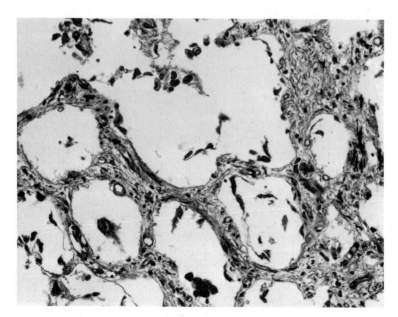

Figure 7-5. Interstitial fibrosis (Trichrome, original magnification ×200). Diffuse interstitial widening is caused by fibrosis due to scleroderma. Inflammation is minimal. Epithelial desquamation is a postmortem artifact. (Courtesy of Leslie A. Litzky, M.D.)

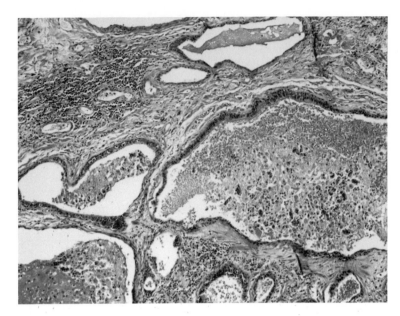

Figure 7-6. Honeycomb, end-stage lung (hematoxylin and eosin, original magnification ×200). Normal lung architecture is destroyed. Note interstitial fibrosis and formation of nonfunctional, irregular air spaces lined by metaplastic epithelium. Mucus, neutrophils, and macrophages have accumulated within the air spaces. (Courtesy of Leslie A. Litzky, M.D.)

of neutrophils and eosinophils, which are not normally recovered in the fluid, usually reflects a fibrotic or destructive alveolar process.

BLOOD VESSELS

Systemic illnesses characterized by inflammation in blood vessels—*vasculitis*—may involve the lungs. Although pulmonary disease secondary to small vessel vasculitis is uncommon, some vasculitides (e.g., Wegener granulomatosis) preferentially involve the lung. In addition, vasculitis may also be a prominent part of pulmonary involvement in collagen vascular diseases, sarcoidosis, and necrotizing infections (e.g., tuberculosis and aspergillosis). Finally, infarction of pulmonary vessels due to disease of the vasa vasorum may lead to inflammation, fibrosis, and destruction of alveolar walls.

SMALL AIRWAYS

In some interstitial lung diseases, the small airways or bronchioles constitute an important site of inflammation. *Bronchiolitis obliterans with organizing pneumonia* is an example of an interstitial lung disease involving the bronchioles. This condition is characterized by bronchiolar inflammation and formation of plugs of mucus and inflammatory exudate that obstruct the bronchiole lumen. Sarcoidosis is also associated with bronchiolar involvement.

FUNCTIONAL CHANGES IN INTERSTITIAL LUNG DISEASES

The interstitial lung diseases produce well-defined alterations in pulmonary function tests (Table 7-3). Although not all abnormalities described in the following sections are present in all patients with interstitial lung disease, the

TABLE 7-3. *PULMONARY FUNCTION ABNORMALITIES IN INTERSTITIAL LUNG DISEASES*

MEASUREMENT	ABNORMALITY
Lung volumes	Decreased
Spirometry	Normal or decreased if small airway disease present
Diffusing capacity	Decreased
Exercise testing	Decreased tidal volume Increased respiratory rate Decreased arterial P_{O_2} Decreased maximal oxygen uptake

patterns of abnormalities reviewed are common. In addition, pulmonary function tests are of practical value in screening for these disorders and assessing their course.

LUNG VOLUMES

The pathophysiologic hallmark of the interstitial lung disorders is restriction (see Chap. 4). Restriction is manifested by a decrease in lung volumes, including TLC, FRC, RV, and VC (Fig. 7-7). The underlying mechanism is based on decreased lung compliance due to thickening of alveolar walls as a consequence of inflammation and fibrosis. In addition, air space volume is reduced because of an influx of inflammatory cells and exudation of fluid. Changes in the alveolar walls and air spaces cause a shift in the compliance curve downward and to the right; an increased pressure is required to inflate the lung to any given lung volume (Fig. 7-8).

In addition to parenchymal disease, other factors may be operative in reducing lung volumes in the interstitial disorders. For example, some systemic illnesses (e.g., collagen vascular diseases) may result in weakness of skeletal muscles, including the respiratory muscles (Fig. 7-9).

The differentiation between reduced lung volumes caused by respiratory

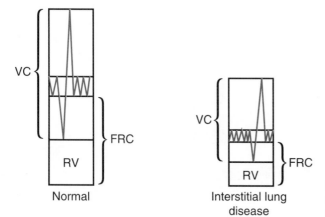

Figure 7-7. Lung volume changes in interstitial lung disease. See text for details.

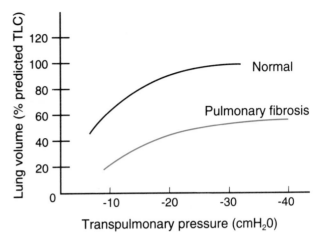

Figure 7-8. Lung compliance in pulmonary fibrosis. The curve is shifted downward and to the right. See text for details.

muscle weakness and parenchymal lung disease is not always easy. Measurement of pulmonary compliance may be helpful. Pulmonary compliance is normal in the presence of muscle weakness, but it is reduced with parenchymal lung disease. In addition, RV may be preserved in muscle weakness, because this measurement is independent of muscle strength. Hence, a reduced VC and normal RV should raise suspicion of respiratory muscle weakness.

Corticosteroids, which are used commonly in the treatment of a variety of interstitial lung diseases, can also be an important cause of muscle weakness. Long-term, high-dose corticosteroid treatment may induce muscle weakness, which can be confused with progressive interstitial lung disease if only lung volumes are measured.

Finally, pleural disease may coexist with certain interstitial lung disorders (e.g., asbestosis or rheumatoid lung disease). Because significant pleural disease limits lung expansion, total lung capacity may be reduced.

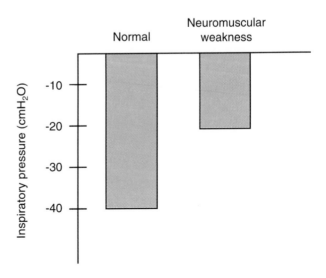

Figure 7-9. Maximal inspiratory force in neuromuscular weakness.

SPIROMETRY

Normally, airflow rates are preserved in interstitial lung disorders. Increased lung stiffness stents open the small airways and may actually increase airflow rates at low lung volumes. Because lung inflation is limited, however, VC is reduced. The FEV_1 is also reduced; $FEV_1/FVC\%$ is normal or increased (Fig. 7-10).

Although normal airflow rates in interstitial lung disorders are expected, some conditions produce reduced airflow because of abnormalities in small airways (e.g., sarcoidosis and chronic beryllium disease). Test results of small airway function, such as volume of isoflow and $FEF_{25\%-75\%}$ (see Chap. 4), are frequently abnormal. Occasionally, airway obstruction may be the major manifestation of interstitial lung disease.

GAS EXCHANGE

As a consequence of the pathologic changes in alveolar walls, air spaces, blood vessels, and small airways, hypoxemia is a major manifestation of interstitial lung disease. The patchy nature of most interstitial disorders is responsible for abnormal ventilation–perfusion relationships (see Chap. 9). Because the oxyhemoglobin dissociation curve is *curvilinear* (see Chap. 10), increased oxygen delivery to areas where ventilation is high relative to perfusion cannot compensate for decreased oxygen delivery to areas where ventilation is low relative to perfusion (see Chap. 13). To compensate for the hypoxemia of poorly ventilated regions, total minute ventilation must increase. In contrast, the *linear* carbon dioxide–hemoglobin dissociation curve (see Chap. 10) results in decreased carbon dioxide elimination in areas where ventilation is low relative to perfusion, compensating for the increased carbon dioxide elimination in areas where ventilation is high relative to perfusion. Thus, the increased minute ventilation required to maintain arterial oxygen levels causes arterial carbon dioxide levels to fall.

Gas exchange in interstitial disorders also may be impaired because of thickening of the diffusion pathway (see Chap. 9). Fluid in the air spaces and thickening of the alveolar walls due to inflammation or fibrosis increase the

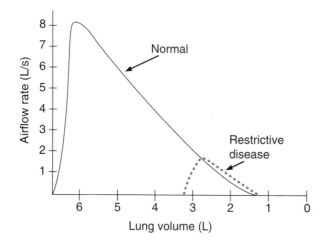

Figure 7-10. Flow–volume curve in restrictive lung disease. Lung volume is reduced. Airflow rates are maintained or increased.

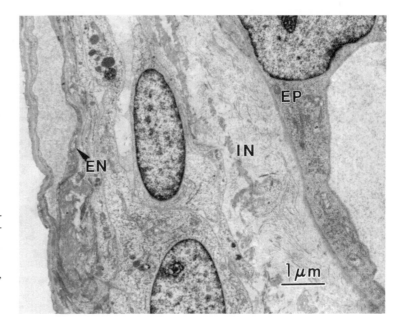

Figure 7-11. Electron micrograph (original magnification ×15,000) showing thickened alveolar wall in a patient in the reparative phase of the adult respiratory distress syndrome (see Chap. 14). The interstitial space is markedly increased. IN, interstitium; EN, endothelial cell; EP, type I pneumocyte (epithelial cell). (Courtesy of Giuseppe G. Pietra, M.D.)

distance that oxygen must diffuse to reach the capillaries (Fig. 7-11). In healthy subjects, blood in the pulmonary capillaries is fully oxygenated after traversing only the first third of the distance through the capillary. In the absence of severe interstitial lung disease, hypoxemia at rest secondary to diffusion abnormalities usually does not occur.

Measurement of diffusion of a gas into and out of the alveolar capillaries is best estimated by the single-breath diffusing capacity for carbon monoxide (DLCO), as discussed in Chapter 9. Because DLCO measures abnormalities related not only to thickening of the membrane, but also to changes in lung surface area and capillary volume, abnormalities in this measurement may reflect pathophysiologic changes in any of these three elements. DLCO is a very sensitive test for assessing interstitial lung disease.

EXERCISE TESTING

Early in the course of interstitial lung disease, patients may notice shortness of breath only on exertion. As the disease progresses, shortness of breath at rest develops. Exercise testing is one of the most sensitive means of monitoring the severity of the interstitial diseases (see Chap. 19).

Exercise decreases the transit time of red blood cells in the alveolar capillaries, reducing the time available for diffusion of oxygen. If a thickened diffusion pathway is present, hypoxemia due to diffusion limitation may be observed selectively during exercise. The degree of hypoxemia correlates with the decrease in red blood cell transit time (see Chap. 9).

Exercise testing also may demonstrate a second physiologic abnormality in interstitial lung diseases: an inability to increase tidal volume during exercise. Because most interstitial lung diseases are characterized by limited lung expansion, tidal volume fails to increase normally with exercise. To increase minute ventilation, the respiratory rate rises excessively. A marked increase in respiratory rate, accompanied by only a small increase in tidal volume, is characteristic of these disorders. The resultant rapid, shallow breathing pattern is inefficient because it produces an increase in dead space ventilation (see Chap. 3).

Normally, as tidal volume increases, the proportion of ventilation to anatomic dead space decreases. With a limited increase in tidal volume, the relative decrease in dead space ventilation does not occur. Hence, exercise tolerance is limited not only because tidal volume and minute ventilation are limited, but also because ventilation is inefficient.

Finally, exercise tolerance may be limited in interstitial lung diseases because of development of pulmonary hypertension secondary to vasculitis, destruction of lung parenchyma, or hypoxemia. In the face of an increase in cardiac output during exercise, pulmonary artery pressure rises. The rise limits cardiac output if the right ventricle cannot augment its force of contraction to maintain flow through the pulmonary circulation (see Chap. 12); left-sided cardiac output is limited because of decreased left atrial filling. Hence, exercise intolerance in interstitial lung disease may be the result of limitations in ventilation, diffusion, and cardiac output.

SELECTED READING

Banks DE. Immunologically mediated lung disease. Immunol Allerg Clin North Am 12:205–489, 1992.

Crystal RG, Ferrans VJ. Reactions of the interstitial space to injury. In: Fishman AP, ed. Pulmonary Diseases and Disorders, 2nd ed. New York: McGraw-Hill, 1988:711–738.

Fanburg BL. Sarcoidosis and Other Granulomatous Diseases of the Lung. New York: Marcel Dekker, 1983.

Jackson LK, Fulmer JD. Structural–functional features of the interstitial lung diseases. In: Fishman AP, ed. Pulmonary Diseases and Disorders, 2nd ed. New York: McGraw-Hill, 1988:739–754.

Lynch JP, DeRemee RA. Immunologically Mediated Pulmonary Diseases. Philadelphia: JB Lippincott, 1991.

Merchant JA. Occupational Respiratory Diseases. Department of Health and Human Services (NIOSH) Publication No. 86-102. Washington, DC: U.S. Government Printing Office, 1986.

Schwartz MI, King TE. Interstitial Lung Disease. Philadelphia: BC Decker, 1988.

Lippincott's Pathophysiology Series: Pulmonary Pathophysiology, edited by Michael A. Grippi. J. B. Lippincott Company, Philadelphia © 1995.

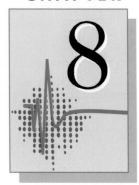

Clinical Presentations: Mechanics and Obstructive and Restrictive Disorders

Michael A. Grippi

Many of the physiologic principles highlighted in the preceding chapters serve as the basis for a variety of tests used in the clinical evaluation of known or suspected lung disease. The following three cases highlight the mechanical alterations that exist within the spectrum of obstructive and restrictive pulmonary disorders. Each is based on aspects of pathophysiology discussed previously. Punctuating information gathered as part of the routine clinical evaluation are brief interpretations of the data. As additional tests are performed or supplemental clinical details obtained, further interpretation is provided.

CASE 1

The patient is a 45-year-old man with a 6-month history of progressive shortness of breath, nonproductive cough, generalized weakness, and fatigue.

Physical examination shows the patient to be seated bolt upright. He is markedly short of breath. Cyanosis of the lips and nail beds is present. There is no digital clubbing. Diffuse, moist rales are audible throughout the chest.

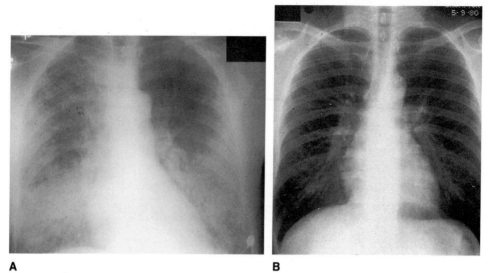

A   **B**

Figure 8-1. Case 1: chest radiographs. **(A)** Patient's posteroanterior chest radiograph. **(B)** Posteroanterior chest radiograph of a healthy subject for comparison.

Chest radiography is performed (Fig. 8-1A; for comparison, a normal chest radiograph is shown in Fig. 8-1B). Arterial blood gases, obtained while the patient was breathing room air, are as follows:

Pa_{O_2} (mmHg)	36
Pa_{CO_2} (mmHg)	33
pH	7.47
[HCO_3^-] (mEq/L)	24

The patient has a chronic history of cough, dyspnea, and systemic symptoms, including weakness and fatigue. He is cyanotic, indicating the presence of deoxygenated hemoglobin (see Chap. 10). Rales are heard throughout the lung fields, consistent with alveolar or interstitial fluid or fibrosis. The chest radiograph shows diffuse infiltrates. Arterial blood gases demonstrate hypocapnia and severe hypoxemia. None of these findings, individually or collectively, establishes a specific diagnosis.

Pulmonary function tests, including measurement of lung volumes and spirometry, are performed (Fig. 8-2).

Lung volumes (TLC, FRC, and RV) are moderately reduced, consistent with a restrictive abnormality.

The following parameters should be calculated from the expiratory spirogram shown in Figure 8-2B: FVC (predicted = 3.9 L), FEV_1 (predicted = 3.3 L), FEV_1/FVC% (predicted >70%), FEV_3/FVC% (predicted >95%), and $FEF_{25\%-75\%}$ (predicted = 2.5 L/s).

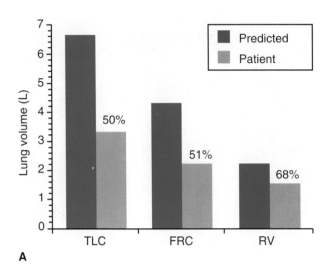

A

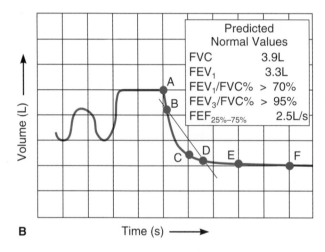

B

Figure 8-2. Case 1: pulmonary function tests. (**A**) Lung volumes and predicted normal values. Percentages indicate patient's results relative to predicted. (**B**) Expiratory spirogram. Scale: 1 second/block on horizontal axis; 1 liter/block on vertical axis. See text for details.

The FEV_1, the volume exhaled during the first second of the forced expiratory vital capacity maneuver (see Fig. 8-2B, interval A–C), is measured as 2.5 L.

To measure the $FEV_1/FVC\%$, the FVC must first be determined. The FVC is the total amount of gas exhaled during the forced expiratory vital capacity maneuver (see Fig. 8-2B, interval A–F); this is measured as 3.0 L. Therefore, the $FEV_1/FVC\%$ is 2.5/3.0, or 83%.

The $FEV_3/FVC\%$ is determined in the same way as the $FEV_1/FVC\%$. The FEV_3 is approximately 2.9 L (see Fig. 8-2B, interval A–E). Therefore, the $FEV_3/FVC\%$ is 2.9/3.0, or 97%.

The $FEF_{25\%-75\%}$ is the expiratory flow rate between 25% and 75% of the exhaled vital capacity; it is calculated as the slope of the expiratory spirogram between these two volume points (see Fig. 8-2B, slope of line BD). As measured in Figure 8-2B, the $FEF_{25\%-75\%}$ is 1.8 L/1.1 s or 1.64 L/s.

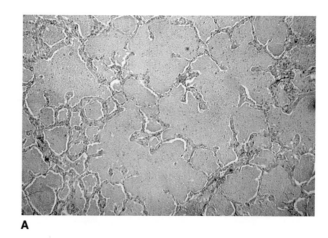

A

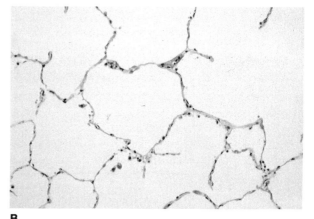

Figure 8-3. Case 1: tissue sections. **(A)** Patient's lung biopsy. **(B)** Section of healthy lung shown for comparison (hematoxylin–eosin, original magnifications ×100). (Panel B courtesy of Leslie A. Litzky, M.D.)

B

The pattern of abnormality indicated by spirometry is restrictive because the FEV_1 and FVC are reduced and the $FEV_1/FVC\%$ is normal. Hence, spirometry and lung volumes show consistent results.

In order to establish a definitive diagnosis, a lung biopsy is performed (Fig. 8-3A; for comparison, a normal lung section is shown in Fig. 8-3B).

The lung biopsy shows the alveolar spaces filled with material that displaces gas from the lungs, accounting for the "restrictive" nature of the disorder. Because the lungs contain less air and are unable to inflate and deflate fully, vital capacity and lung volumes are reduced.

Based on the pathologic findings, the patient undergoes whole lung lavage, a procedure in which each lung, in sequence, is "washed" repeatedly with saline administered through a tube placed in the main bronchi.

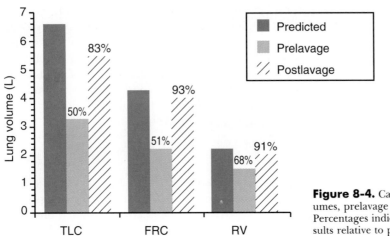

Figure 8-4. Case 1: lung volumes, prelavage and postlavage. Percentages indicate patient's results relative to predicted.

Arterial blood gas results, obtained after lavage while the patient was breathing room air, are as follows:

Pa_{O_2} (mmHg)	71
Pa_{CO_2} (mmHg)	39
pH	7.43
$[HCO_3^-]$ (mEq/L)	26

Lung volumes are determined after lavage (Fig. 8-4; normal predicted values and prelavage results are shown for comparison). A repeat chest radiograph is obtained (Fig. 8-5).

The lung biopsy establishes the diagnosis of pulmonary alveolar proteinosis, an uncommon disorder in which surfactant-like material accumu-

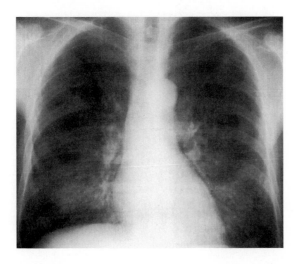

Figure 8-5. Case 1: posteroanterior chest radiograph, postlavage.

lates within alveolar spaces, producing symptoms of dyspnea and cough, as well as restrictive pulmonary physiology. Lung lavage promotes removal of the material from alveoli, resulting in a return of lung volumes toward normal. The postlavage chest radiograph shows marked improvement.

Repeated lung biopsies are not a practical way of assessing disease activity. Pulmonary function tests and arterial blood gas measurements, however, permit safe and reliable evaluation of the physiologic effects of the disease and the extent of pulmonary involvement.

CASE 2

The patient is a 44-year-old woman with rheumatoid arthritis (RA). She was treated initially with nonsteroidal antiinflammatory drugs and then with corticosteroids. One year later, her arthritis worsened and she complained of dyspnea on exertion. She was then switched to gold therapy for her arthritis. Over the past 2 years, the patient's exertional dyspnea has progressed, although she is not short of breath at rest. A nonproductive cough also has developed.

Physical examination reveals a thin woman in no acute distress. Chest examination shows normal diaphragm excursion bilaterally and dry, bibasilar rales. Examination of the heart is normal. No cyanosis, clubbing, or edema are present.

A chest radiograph is obtained (Fig. 8-6). Arterial blood gases, obtained while the patient was breathing room air, are as follows:

Pa_{O_2} (mmHg)	77
Pa_{CO_2} (mmHg)	38
pH	7.42
$[HCO_3{}^-]$ (mEq/L)	24
% Hemoglobin saturation	96

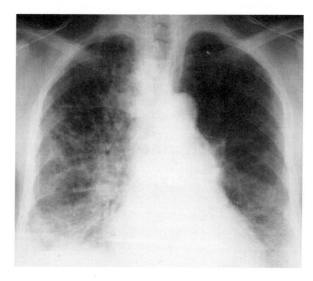

Figure 8-6. Case 2: postero-anterior chest radiograph.

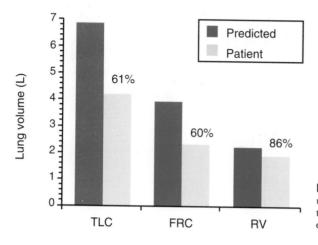

Figure 8-7. Case 2: lung volumes. Percentages indicate patient's results relative to predicted.

The chest radiograph shows interstitial lung disease. Arterial blood gases reveal a mild reduction in Pa_{O_2}.

RA is associated with a variety of pleuropulmonary manifestations. Diffuse interstitial fibrosis (see Chap. 7) occurs in up to 5% of patients with RA. Pulmonary involvement is about twice as common in men as in women, with the most frequent onset in the fifth decade or later. Usually, pulmonary fibrosis appears after the arthritis has developed; however, in about 15% of cases the pulmonary manifestations may precede the arthritis by as long as 5 years. Other pulmonary manifestations of RA include lung nodules and exudative pleural effusions. Rarely, pulmonary arteritis, pulmonary hypertension (see Chap. 12), or bronchiolitis (see Chap. 7) may develop.

Pulmonary function tests are performed. The diffusing capacity (D_{LCO}) is 10 ml/minute/mmHg (predicted normal, 23 ± 7). Lung volumes are measured (Fig. 8-7) and a flow–volume loop is obtained (Fig. 8-8). Subsequently, a pressure–volume curve is determined (Fig. 8-9).

The lung volumes and D_{LCO} are reduced due to interstitial fibrosis. The progression of the patient's lung disease may be related to the total duration of her RA. Gold therapy also has been associated with diffuse interstitial fibrosis, which appears to resolve slowly after discontinuing the agent. Healing may be accelerated after administration of corticosteroids. The patient's dyspnea got worse because of progression of her interstitial fibrosis.

Although the patient's flow–volume loop is much smaller than the predicted loop, at any given thoracic gas volume, the maximal expiratory airflow rate is actually higher than predicted. This is quite typical of interstitial fibrosis because the airways are tethered open, rather than collapsed, during an expiratory maneuver (see Chaps. 2 and 4). The calculated FEV_1/FVC% is 88%, which is greater than predicted. There is no evidence of obstructive airway disease.

The pressure–volume curve indicates that lung compliance is re-

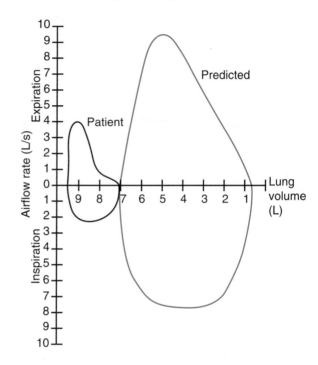

Figure 8-8. Case 2: Flow–volume loop compared with predicted.

duced. A greater transpulmonary pressure is required for lung inflation to a given volume; the lungs are stiff.

As a final step in the evaluation, arterial blood gases are obtained while the patient is breathing room air during exercise. The results are as follows:

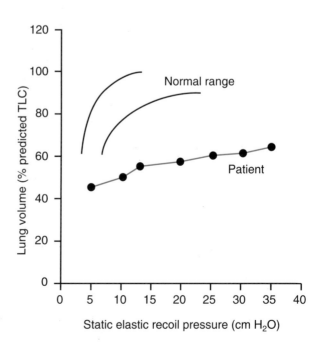

Figure 8-9. Case 2: pressure–volume curve compared with normal range.

Pa_{O_2} (mmHg)	65
Pa_{CO_2} (mmHg)	37
pH	7.38
$[HCO_3^-]$ (mEq/L)	22
% Hemoglobin saturation	92

A drop in Pa_{O_2} or "desaturation" during exercise is noted and probably occurs for two reasons: (1) ventilation–perfusion mismatching (see Chap. 13) and (2) abnormal diffusion of O_2 from alveoli into the capillaries (see Chap. 9). Exercise significantly increases cardiac output, and the redistribution of the increased blood flow through the abnormal pulmonary vascular bed may produce ventilation–perfusion mismatching.

Although the presence of a diffusion barrier may not be a significant cause of hypoxemia at rest in this patient, it may be important during exercise. During exertion, there is a rapid transit of blood through the pulmonary capillaries, decreasing the amount of time available for O_2 in alveoli to equilibrate with blood in adjacent capillaries. In addition, surface area for diffusion is reduced, as suggested by the reduced D_{LCO}.

CASE 3

The patient is a 37-year-old truck driver admitted to the hospital for progressive shortness of breath. At 25 years of age, he noted a decrease in exercise tolerance and experienced episodes of shortness of breath. At 31 years of age, a chest radiograph showed hyperinflation and lower lobe bullae (cystic collections of air within the lung parenchyma). By 37 years of age, the patient was totally disabled by his lung disease. He has been admitted frequently to the hospital for increasing shortness of breath. He has smoked one pack of cigarettes daily for 25 years. A younger brother began showing similar symptoms at 31 years of age. Neither parent has symptoms of lung disease.

Physical examination reveals a thin man in moderate respiratory distress. Clubbing and cyanosis are absent. Examination of the chest shows a marked increase in anteroposterior diameter, hyperresonant lung fields, low diaphragms, distant breath sounds, and occasional expiratory wheezing. The heart examination is normal. No peripheral edema is noted.

A chest radiograph is obtained (Fig. 8-10). Arterial blood gases, obtained while the patient was breathing room air, are as follows:

Pa_{O_2} (mmHg)	71
Pa_{CO_2} (mmHg)	40
pH	7.42
$[HCO_3^-]$ (mEq/L)	26

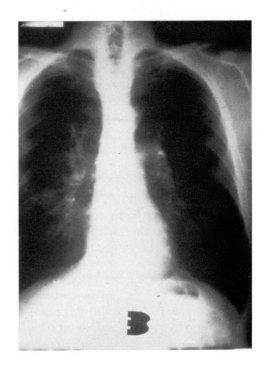

Figure 8-10. Case 3: posteroanterior chest radiograph.

Although the patient has a significant smoking history, his shortness of breath developed at an early age and has been rapidly progressive. The early onset and family history of a brother with similar symptoms suggest the possibility of a heritable disorder, such as α_1-antitrypsin deficiency.

Physical examination of the chest is consistent with hyperinflation and airway obstruction. The chest radiograph shows hyperinflated lung fields. Arterial blood gases reveal mild hypoxemia.

Pulmonary function tests are performed, including measurements of lung volume (Fig. 8-11), spirometry, and airway resistance; the latter two are determined before and after administration of an inhaled bronchodilator. The results, along with predicted normal values, are as follows:

	Predicted Normal	Prebroncho-dilator	Postbroncho-dilator
FEV_1 (L)	3.8	0.6	0.7
FVC (L)	4.8	1.4	1.7
FEV_1/FVC%	>70	44	40
FEV_3/FVC%	>97	83	75
$FEF_{25\%-75\%}$ (L/s)	4.0	0.4	0.4
Raw (cm H_2O/L/s)	0.8	3.4	3.0

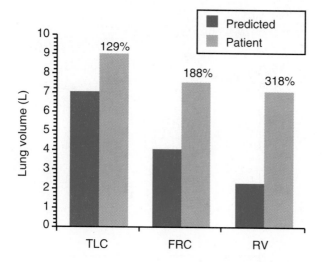

Figure 8-11. Case 3: lung volumes. Percentages indicate patient's results relative to predicted.

The differential diagnosis includes (congenital) bullous disease, asthma, and early-onset emphysema. Residual volume is markedly increased. Expiratory airflow rates are decreased, and airway resistance is elevated. The FVC increased and airway resistance decreased slightly after administration of a bronchodilator, suggesting resolution of some bronchospasm. Pulmonary function is still markedly abnormal, however, indicating that the disease is largely irreversible.

An expiratory flow–volume curve (Fig. 8-12) and pressure–volume curve (Fig. 8-13) are obtained.

The flow–volume curve indicates a rapid decrease in expiratory airflow shortly after the onset of expiration. This finding is the result of airway compression secondary to the positive pleural pressure created by the expiratory effort (see Chaps. 2, 4, and 6). During inspiration, airway compres-

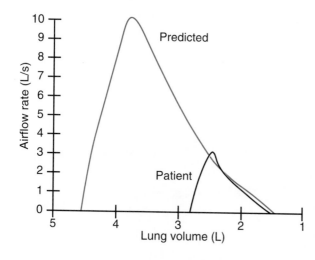

Figure 8-12. Case 3: expiratory flow–volume curve compared with predicted.

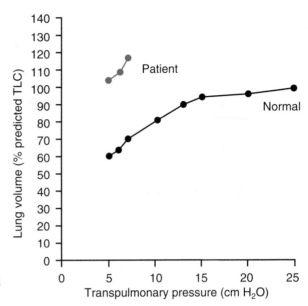

Figure 8-13. Case 3: pressure–volume curve compared with normal.

sion does not occur, and the limiting factor for inspiratory flow is the pressure generated by inspiratory muscles. The curve is shifted to the right because of lung hyperinflation.

The pressure–volume curve is displaced upward and to the left, indicating elevated lung compliance, a finding best explained by destruction of lung tissue and loss of elastic recoil.

A serum protein electrophoresis is performed.

A serum protein electrophoresis is performed to evaluate for possible α_1-antitrypsin deficiency (see Chap. 6); it reveals an absent α_1-globulin band. A quantitative α_1-antitrypsin level of 7 μmol/L is obtained (normal, 20–55 μmol/L).

α_1-Antitrypsin deficiency is a recessively inherited, genetic disease manifested by childhood cirrhosis or premature emphysema in young adults. These two phenotypic expressions usually are not seen in the same patient, however. Although emphysema occurs in some, but not all, patients with α_1-antitrypsin deficiency, cigarette smoking greatly increases the frequency of clinically significant lung disease.

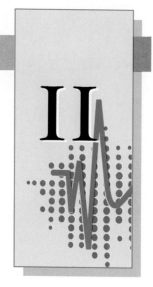

GAS EXCHANGE AND TRANSPORT

II

Lippincott's Pathophysiology Series: Pulmonary Pathophysiology, edited by Michael A. Grippi. J. B. Lippincott Company, Philadelphia © 1995.

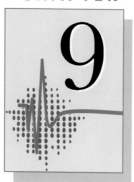

Gas Exchange in the Lung

Michael A. Grippi

The preceding chapters focus on mechanical properties of the airways and lung parenchyma that determine gas movement into and out of alveoli. Gas exchange across the alveolar–capillary membrane, that is, the uptake of oxygen and elimination of carbon dioxide, represents a function critical to tissue metabolism.

This chapter addresses oxygen and carbon dioxide movement across the alveolar–capillary membrane, in plasma, and in red blood cells. After a brief review of the basic principles of the physics of gases, diffusion and the diffusing capacity of the lung are examined. Alterations in diffusing capacity in disease states are highlighted and related to the underlying pathophysiology.

BASIC CONCEPTS

An understanding of several basic concepts related to the physics of gases is important in considering oxygen and carbon dioxide exchange in the lung. Key among these concepts are fractional concentration and partial pressure, topics initially introduced in Chapter 3 and summarized here (Fig. 9-1).

FRACTIONAL CONCENTRATION OF A GAS

The kinetic energy of all molecules of atmospheric gas creates *atmospheric* or *barometric pressure* (PB). PB varies inversely with altitude; at sea level, PB is 760 mmHg. This pressure refers to an actual or *absolute* measurement, rather than

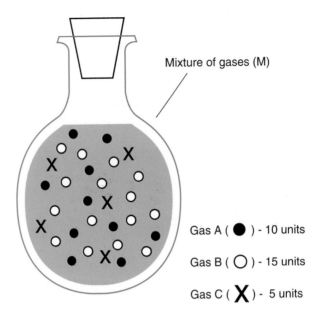

Mixture of gases (M)

Gas A (●) - 10 units

Gas B (○) - 15 units

Gas C (**X**) - 5 units

Calculation of Fractional Concentrations	Calculation of Partial Pressures
$$F_MA = \frac{10}{10 + 15 + 5} = 0.33$$	$$P_MA = F_MA \cdot (P_B - 47 \text{ mm Hg})$$ $$= 0.33 \cdot (760 - 47)$$ $$= 235.3 \text{ mm Hg}$$
$$F_MB = \frac{15}{10 + 15 + 5} = 0.50$$	$$P_MB = F_MB \cdot (P_B - 47 \text{ mm Hg})$$ $$= 0.50 \cdot (760 - 47)$$ $$= 356.5 \text{ mm Hg}$$
$$F_MC = \frac{5}{10 + 15 + 5} = 0.17$$	$$P_MC = F_MC \cdot (P_B - 47 \text{ mm Hg})$$ $$= 0.17 \cdot (760 - 47)$$ $$= 121.2 \text{ mm Hg}$$

Figure 9-1. Fractional concentration and partial pressure of a gas. A "dry" mixture (M), comprising gases A, B, and C, is inside the sealed container. The fractional concentration of each gas is the number of molecules (or units) of the gas divided by the total number of molecules (or units) in the mixture. The partial pressure of each gas is the product of the gas's fractional concentration and the difference between barometric pressure (P_B) and water vapor presure (47 mmHg). In the example shown, P_B is 760 mmHg—barometric pressure at sea level.

a *relative* measurement, as is the case for the pressures considered in Chapter 2. Customarily, alveolar, airway, and pleural pressures are expressed relative to atmospheric and are known as *gauge pressures*. When gauge pressures are considered, atmospheric pressure is zero (i.e., zero gauge pressure).

   Atmospheric air is a mixture of several gases: nitrogen, oxygen, argon, carbon dioxide, and water vapor. The amounts of argon and carbon dioxide are minimal, and water vapor pressure under normal ambient conditions is small. Therefore, for practical purposes, atmospheric air can be considered a mixture of 21% oxygen and 79% nitrogen. That is, F_{IO_2} is 0.21 and F_{IN_2} is 0.79, where F_{IO_2} and F_{IN_2} represent the *fractional concentrations* of oxygen and nitrogen, respectively.

When "dry" atmospheric air is inhaled, it is warmed to body temperature (37°C) and becomes fully saturated with water vapor. Under these circumstances, water vapor pressure is significant, as described below.

PARTIAL PRESSURE OF A GAS

As noted in Chapter 3, in a mixture of gases, the kinetic energy of each gas creates a pressure known as the gas's *partial pressure*. In a mixture of gases within a container, the sum of the individual partial pressures of the gases is the total pressure exerted by the gas mixture (*Dalton's law*). For atmospheric air:

$$P_B \quad = P_{O_2} + P_{CO_2} + P_{N_2} + P_{H_2O} \qquad [9\text{-}1]$$

where

$$
\begin{aligned}
P_{O_2} &= \text{partial pressure of } O_2 \\
P_{CO_2} &= \text{partial pressure of } CO_2 \\
P_{N_2} &= \text{partial pressure of } N_2 \\
P_{H_2O} &= \text{partial pressure of water vapor}
\end{aligned}
$$

The water vapor pressure in inspired air that is warmed to body temperature and fully humidified is 47 mmHg. Conventionally, the fractional concentration of a gas is calculated after water vapor pressure has been subtracted (i.e., as "dry gas"). The partial pressure of gas X in a mixture of inspired gases—P_{IX}—is the product of the gas's fractional concentration (F_{IX}) and the total pressure of the dry mixture ($P_B - 47$):

$$P_{IX} = F_{IX} \cdot (P_B - 47) \qquad [9\text{-}2]$$

DIFFUSION OF GASES

As discussed in Chapter 1, from an anatomic standpoint, the alveolar–capillary membrane is ideally suited for the movement of gases between alveolar spaces and pulmonary capillaries. The expansive alveolar surface area and extensive network of interfacing capillaries optimize the opportunity for O_2 uptake and CO_2 elimination.

Gas movement across the alveolar–capillary membrane occurs by diffusion, as described by *Fick's law* (Fig. 9-2). According to Fick's law, the rate of gas transfer across a tissue plane or "membrane" (e.g., the alveolar–capillary membrane) is directly proportional to: (1) the difference in partial pressure of the gas on the two sides of the membrane and (2) a constant for the membrane known as the *diffusing capacity* (D_M):

$$\dot{V}_G = D_M \cdot (P_1 - P_2) \qquad [9\text{-}3]$$

where

$$
\begin{aligned}
\dot{V}_G &= \text{rate of gas movement across a tissue plane} \\
P_1 &= \text{partial pressure of gas on one side of tissue plane} \\
P_2 &= \text{partial pressure of gas on other side of tissue plane}
\end{aligned}
$$

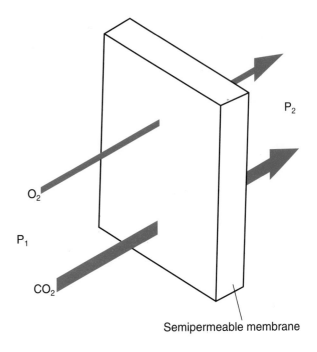

Figure 9-2. Fick's law. The rate of transfer of a gas across a membrane ($\dot{V}_G$) is determined by the membrane's surface area and thickness, the gas's molecular weight (MW) and solubility (α) in the membrane, and the partial pressure difference of the gas across the membrane ($P_1 - P_2$). $\dot{V}_G$ increases with increases in area, gas solubility, and partial pressure difference; $\dot{V}_G$ decreases with increases in membrane thickness and molecular weight of the gas.

$$\dot{V}_G \; \alpha \; \frac{\text{Area}}{\text{Thickness}} \cdot \frac{\text{Solubility}}{\sqrt{\text{MW}}} \cdot (P_1 - P_2)$$

D_M, in turn, comprises several components, including tissue solubility of the gas (α), tissue plane area (A), tissue plane thickness (d), and molecular weight of the gas (MW):

$$D_M = k \cdot \frac{A}{d} \cdot \frac{\alpha}{\sqrt{MW}} \qquad [9\text{-}4]$$

where k is a constant.

Substitution of equation [9-4] into equation [9-3] yields the following:

$$\dot{V}_G = k \cdot \frac{A}{d} \cdot \frac{\alpha}{\sqrt{MW}} \cdot (P_1 - P_2) \qquad [9\text{-}5]$$

From equation [9-5] it is evident that, for a given gas, the rate of its diffusion across the alveolar–capillary membrane increases with: (1) increases in membrane surface area, gas solubility, and gas pressure gradient across the membrane; and (2) decreases in tissue thickness and molecular weight of the gas. The effect of changes in these variables on gas transfer is intuitively clear. Diffusion is enhanced if there is more "available" membrane (increased membrane surface area) and the diffusion path length is reduced (reduced membrane thickness). Diffusion is also augmented if there is a greater "driving pressure" (greater pressure gradient across the membrane, $P_1 - P_2$) and if the solubility of the gas in the membrane through which it is diffusing is increased (higher α). Finally, the lighter the gas (the lower the molecular weight), the faster is its diffusion.

For the lung as a whole, the term, D_L—the *diffusing capacity of the lung*—is substituted for D_M (see later).

DIFFUSION AND PERFUSION LIMITATIONS TO GAS MOVEMENT ACROSS THE ALVEOLAR–CAPILLARY MEMBRANE

Thus far, the discussion has focused on diffusion as an instantaneous process, occurring when alveolar gas and an aliquot of pulmonary blood interface across alveolar walls. However, blood *flows* through the capillaries, creating special considerations. In particular, there is a *finite* time for gas transfer. Whether this time is sufficient for full equilibration of partial pressures across the alveolar–capillary membrane depends on several physiologic variables.

Under normal resting conditions, the transit time of a red blood cell through a pulmonary capillary is about 0.75 second. All of the factors included in equation [9-5] determine whether this time is sufficient to allow complete gas transfer from alveoli to the red blood cell. For any gas diffusing across a lung of constant surface area, and along a diffusion path of fixed length, the primary determinant of the diffusion rate is the partial pressure gradient for the gas across the membrane ($P_1 - P_2$). Furthermore, at a constant (or nearly constant) partial pressure in the alveolus, the pressure gradient is determined by the gas's partial pressure in capillary blood, which, in turn, depends on the dynamics between the gas dissolved in plasma and in red blood cells, bound to hemoglobin. The physiology of two gases, carbon monoxide (CO) and nitrous oxide (N_2O), serve as useful models for the analysis of diffusion (Fig. 9-3).

As inspired CO diffuses across the alveolar–capillary membrane, it moves rapidly into red blood cells and binds avidly, yet reversibly, to hemoglobin. As a consequence, there is virtually no increase in the partial pressure of CO in the plasma. Consequently, ($P_1 - P_2$) remains maximal, with no development of "back pressure." Under these circumstances, the amount of CO taken up in the circulation depends on the diffusion characteristics of the alveolar–capillary membrane, not on the amount of capillary blood. Therefore, CO uptake is *diffusion limited* (see Fig. 9-3A).

In contrast to CO, inspired N_2O does not combine with hemoglobin. Rather, as N_2O moves from alveoli into blood, the amount dissolved in plasma increases, and the partial pressure of the gas rises. Because of the resultant "back pressure," further uptake of N_2O is limited. In fact, alveolar and blood partial pressures of N_2O equilibrate by the time the red blood cell has traversed the first quarter of its route through the alveolar capillary. Thereafter, no additional N_2O is taken up because ($P_1 - P_2$) is zero. The amount of N_2O taken up depends entirely on the rate of pulmonary blood flow, not on the diffusion characteristics of the alveolar–capillary membrane. N_2O transfer is *perfusion limited* (see Fig. 9-3B).

The physiology of O_2 movement across the alveolar–capillary membrane is intermediate to that of CO and N_2O. Although O_2 does combine with hemoglobin, it does so much less avidly than CO. The partial pressure of O_2 in blood flowing through pulmonary capillaries is equal to the alveolar partial pressure of O_2 by the time the red blood cell traverses approximately one third of the capillary length. Consequently, as for N_2O, the diffusion of O_2 is normally perfusion limited. In a variety of disease states, however, equilibration of alveolar and

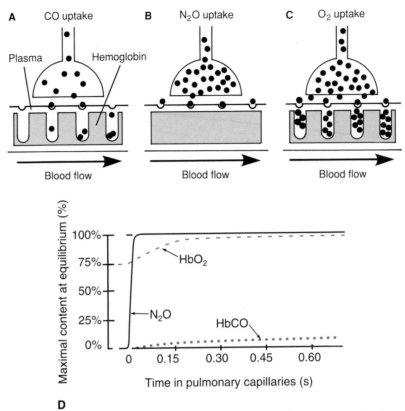

Figure 9-3. Diffusion-limited and perfusion-limited gas transfer from alveoli to blood. **(A)** CO transfer is diffusion limited. Because CO is rapidly and avidly bound to hemoglobin, no CO back pressure develops, and the pressure gradient for CO diffusion remains maximal. Gas transfer rate depends on the pressure gradient, membrane characteristics, and physical properties of the gas. **(B)** N_2O transfer is perfusion limited. As N_2O builds up in the plasma (N_2O is not bound to hemoglobin), blood becomes saturated with the gas, limiting further transfer. Additional gas transfer depends on continued blood flow to replace saturated plasma. **(C)** O_2 transfer is intermediate to diffusion-limited and perfusion-limited gases. **(D)** Maximal blood N_2O content is achieved quickly; maximal O_2 content is achieved less rapidly. CO content remains limited, even by the time the aliquot of blood traverses the entire length of the capillary. See text for details. (Modified from Forster RE II, Dubois AB, Briscoe WA, Fisher AB. Measurement of pulmonary diffusing capacity. In: The Lung, Physiologic Basis of Pulmonary Function Tests, 3rd ed. Chicago: Year Book Medical Publishers, 1986:198.)

blood partial pressures of O_2 may be delayed (relative to red blood cell capillary transit time), resulting in a diffusion limitation, as well (see Fig. 9-3C).

DIFFUSION ALONG THE COURSE OF THE PULMONARY CAPILLARY

As noted, blood flowing along the pulmonary capillary is fully oxygenated by the time it is one third the way along the course of the capillary. The mixed venous oxygen tension of 40 mmHg (see Chap. 10) rises to approximately alveolar oxygen tension (100 mmHg) in 0.25 second. Even with significant diffusion impairment (e.g., secondary to thickening of the alveolar–capillary membrane), equilibration of oxygen tension between capillary blood and alveolar gas is com-

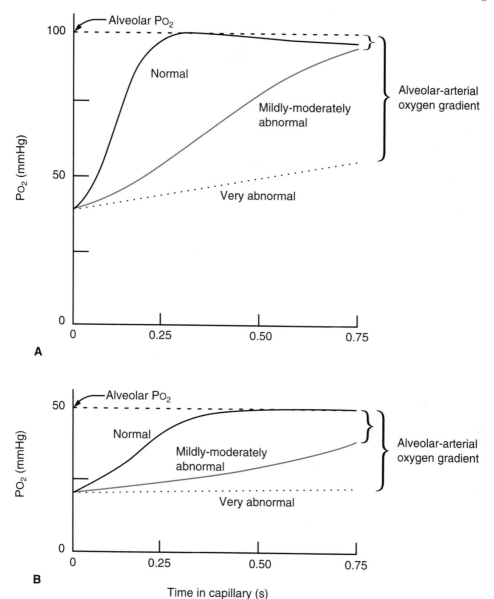

Figure 9-4. Equilibration of alveolar and pulmonary capillary Po₂. (A) In a healthy subject breathing room air, equilibration of alveolar and pulmonary capillary Po₂ occurs before the red blood cell has completed one third of its journey through the capillary. In mild lung disease, sufficient pulmonary reserve may permit equilibration before the cell completes its transit through the capillary; in severe lung disease, equilibration time may be insufficient. During exercise, as capillary transit time is shortened, equilibration may not take place, even in the presence of mild disease. (B) Effect of alveolar hypoxia. Breathing a hypoxic gas mixture or ascending to altitude creates an alveolar–arterial oxygen gradient at rest, even in the presence of only mild lung disease. (Modified from West JB. Diffusion. In: Respiratory Physiology: The Essentials, 4th ed. Baltimore: Williams & Wilkins, 1990:25.)

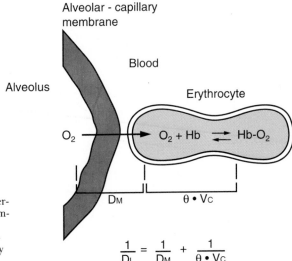

Figure 9-5. Resistances to diffusion. 1/D_L may be viewed as the overall resistance to diffusion. The overall resistance comprises two components: (1) the membrane component (1/D_M) and (2) the red blood cell component (1/$\theta \cdot V_c$). The latter depends on the reaction rate of the gas with hemoglobin (θ) and capillary blood volume (V_c).

plete by the time the aliquot of blood concludes its passage through the capillary. On the other hand, with significant diffusion impairment, end-capillary P_{O_2} may be significantly lower than alveolar P_{O_2}; that is, there is an *alveolar–arterial oxygen gradient* (Fig. 9-4A).

Another pathophysiologic mechanism that may limit diffusion in the lung is highlighted by administration of hypoxic gas mixtures or ascent to high altitude. The resulting *alveolar hypoxia* produces a drop in mixed venous P_{O_2} and in the diffusion gradient for O_2 from alveoli to capillary blood (see Fig. 9-4B). As a consequence, end-capillary P_{O_2} is substantially below arterial. The effect is accentuated during exercise, which reduces red blood cell capillary transit time.

MOVEMENT OF OXYGEN INTO RED BLOOD CELLS AND HEMOGLOBIN BINDING

As described by a modification of equation [9-3], the diffusing capacity of the lung, D_L, is defined as the rate of gas flow across the lung ($\dot{V}_G$) divided by the pressure gradient for flow ($P_1 - P_2$):

$$D_L = \frac{\dot{V}_G}{P_1 - P_2} \qquad [9\text{-}6]$$

Conceptually, movement of gas across the alveolar–capillary membrane can be compared with the flow of electricity in a circuit, described by Ohm's law. The resistance to gas transfer is the quotient of the driving pressure for gas flow (analogous to voltage) and rate of gas flow (analogous to current). Because flow ($\dot{V}_G$) divided by the pressure gradient ($P_1 - P_2$) equals D_L, 1/D_L can be viewed as the resistance to gas flow.

The overall resistance to gas flow actually comprises two individual components: (1) membrane resistance and (2) the resistance represented by the reaction of O_2 with hemoglobin. Furthermore, membrane resistance may be considered to comprise the individual resistances of the alveolar wall and the red blood cell membrane (Fig. 9-5). Hence,

$$\frac{1}{D_L} = \frac{1}{D_M} + \frac{1}{\theta \cdot V_c}$$

[9-7]

where

D_L = diffusing capacity of the lung
D_M = diffusing capacity of the membrane, including the red blood cell membrane
θ = reaction rate of O_2 with hemoglobin
V_c = capillary blood volume

As equation [9-7] indicates, diffusion across the lung rises with an increase in either membrane diffusing capacity or capillary blood volume. Capillary blood volume rises with increased pulmonary blood flow (e.g., during exercise), increased transmural pulmonary artery pressure, and capillary "recruitment" (see Chap. 12).

MEASUREMENT OF DIFFUSING CAPACITY

Based on the physiologic principles outlined earlier, carbon monoxide is a useful gas for determining the diffusing capacity of the lung. Three carbon monoxide-based methods for measuring D_{LCO} are used clinically: (1) steady-state method, (2) single-breath method, and (3) rebreathing method. The single-breath method is the most commonly used and is described briefly.

With the single-breath method, the subject inhales a gas mixture containing a low concentration of CO and a tiny amount of the inert tracer gas, helium (Fig. 9-6). At end-inspiration, the subject holds his or her breath for 10 seconds. During exhalation, the expired gas is analyzed for CO and helium concentrations. During the breath-hold period, some CO diffuses from alveoli into blood; the amount can be calculated from measurements of the CO concentration in alveolar gas at the beginning and end of the 10-second interval. The gradient for CO diffusion is the difference between mean alveolar P_{CO} and mean pulmonary capillary P_{CO}; mean pulmonary capillary P_{CO} is negligible and can be assumed to be zero (see section on Diffusion of Gases, earlier).

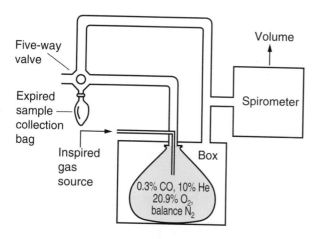

Five-way valve

Expired sample collection bag

Inspired gas source

Volume

Spirometer

Box

0.3% CO, 10% He 20.9% O_2, balance N_2

Figure 9-6. Single-breath technique for measurement of D_{LCO}. The circuit consists of a spirometer, a valve, a bag in a box, and a sample-collecting bag. The bag in the box serves as a reservoir to hold the test gas. The volume of air removed from it during the single inspiration is recorded on the spirometer. See text for details. (From Grippi MA, Metzger LF, Krupinski AV, Fishman AP. Pulmonary function testing. In: Fishman AP, ed. Pulmonary Diseases and Disorders. New York: McGraw-Hill, 1988:2496.)

The mean alveolar concentration of CO at the beginning of the breath-hold is determined from the dilution of inspired helium. Because helium is inert and is not taken up by lung tissue or blood, the decrease in helium concentration from its initial, known value is proportional to the lung volume (plus machine circuit volume) into which the CO is distributed—the "alveolar" volume:

$$F_{ACO_{initial}} = \frac{F_{EHe}}{F_{IHe}} \cdot F_{ICO} \qquad [9-8]$$

where

$F_{ACO_{initial}}$ = alveolar concentration of CO at start of breath-hold
F_{EHe} = expired fractional concentration of He
F_{IHe} = inspired fractional concentration of He
F_{ICO} = inspired fractional concentration of CO

Hence, by measuring the amount of CO transferred across the lung per unit time ($\dot{V}_G$), the mean alveolar CO concentration (P_1), and the mean capillary CO concentration (P_2, assumed to be 0), D_{LCO} can be calculated using equation [9-3].

In clinical practice, D_{LCO} is actually calculated from the following equation:

$$D_{LCO} = \left[\frac{V_A \cdot 60}{(P_B - 47) \cdot time} \right] \cdot \left[\ln \frac{F_{ACO_{initial}}}{F_{ACO_{final}}} \right] \qquad [9-9]$$

where

V_A = alveolar volume
P_B = barometric pressure
time   = time of breath-hold
$F_{ACO_{initial}}$ = alveolar concentration of CO at start of breath-hold
$F_{ACO_{final}}$ = alveolar concentration of CO at end of breath-hold

FACTORS THAT AFFECT D_{LCO}

A variety of factors which affect the diffusing capacity (Table 9-1) must be considered when interpreting the D_{LCO} as a measure of lung function.

TABLE 9-1. *FACTORS THAT AFFECT D_{LCO}*

INCREASE D_{LCO}	DECREASE D_{LCO}
Increases in:	Increase in alveolar P_{O_2}
Body size	Most lung diseases
Lung volume	Increasing age after 20 years
Alveolar P_{CO_2}	
Male sex	
Supine position	
Exercise	
Increasing age to 20 years	

BODY SIZE

D_{LCO} increases with increasing body size, as reflected in body weight, height, and body surface area.

AGE AND SEX

Age and sex also affect D_{LCO}. D_{LCO} increases in childhood and reaches a maximal value at about 20 years of age. Thereafter, D_{LCO} declines by about 2% per year. For comparable age and body size, women have a lower D_{LCO} than men by approximately 10%.

LUNG VOLUME

D_{LCO} increases with increasing lung volume, perhaps because of an increase in capillary blood volume or in the membrane component of the term (D_M). The ratio of D_{LCO} to alveolar volume (Krogh's constant) is a useful index in patients with hyperinflated lungs (e.g., due to emphysema), where lung volume changes may obscure the principal effect of the disease on gas exchange. "Normalization" of the D_{LCO} by relating it to lung volume factors out the hyperinflation of emphysema and permits interpretation of D_{LCO} as a purer measure of gas exchange.

EXERCISE

D_{CLO} increases during exercise. Presumably, the increase reflects an increase in contact area of the pulmonary capillaries with alveolar gas because of dilation of vessels or opening of capillaries previously closed (blood vessel recruitment).

BODY POSITION

D_{LCO} is higher in the supine than sitting position; D_{LCO} is higher in the sitting than standing position. The changes may reflect alterations in capillary blood volume in the three positions.

ALVEOLAR P_{O_2} AND P_{CO_2}

Finally, increases in alveolar P_{O_2} result in reductions in D_{LCO} because O_2 competes with CO for binding to hemoglobin. Increases in alveolar P_{CO_2} result in increases in D_{LCO}.

D_{LCO} IN DISEASE

A wide variety of diseases affect D_{LCO}. The basis for alterations in the measurement depends on the underlying pathophysiology (Table 9-2).

CHRONIC OBSTRUCTIVE PULMONARY DISEASE

D_{LCO} is reduced in chronic obstructive pulmonary disease. Reductions are greater in emphysema than chronic bronchitis, and measurement of D_{LCO} has

TABLE 9-2. *CHANGES IN D_{LCO} IN DISEASE*	
DISEASE	**EFFECT ON D_{LCO}**
Chronic obstructive pulmonary disease (especially emphysema)	Decrease
Restrictive pulmonary parenchymal disease	Decrease
Pulmonary edema	Decrease
Pulmonary vascular disease	Decrease
Pulmonary hemorrhage	Increase
Polycythemia	Increase
Anemia	Decrease

been advocated as a useful test for distinguishing between these two disorders (see Chap. 6). Reductions in D$_{LCO}$ in emphysema reflect loss of alveolar–capillary surface area and reduced alveolar capillary blood volume.

RESTRICTIVE PULMONARY DISORDERS

The restrictive pulmonary disorders include a variety of processes affecting the respiratory neuromuscular apparatus, chest wall, pleural space, and lung parenchyma (see Chaps. 4 and 7). Although neuromuscular diseases and disorders of the chest wall may have secondary effects on the lung parenchyma and, thereby affect D$_{LCO}$, D$_{LCO}$ is usually normal. In contradistinction, parenchymal lung diseases that produce a restrictive pattern on pulmonary function testing are usually accompanied by a reduction in D$_{LCO}$.

The large number of interstitial lung diseases are characterized by several common pathologic features: interstitial edema, fibrosis, and capillary destruction (see Chap. 7). Hence, there may be increased diffusion pathway thickness, loss of capillaries, reduced capillary blood volume, and an imbalance between alveolar ventilation and capillary perfusion. These factors, individually or collectively, reduce D$_{LCO}$.

PULMONARY EDEMA

Flooding of alveoli with fluid due to cardiogenic or noncardiogenic pulmonary edema (see Chap. 14) increases diffusion distance and decreases D$_{LCO}$.

PULMONARY VASCULAR DISEASE

A variety of pulmonary vascular diseases affect D$_{LCO}$. Thrombotic or embolic occlusion of a branch of the pulmonary artery reduces D$_{LCO}$. Similarly, occlusion of the pulmonary capillary bed due to vasculitis decreases D$_{LCO}$. Pulmonary hypertension, per se, does not affect D$_{LCO}$. If the pulmonary hypertension is severe, however, D$_{LCO}$ may be reduced because of pulmonary capillary obliteration (see Chap. 12).

PULMONARY HEMORRHAGE

Acute alveolar hemorrhage is accompanied by an *increase* in D$_L$CO. The additional hemoglobin in alveolar spaces serves as a sink for CO, resulting in greater CO transfer during the measurement. Chronic, recurrent alveolar hemorrhage is associated with pulmonary fibrosis and a *reduced* D$_L$CO.

POLYCYTHEMIA AND ANEMIA

An increase in hematocrit (polycythemia) increases D$_L$CO through an increase in capillary red blood cells (more CO "sinks"), whereas a decrease in hematocrit (anemia) reduces D$_L$CO. Abnormalities in hematocrit must be mathematically accounted for in interpreting the D$_L$CO properly as a measure of lung function; the correction is made by applying clinically derived correction equations to the measured D$_L$CO.

CO$_2$ EXCHANGE IN THE LUNG

Because the solubility of CO$_2$ in tissues is approximately 20 times that of O$_2$, the rate of diffusion of CO$_2$ across the alveolar–capillary membrane is 20 times as fast as that of O$_2$. Hence, there is a great deal of reserve built into the system, and mild abnormalities of the lung parenchyma may not be accompanied by an arterial–alveolar gradient for CO$_2$.

With moderate or severe thickening of the alveolar–capillary membrane, CO$_2$ transfer from blood to alveolus may be limited. Indeed, when D$_L$CO is reduced to approximately 25% of normal, CO$_2$ transfer is impaired, and an arterial–alveolar CO$_2$ gradient develops.

SELECTED READING

Cotes JE, Dabbs JM, Elwood PC, Hall AM, McDonald A, Saundres MJ. Iron deficiency anemia: Its effect on transfer factor for the lung (diffusing capacity) and ventilation and cardiac frequency during sub-maximal exercise. Clin Sci 42:325–335, 1972.

Filley GF, MacIntosh DJ, Wright GW. Carbon monoxide uptake and pulmonary diffusing capacity in normal subjects at rest and during exercise. J Clin Invest 33:530–539, 1954.

Forster RE. Exchange of gases between alveolar air and pulmonary capillary blood: Pulmonary diffusion capacity. Physiol Rev 37:391–452, 1957.

Krogh M. The diffusion of gases through the lungs of man. J Physiol 49:271–300, 1915.

Ogilvie CM, Forster RE, Blakemore WS, Morton JW. A standardized breath holding technique for the clinical measurement of the diffusing capacity of the lung for carbon monoxide. J Clin Invest 36:1–17, 1957.

Roughton FJW, Forster RE. Relative importance of diffusion and chemical reaction rates in determining the rate of exchange of gases in the human lung, with special reference to true diffusing capacity of pulmonary membrane and volume of blood in the lung capillaries. J Appl Physiol 11:290–302, 1957.

Lippincott's Pathophysiology Series: Pulmonary Pathophysiology, edited by Michael A. Grippi. J. B. Lippincott Company, Philadelphia © 1995.

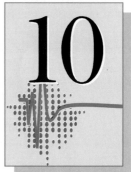

Gas Transport To and From Peripheral Tissues

Gregory Tino and Michael A. Grippi

Alveolar gas exchange entails a series of complex physiologic interactions. Critical events taking place at the alveolar–capillary membrane are described in Chapter 9. Other processes, such as erythrocyte transport and unloading of O_2 in peripheral tissues and concurrent removal of CO_2, are equally important. Hence, integrated function of the lungs, cardiovascular system, and blood characterizes normal respiration. This chapter focuses on erythrocyte and hemoglobin physiology and biochemistry, particularly as they affect O_2 and CO_2 binding, O_2 and CO_2 transport in blood, and acid–base physiology.

ERYTHROCYTE PHYSIOLOGY AND BIOCHEMISTRY

Often lost in the intricacies of gas exchange is the role of the erythrocyte, a cell largely responsible for transporting O_2 to peripheral tissues and for removing metabolically produced CO_2. The erythrocyte is derived from undifferentiated bone marrow progenitor cells. As the cell matures, it loses its nucleus, ribosomes, and mitochondria. As a consequence, the erythrocyte is incapable of many common mammalian cellular functions, including cell division, oxidative phosphorylation, and protein synthesis. For energy production, the erythrocyte relies almost exclusively on glucose metabolized by way of the Embden–Meyerhoff pathway or hexose monophosphate shunt.

THE ERYTHROCYTE MEMBRANE

The erythrocyte cell membrane imparts many of the properties that allow the cell to serve as an effective O_2 carrier. The cell membrane is pliable, permitting the cell to traverse small capillaries; its durability allows the cell to withstand turbulent flow in larger blood vessels.

The cell membrane is a typical lipid bilayer, containing phospholipids, unesterified cholesterol, and glycolipids interspersed with proteins. Membrane proteins subserve important functions, including calcium homeostasis, anion exchange, and maintenance of cell volume. These proteins also serve as essential membrane channels and as cell surface receptors.

HEMOGLOBIN

The most important intracellular protein for O_2 and CO_2 transport is hemoglobin (Hb). Each molecule of hemoglobin consists of a *globin* protein and *heme*, which is a complex of iron and porphyrin (Fig. 10-1).

The globin protein is a tetramer of polypeptide chains, including alpha (α) and nonalpha types. Hemoglobin A (HbA), the major adult hemoglobin, contains two α and two beta (β) chains and is designated $\alpha_2\beta_2$. The minor adult hemoglobin, HbA_2, contains two α and two delta (δ) chains ($\alpha_2\delta_2$).

As with other proteins, the amino acid sequence of the globin chains determines the protein's primary structure; the chains' helical arrangement confers the protein's secondary structure. Each α subunit of HbA consists of 141 amino acids arranged in 8 helices. Each β chain consists of 196 amino acids arranged in 7 helices.

The folding of the protein helices into a three-dimensional shape confers the protein's tertiary structure—the state of lowest possible energy and maximal stability. Hydrophobic interactions between the hydrocarbon moieties of polypeptide side chains govern this tertiary arrangement.

The quaternary globin structure, the final level of organization of the hemoglobin molecule, is intricate; it is determined primarily by noncovalent bonding between polypeptide chains. The quaternary state undergoes significant conformational shifts during a variety of erythrocyte functions, including O_2 binding.

The other major component of hemoglobin, heme, consists of a single

Figure 10-1. Structure of hemoglobin. A molecule of hemoglobin is composed of two α and two β chains. Each chain contains a heme moiety, which houses ferrous iron to which O_2 binds. Conformational changes among the subunits as O_2 binding occurs facilitate additional O_2 loading. See text for details. (From: Schrier SL. Hematology. Scientific American Medicine 2:7, 1988.)

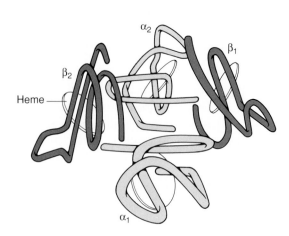

ferrous ion (Fe^{2+}) chelated in a porphyrin ring (protoporphyrin IX). O_2 binds directly to the heme moiety housed within the helical structure of each globin polypeptide chain. Each heme ion avidly, and reversibly, binds a single O_2 molecule, allowing a maximum of four O_2 molecules to bind to each molecule of hemoglobin. Hemoglobin loaded with a full complement of O_2 is known as *oxyhemoglobin*; hemoglobin without O_2 or with incomplete O_2 binding is *deoxygenated hemoglobin*.

The unique arrangement of heme and protein molecules in human hemoglobin is critical for the reversible binding of O_2. In its isolated ionic form, ferrous heme binds O_2 irreversibly, producing oxidized, ferric heme (Fe^{3+}). This complex precludes O_2 unloading at the tissue level. In the intact hemoglobin molecule, the association of O_2 with ferrous heme causes significant conformational changes in both the tertiary and quaternary globin structure, preventing ferric ion formation. The end result is *reversible* O_2 binding by hemoglobin—a step that is critical for O_2 release, uptake, and utilization in peripheral tissues.

OXYGEN TRANSPORT

As discussed in Chapter 9, the binding of O_2 to hemoglobin is driven by the difference in Po_2 between alveoli and erythrocytes. As O_2 traverses the alveolar capillaries, O_2-depleted venous blood provides a "sink" for O_2 binding, promoting movement of O_2 into the erythrocyte. O_2 is transported in arterial blood in two forms: bound to hemoglobin within erythrocytes and dissolved in plasma.

HEMOGLOBIN-BOUND OXYGEN

The principal form in which O_2 is transported is oxyhemoglobin. Each gram of hemoglobin can bind maximally 1.34 ml of O_2. Hence, the *oxygen carrying capacity* of blood is directly dependent on the hemoglobin concentration:

$$\text{Oxygen carrying capacity} = [Hb] \cdot 1.34 \text{ ml } O_2/g \text{ Hb/dl blood} \quad \text{[10-1]}$$

In a healthy person with a hemoglobin of 15 g/dl, the oxygen carrying capacity is 20.1 ml O_2/dl of blood.

A key determinant of the actual amount of O_2 bound to hemoglobin is the *oxygen saturation* of arterial blood (Sao_2), which expresses the relationship between the amount of oxygen bound to hemoglobin and the oxygen carrying capacity:

$$Sao_2 = \frac{\text{oxygen bound to Hb}}{O_2 \text{ carrying capacity}} \cdot 100\% \quad \text{[10-2]}$$

According to the *oxyhemoglobin dissociation curve*, which relates Sao_2 to Pao_2, Sao_2 is approximately 97% when Pao_2 is 100 mmHg (Fig. 10-2). In mixed venous blood, which has a Po_2 of 40 mmHg, Sao_2 is about 75%.

DISSOLVED OXYGEN

Blood contains a small amount of O_2 dissolved in plasma, rather than bound to hemoglobin. According to Henry's law, the amount of dissolved O_2 is

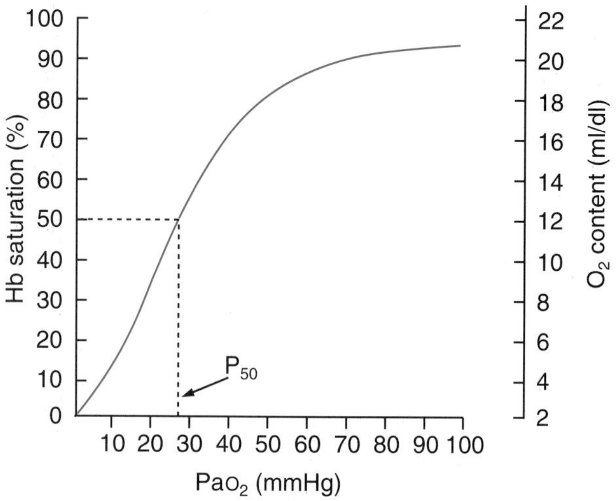

Figure 10-2. Oxyhemoglobin dissociation curve. Hemoglobin saturation is plotted against Pa_{O_2}. Corresponding O_2 content, assuming a hemoglobin of 15 g/dl, is shown along the right-hand y-axis. The Pa_{O_2} at which hemoglobin is 50% saturated—the P_{50}—is normally 26.6 mmHg.

proportional to the partial pressure of O_2 and its solubility coefficient. In general, the solubility of O_2 in blood ($\propto$) is very low; only 0.0031 ml of O_2 is dissolved per dl of blood per mmHg. Expressed differently, at a Pa_{O_2} of 100 mmHg, 100 ml of arterial blood contains only 0.31 ml of dissolved O_2. The amount of dissolved O_2 in blood is calculated as:

$$\text{Dissolved } O_2 = Pa_{O_2} \cdot 0.0031 \text{ ml } O_2/\text{dl blood/mmHg} \quad [10\text{-}3]$$

OXYGEN CONTENT

The *oxygen content* of blood (Ca_{O_2}) is the sum of hemoglobin-bound O_2 and dissolved O_2:

$$Ca_{O_2} = [\text{Hb-bound } O_2] + [\text{dissolved } O_2] \quad [10\text{-}4]$$

Equation [10-4] may be expanded to:

$$Ca_{O_2} = [(O_2 \text{ carrying capacity})(Sa_{O_2})] + [(Pa_{O_2})(0.0031)] \quad [10\text{-}5]$$

or:

$$Ca_{O_2} = [(1.34)[\text{Hb}](Sa_{O_2})] + [(Pa_{O_2})(0.0031)] \quad [10\text{-}6]$$

Obviously, Ca_{O_2} depends greatly on the fraction of O_2 bound to hemoglobin. The O_2 content of blood changes little with variations in Pa_{O_2} as long as Sa_{O_2} is well maintained. Changes in hemoglobin concentration, however, portend much larger changes in Ca_{O_2}. Normal Ca_{O_2} is 19.8 ml O_2/dl of blood, assuming a Pa_{O_2} of 100 mmHg, a hemoglobin concentration of 15 g/dl, and an Sa_{O_2} of 97%. Modest anemia (e.g., a hemoglobin of 12 g/dl), in the setting of a normal Pa_{O_2}, results in a Ca_{O_2} of only 16 ml O_2/dl.

OXYHEMOGLOBIN DISSOCIATION CURVE

As noted, hemoglobin's affinity for O_2 increases as successive molecules of O_2 bind, imparting a sigmoid or S-shape to the oxyhemoglobin dissociation curve (see Fig. 10-2). This curve relates SaO_2 to PaO_2 and is a useful construct for analyzing O_2 transport to peripheral tissues.

The upper portion of the curve ($PaO_2 > 60$ mmHg) is flat, indicating that SaO_2 and, therefore, CaO_2, remain relatively constant, despite significant fluctuations in PaO_2. Furthermore, an increase in CaO_2 or O_2 transport over this range can be accomplished only by an increase in hemoglobin concentration (e.g., from a blood transfusion) or an increase in O_2 dissolved in plasma (e.g., from an increase in PaO_2 by administration of supplemental O_2).

The steep middle and lower portions of the curve illustrate that although SaO_2 drops when PaO_2 falls below 60 mmHg, O_2 loading onto hemoglobin continues, because a concentration gradient for O_2 between alveoli and capillaries persists. Under these circumstances, peripheral tissues may continue to extract large amounts of O_2, despite decrements in capillary PO_2.

The PaO_2 at which hemoglobin is 50% saturated (at 37°C and pH of 7.4) is known as the P_{50}. The P_{50} is a conventional measure of hemoglobin affinity for O_2. The P_{50} of human blood is normally 26.6 mmHg; however, it can change under a variety of metabolic and physiologic conditions characterized by changes in O_2–hemoglobin binding.

In general, as hemoglobin's affinity for O_2 diminishes, O_2 is more readily unloaded at the tissue level, and vice-versa. An increase in the P_{50} denotes a rightward shift of the oxyhemoglobin curve (Fig. 10-3). The affinity of hemoglobin is decreased, indicating that a higher PaO_2 is necessary to maintain SaO_2 constant. The lower O_2 affinity signals enhanced O_2 release to tissues.

Conversely, a leftward shift in the curve, denoted by a decreased P_{50}, indicates increased hemoglobin affinity for O_2 and less O_2 release to peripheral tissues. Several important factors affect the P_{50} and position of the oxyhemoglobin dissociation curve.

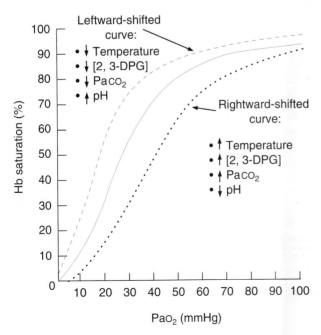

Figure 10-3. Shifts in oxyhemoglobin dissociation curve caused by changes in temperature, concentration of 2,3-DPG, $PaCO_2$, and pH. Rightward shift indicates an increase in P_{50} and diminished affinity of hemoglobin for O_2; O_2 release is enhanced. Leftward shift indicates a decrease in P_{50} and increased affinity of hemoglobin for O_2; O_2 release is diminished.

Hydrogen Ion Concentration

Changes in hemoglobin affinity for O_2 with variations in intracellular hydrogen ion concentration constitute the *Bohr effect*. Decreases in pH shift the curve to the right; increases in pH shift the curve to the left.

Consideration of changes in CO_2 and hydrogen ion levels in the lung and in peripheral tissues facilitates analysis of the effect of pH on the curve. In metabolizing peripheral tissues, the CO_2 produced diffuses into the circulation at the capillary level. As tissue P_{CO_2} rises, hydrogen ion concentration increases and tissue pH falls. Hemoglobin's affinity for O_2 decreases, promoting O_2 release. In the lung, P_{CO_2} is reduced and pH increased; the affinity of hemoglobin for O_2 increases, promoting O_2 binding to hemoglobin.

Carbon Dioxide Concentration

Carbon dioxide exerts a dual effect on the oxyhemoglobin dissociation curve. First, CO_2 concentration influences intracellular pH—the Bohr effect, as described previously. Second, CO_2 accumulation results in the generation of *carbamino compounds* through chemical interaction between CO_2 and amino groups of hemoglobin. These carbamino compounds serve as allosteric effectors of the hemoglobin molecule and directly affect O_2 binding. Low levels of carbamino compounds cause a rightward shift of the curve and decreased hemoglobin affinity for O_2; release of O_2 to tissues is enhanced. As Pa_{CO_2} increases, a concomitant increase in carbamino compounds shifts the curve to the left, enhancing O_2 binding by hemoglobin.

Concentration of Organophosphates

Organophosphates, particularly 2,3-diphosphoglycerate (2,3-DPG), are generated in erythrocytes during glycolysis. Organophosphates are present in concentrations several times greater than that of adenosine triphosphate, a major energy source in other human cells. The erythrocyte relies on 2,3-DPG because it has no mitochondria for oxidative phosphorylation. The production of 2,3-DPG increases during hypoxemia, presumably representing an important adaptive mechanism. A number of conditions resulting in diminished peripheral O_2 availability, such as anemia, acute blood loss, chronic lung disease, congestive heart failure, high altitude, and right-to-left shunts (see Chaps. 12 and 13), are characterized by increased organophosphate production within erythrocytes. This diminished affinity of hemoglobin for O_2 enhances O_2 release to tissues. Conversely, the low level of 2,3-DPG seen in certain pathologic states, such as septic shock and hypophosphatemia, causes a leftward shift in the curve.

Temperature

The effect of body temperature on the oxyhemoglobin dissociation curve is neither as dramatic, nor clinically significant, as the factors described previously. Hyperthermia causes an increase in P_{50}, that is, a shift in the curve to the right—a favorable adaptive response, given the increased cellular demand for O_2 during fever. Hypothermia causes a decrease in P_{50}, that is, a leftward shift in the curve.

Carbon Monoxide

Carbon monoxide, a gas used routinely in measuring the diffusing capacity of the lung (see Chap. 9), diffuses rapidly across the alveoli and binds directly to hemoglobin at oxygen-binding sites. CO, however, binds with a 240-fold greater affinity than O_2. CO bound to hemoglobin—*carboxyhemoglobin*—impairs peripheral tissue oxygenation through two mechanisms: (1) CO directly decreases oxygen carrying capacity by decreasing the amount of hemoglobin available for O_2 binding; and (2) CO lowers the P_{50} and shifts the oxyhemoglobin dissociation curve to the left. An important clinical correlate is that severe tissue hypoxia may occur in the setting of high levels of carboxyhemoglobin, despite measurement of a normal Pao_2.

Methemoglobinemia

Oxidation of the iron moiety of hemoglobin from the ferrous to ferric state generates *methemoglobin*. Normally, methemoglobin makes up less than 3% of the total hemoglobin in healthy humans; low levels are maintained by intracellular enzymatic reductive pathways. Methemoglobinemia may occur as a consequence of congenital deficiencies in these reductive enzymes or from production of abnormal hemoglobin molecules resistant to enzymatic reduction (e.g., hemoglobin M). Oxidant drugs (e.g., antimalarials, phenacetin, dapsone, and local anesthetics) may also cause methemoglobinemia by accelerating iron oxidation.

Methemoglobin causes a leftward shift in the oxyhemoglobin dissociation curve, inhibiting release of O_2 to peripheral tissues.

Other Abnormal Hemoglobins

Many genetic variations of the hemoglobin molecule have been described in which the molecule's affinity for O_2 is unaltered. Fetal hemoglobin (HbF), however, is a notable exception.

Hemoglobin F has two gamma (γ) chains, rather than the β chains characteristic of HbA. The oxyhemoglobin dissociation curve for HbF is shifted to the left, possibly because of the inability of 2,3-DPG to bind to the γ chains, thereby maintaining the hemoglobin's high affinity for O_2. This is of significant advantage during fetal life, when Pao_2 is low; placental uptake of O_2 is enhanced by the avidity of HbF for O_2.

OXYGEN DELIVERY AND TISSUE OXYGEN UTILIZATION

Thus far, the discussion has focused on determinants of *oxygen content*, that is, the amount of O_2 bound to hemoglobin and dissolved in plasma. For metabolizing peripheral tissues, however, the key physiologic variable is *oxygen delivery*—the amount of O_2 transported to tissues per unit time. To maintain aerobic metabolism and prevent genesis of lactic acid through anaerobic mechanisms, peripheral tissues must receive a continuous supply of O_2. Furthermore, the circumstances that determine the adequacy of the O_2 supply vary widely and include rest, exercise, hypercatabolic states, and infection.

SYSTEMIC OXYGEN DELIVERY

Oxygen delivery to peripheral tissues is determined by the quantity of O_2 in each aliquot of blood and the blood flow. Although blood flow to individual organs varies, overall blood flow to peripheral tissues is represented by cardiac output (C.O.). Hence, *systemic oxygen delivery*, Do_2, is calculated as:

$$Do_2 = \text{C.O. (L/min)} \cdot O_2 \text{ content (ml/L)} \tag{10-7}$$

O_2 content is the sum of hemoglobin-bound O_2 and O_2 dissolved in plasma. Therefore, equation [10-7] can be rewritten as:

$$Do_2 = \text{C.O.} \cdot ([(Hb) \cdot 1.34 \cdot \% \text{ saturation}] + [0.0031 \cdot Pao_2]) \tag{10-8}$$

TISSUE OXYGEN UTILIZATION AND ARTERIOVENOUS OXYGEN DIFFERENCE

Under normal basal circumstances, an adult of average size consumes approximately 250 ml of O_2 per minute; however, the individual rates of O_2 utilization by different tissues vary considerably.

The fractional distribution of the cardiac output to organ systems differs during rest and exercise and in disease states. Furthermore, *tissue oxygen extraction* varies among organ systems. For example, although heart muscle receives only a small fraction of the cardiac output, it extracts nearly all the O_2 delivered. Indeed, measurement of O_2 content of venous blood leaving heart muscle (as measured in the coronary sinus) reveals a large *arteriovenous oxygen difference*.

Without placement of a catheter directly into the veins draining an organ, the arteriovenous O_2 difference across the organ and, hence, the organ's *oxygen utilization*, cannot be calculated. In clinical practice, however, passage of a catheter through the right side of the heart permits sampling of blood in the right ventricle or pulmonary artery and measurement of *mixed venous oxygen content* or *saturation*. The technique and commonly performed measurements are described in Chapter 12. The O_2 content of mixed venous blood represents the "weighted average" of venous blood from all organs, including those with low and high levels of O_2 extraction.

FICK PRINCIPLE

From the previous discussion, it is evident that there is a tight coupling among arterial O_2 content, cardiac output, tissue O_2 utilization, and mixed venous O_2 content. Certain disorders, such as the adult respiratory distress syndrome (see Chap. 14) and sepsis, are characterized by an "uncoupling" between peripheral tissue O_2 utilization and O_2 delivery; O_2 utilization declines when O_2 delivery falls below a threshold.

The relationship among these variables is expressed by the *Fick principle,* which states that O_2 consumption (volume per minute) is the product of cardiac output and arteriovenous O_2 difference:

$$\dot{V}o_2 = \text{C.O.} \cdot (Cao_2 - C\bar{v}o_2) \tag{10-9}$$

where

$$Cao_2 = \text{arterial } O_2 \text{ content (ml } O_2/dl)$$
$$C\bar{v}o_2 = \text{mixed venous } O_2 \text{ content (ml } O_2/dl)$$

Analysis of the Fick equation reveals that an increased O_2 demand, in the setting of a fixed cardiac output, results in an increased arteriovenous O_2 difference. Conversely, a reduced metabolic demand, with a fixed cardiac output, results in a reduced arteriovenous O_2 difference. Hence, mixed venous O_2 content and, therefore, mixed venous O_2 saturation and Po_2, depend on tissue O_2 extraction and O_2 delivery.

For a healthy person of average size, who has a cardiac output of 5 L/minute and an O_2 consumption of 250 ml/minute, the arteriovenous O_2 difference is calculated using equation [10-9]:

$$250 \text{ ml/min} = 5 \text{ L/min} \cdot (Cao_2 - C\bar{v}o_2) \qquad [10\text{-}10]$$

$$(Cao_2 - C\bar{v}o_2) = 50 \text{ ml } O_2/L = 5 \text{ ml/dl} \qquad [10\text{-}11]$$

If the subject has a hemoglobin of 15 g/dl and a normal arterial O_2 saturation, Cao_2 is 20 ml/dl; solving equation [10-11] for $C\bar{v}o_2$ yields a value of 15 ml/dl. Examination of the oxyhemoglobin dissociation curve (for venous blood) reveals a corresponding mixed venous $Po_2(P\bar{v}o_2)$ of 40 mmHg.

In practice, insertion of a right-heart catheter permits measurement of mixed venous O_2 content, which, when combined with measurement of arterial O_2 content derived from arterial blood gases, allows calculation of C.O. using the Fick equation. The rate of O_2 consumption is assumed (250 ml/min); alternatively, O_2 consumption can be measured using a metabolic cart to analyze the concentration of O_2 in expired gas. Pulmonary artery catheters in clinical use actually permit calculation of C.O. using a thermodilution technique, as discussed in Chapter 12.

CARBON DIOXIDE TRANSPORT

Inspired air contains an insignificant amount of CO_2. Therefore, essentially all of the CO_2 in blood is derived from cell metabolism. This section focuses on CO_2 transport, including the multiple forms of CO_2 in blood, and the CO_2 dissociation curve.

TRANSPORT FORMS OF BLOOD CO₂

Carbon dioxide is readily diffusable. In fact, CO_2 is about 20 times as diffusable as O_2. As CO_2 is produced during cell metabolism, it diffuses into capillaries for transport to the lungs. Transport occurs in three principal forms: (1) as dissolved CO_2, (2) as bicarbonate anion, and (3) as carbamino compounds (Fig. 10-4).

Dissolved CO₂

CO_2 is very soluble in plasma, and the amount dissolved is determined by the product of the gas's partial pressure and its solubility coefficient ($\propto = 0.03$ ml/dl blood/mmHg). Approximately 5% of total CO_2 in arterial blood is in the form of dissolved gas.

Bicarbonate Anion

The predominant form of CO_2 (90%) in arterial blood is bicarbonate anion. Bicarbonate anion is created by the reaction of CO_2 with water to form H_2CO_3, which dissociates into hydrogen and bicarbonate ions:

$$CO_2 + H_2O \rightleftarrows H_2CO_3 \rightleftarrows H^+ + HCO_3^- \qquad [10\text{-}12]$$

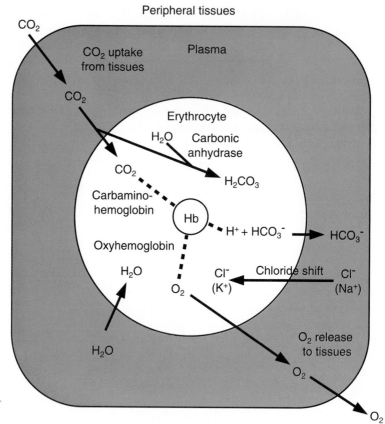

Figure 10-4. CO_2 transport in blood, illustrating formation of HCO_3^- and carbamino compounds, chloride shift, and buffering of H^+. Events depicted occur in the opposite direction in pulmonary capillaries, with uptake of O_2 and release of CO_2. See text for discussion.

Although the reaction of CO_2 and H_2O is very slow in plasma, it occurs rapidly in erythrocytes because of the presence of the intracellular enzyme, *carbonic anhydrase*. Carbonic anhydrase facilitates the reaction of CO_2 and H_2O to form H_2CO_3; the second phase of equation [10-12] is rapid and occurs without catalysis.

As HCO_3^- accumulates within erythrocytes, it diffuses across the cell membrane into plasma. The erythrocyte membrane is relatively impermeable to H^+ and, for that matter, to cations in general; consequently, the hydrogen ions remain intracellular. In preserving electrical neutrality as HCO_3^- diffuses from erythrocytes into plasma, chloride ions move from plasma into erythrocytes, constituting the so-called *chloride shift* (see Fig. 10-4).

The H^+ remaining within the erythrocytes is, in part, buffered by combining with hemoglobin. In peripheral tissues, where CO_2 concentrations are high and significant amounts of H^+ are generated in erythrocytes, H^+ binding is facilitated by the deoxygenation of hemoglobin; reduced hemoglobin is a more avid proton receptor than oxygenated hemoglobin. Hence, the deoxygenation of arterial blood in peripheral tissues promotes H^+ binding through generation of reduced hemoglobin. This enhancement of CO_2 binding to hemoglobin is known as the *Haldane effect* (Fig. 10-5).

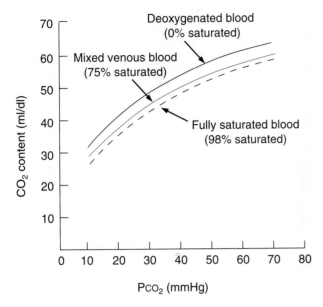

Figure 10-5. Haldane effect. CO_2 binding to hemoglobin is enhanced with deoxygenation of arterial blood. CO_2 content is higher at a given Pco_2 in deoxygenated blood.

Carbamino Compounds

The third form of CO_2 transport in blood is carbamino compounds, formed by the reaction of CO_2 with the terminal amino groups of blood proteins. The major CO_2-binding protein in blood is hemoglobin (in particular, the globin portion of the molecule). The following reaction summarizes the process:

$$Hb{-}NH_2 + CO_2 \rightleftarrows Hb{-}NH \cdot COOH \rightleftarrows Hb{-}NHCOO^- + H^+ \quad [10\text{-}13]$$

The reaction of CO_2 and amino groups occurs rapidly. As is the case for CO_2 binding more readily to reduced hemoglobin, formation of carbamino compounds occurs more easily with the deoxygenated species. Carbamino compounds constitute approximately 5% of the total CO_2 transported in arterial blood.

Finally, with regard to the relative contribution of each of these forms to the *arteriovenous difference* in CO_2 concentration, HCO_3^- constitutes approximately 60%, whereas carbamino compounds and dissolved CO_2 make up approximately 30% and 10%, respectively.

CARBON DIOXIDE–HEMOGLOBIN DISSOCIATION CURVE

The presence of all three forms of CO_2 in blood creates an equilibrium between dissolved CO_2 (Pco_2) and CO_2 chemically combined with other species (see Fig. 10-5).

Unlike the sigmoid-shaped oxyhemoglobin dissociation curve (see Fig. 10-2), the CO_2–hemoglobin dissociation curve is more linear. Of particular physiologic significance is the fact that the total CO_2 content at any given level of Pco_2 depends on the degree of hemoglobin oxygenation (i.e., the Haldane effect).

As unloading of O_2 from hemoglobin occurs in peripheral tissues, hemoglobin binds CO_2 more avidly. Hence, CO_2 content is greater at any given level of tissue P_{CO_2}. It is useful to consider this effect by comparing the CO_2 dissociation curves for fully deoxygenated blood, fully oxygenated blood, and partially oxygenated blood having a P_{O_2} equivalent to mixed venous blood (Fig. 10-6).

In oxygenated arterial blood with a P_{aCO_2} of 40 mmHg, CO_2 content is about 48 ml/dl (Fig. 10-6, point A). As O_2 is unloaded in peripheral tissues, blood leaving the capillaries is approximately 75% saturated with O_2. With a P_{CO_2} of about 46 mmHg, the CO_2 content of mixed venous blood (i.e., blood entering the right ventricle, which represents a mixture of venous blood from all tissue beds) is approximately 53 ml/dl (Fig. 10-6, point B). The increased CO_2 avidity of deoxygenated blood accounts for an additional 2 to 3 ml of CO_2/dl beyond that which could be accommodated without a change in oxyhemoglobin saturation.

Oxygen–Carbon Dioxide Diagram

Interrelationships between O_2 and CO_2 binding and transport in blood are summarized in the O_2–CO_2 diagram, a plot of O_2 and CO_2 contents versus partial pressures of O_2 and CO_2, at varying levels of the other species (Fig. 10-7).

As an example, consider the effect of changes in the level of P_{aCO_2} on O_2 content for a P_{aO_2} of 40 mmHg. With marked hypocapnia (e.g., a P_{aCO_2} of 10 mmHg), a P_{aO_2} of 40 mmHg is associated with an O_2 content of about 18 ml/dl. At a P_{aCO_2} of 40 mmHg, the same P_{O_2} is associated with an O_2 content of 15 ml/dl (Bohr effect).

Now consider the effect of changes in the level of P_{aO_2} on CO_2 content at different levels of P_{aCO_2}. With a P_{aCO_2} of 40 mmHg and a P_{aO_2} of 80 mmHg (e.g., in arterial blood), the CO_2 content is 50 ml/dl. When the P_{aO_2} is 40 mmHg and the P_{aCO_2} is 46 mmHg (e.g., in mixed venous blood), the CO_2 content is about 54 ml/dl (Haldane effect).

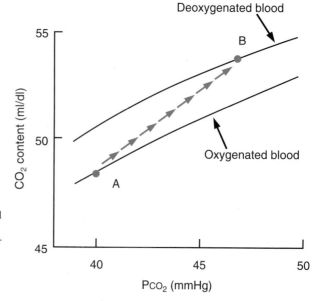

Figure 10-6. CO_2 dissociation curves for oxygenated and deoxygenated blood. As arterial blood with a P_{CO_2} of 40 mmHg (point A) is deoxygenated, its CO_2 binding is enhanced. Mixed venous blood, with a P_{CO_2} of 47 mmHg (point B), carries approximately 6 ml/dl more CO_2 than arterial blood, in part because of this effect. See text for discussion.

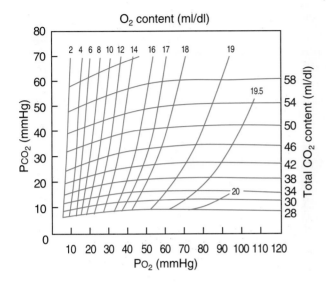

Figure 10-7. Oxygen–carbon dioxide diagram. O_2 and CO_2 contents are not directly proportional to their partial pressures in blood. See text for discussion.

THE LUNG AND ACID–BASE HOMEOSTASIS

In addition to its role in oxygenation and CO_2 elimination, the lung is pivotal in acid–base homeostasis. So-called "fixed acids" are produced by metabolizing tissues and are continually excreted by the kidneys. Normally, about 40 to 80 mEq of fixed acids are removed daily. In the setting of a wide variety of metabolic disorders, such as generation of lactic acid, ketoacidosis, ingestion of poisons (e.g., methanol or ethylene glycol), and renal disease, the kidney's ability to excrete fixed acids may not keep pace with the rate of acid production. Under these circumstances, the lungs compensate, either in the short-term or long-term, to preserve a physiologically acceptable range of pH.

As part of its role in maintaining acid–base homeostasis, the lung is also responsible for excreting approximately 13,000 mEq of carbonic acid daily—a significant acid load that arises from metabolically produced CO_2. Hence, alterations in minute ventilation and, in particular, alveolar ventilation (see Chap. 3), may have profound effects on acid–base balance in health and disease.

PHYSIOLOGIC BUFFER SYSTEMS: THE CO₂–BICARBONATE SYSTEM

The body's buffer systems play a critical role in maintaining a relatively narrow range of pH in which cellular and extracellular physiologic processes operate. The major buffer system is the CO_2–bicarbonate system, which affects extracellular and intracellular body fluids. In addition, intracellular proteins, hemoglobin, plasma proteins, and constituents of bone (e.g., carbonate and collagen) play important roles as buffers. The CO_2–bicarbonate system merits special consideration.

Bicarbonate anion is present in most body fluids and constitutes a large reservoir of buffer referred to as the body's "alkali reserve." Bicarbonate reacts with hydrogen ion to form carbonic acid, which exists in equilibrium with CO_2:

$$H^+ + HCO_3^- \rightleftarrows H_2CO_3 \rightleftarrows H_2O + CO_2 \qquad [10\text{-}14]$$

As noted previously, the conversion of H_2CO_3 to H_2O and CO_2 is catalyzed by the enzyme, carbonic anhydrase. As hydrogen ion is generated from the ingestion or metabolic production of acids (fixed acids), bicarbonate buffer converts the H^+ to H_2CO_3 and, ultimately, to CO_2 and water. The H_2CO_3 constitutes a "volatile acid," because it produces CO_2, a gas that can be eliminated via the lung. Conversely, when CO_2 is produced by cell metabolism, the carbonic acid formed dissociates into H^+ and HCO_3^-.

The pH of the system in which these reactions take place is calculated using the *Henderson-Hasselbalch equation,* which is derived from the expression for the dissociation constant (K_A) for carbonic acid:

$$K_A = \frac{[H^+] \cdot [HCO_3^-]}{[H_2CO_3]}$$ [10-15]

The logarithmic form of equation [10-15] can be written as:

$$\log K_A = \log [H^+] + \log \frac{[HCO_3^-]}{[H_2CO_3]}$$ [10-16]

Because pH is defined as the negative logarithm of the hydrogen ion concentration ($[H^+]$), equation [10-16] can be written as:

$$pH = pK_A + \log \frac{[HCO_3^-]}{[H_2CO_3]}$$ [10-17]

Furthermore, because the equilibrium between CO_2 and H_2CO_3 in plasma favors CO_2 by a factor of 1000 to 1, and because the amount of CO_2 is proportional to its solubility coefficient ($\propto = 0.03$ ml/dl/mmHg), equation [10-17] can be rewritten as:

$$pH = pK_A + \log \frac{[HCO_3^-]}{0.03 \cdot P_{CO_2}}$$ [10-18]

The value of pK_A for the CO_2–bicarbonate buffer system is 6.1. The normal arterial plasma bicarbonate concentration is 24 mEq/L (or 24 mmol/L), and the normal Pa_{CO_2} is 40 mmHg. Therefore, normal arterial pH is 6.1 + log [24]/0.03 · 40 or 7.4.

If the bicarbonate concentration falls and Pa_{CO_2} remains constant, pH falls. Conversely, if the bicarbonate concentration rises and Pa_{CO_2} remains constant, pH rises. On the other hand, if the Pa_{CO_2} changes such that the ratio of bicarbonate to ($\propto \cdot Pa_{CO_2}$) remains at 20, pH is constant at 7.4. A similar analysis holds for primary changes in Pa_{CO_2} in that a rise or fall in Pa_{CO_2}, without an accompanying change in bicarbonate concentration, results in a fall or rise in pH, respectively.

ROLE OF VENTILATION IN ACID–BASE BALANCE

It is clear from the previous considerations that the respiratory system plays a key role in both the *production* of acid–base disturbances and in the *modulation* of changes in pH produced metabolically. In this regard, the relationship between ventilation and Pa_{CO_2}, described in detail in Chapter 3, should be emphasized.

Arterial P_{CO_2} (Pa_{CO_2}) is determined by the rate of CO_2 production ($\dot{V}_{CO_2}$) and the level of minute alveolar ventilation ($\dot{V}_A$):

$$Pa_{CO_2} = K \cdot \frac{\dot{V}_{CO_2}}{\dot{V}_A} \qquad\qquad [10\text{-}19]$$

where K is a constant (see Chap. 3). Hence, changes in $\dot{V}_A$ must keep pace with changes in $\dot{V}_{CO_2}$ if Pa_{CO_2} is to be maintained constant. Conversely, if changes in $\dot{V}_A$ occur with a constant $\dot{V}_{CO_2}$, Pa_{CO_2} will vary; that is, alterations in $\dot{V}_A$ may be *primary* (see section on Primary Acid–Base Disorders, later), rather than secondary to, changes in $\dot{V}_{CO_2}$.

From a "systems" perspective, it is important to recall that alterations in $\dot{V}_A$ are effected primarily by changes in total minute ventilation, $\dot{V}_E$. As discussed in Chapter 3, the relationship between $\dot{V}_E$ and $\dot{V}_A$ is determined by the distribution of the tidal volume between dead space and alveoli—a distribution expressed as the ratio of dead space to tidal volume (V_D/V_T):

$$\dot{V}_A = \dot{V}_E \cdot (1 - V_D/V_T) \qquad\qquad [10\text{-}20]$$

From equation [10-20], it can be seen that the larger is V_D/V_T, the greater the rise in $\dot{V}_E$ necessary to effect a given change in $\dot{V}_A$ and, hence, in Pa_{CO_2}.

DAVENPORT DIAGRAM

The relationship among P_{CO_2}, bicarbonate concentration, and pH may be depicted graphically in the *Davenport diagram* (Fig. 10-8). In Figure 10-8, plasma bicarbonate concentration is plotted against pH at a variety of levels of Pa_{CO_2} (isobars). Corresponding values for pH, bicarbonate concentration, and P_{CO_2} for arterial blood are shown at point A. Point B represents the relationship when carbonic acid is added to blood (e.g., by increasing Pa_{CO_2}). Point C denotes the relationship when carbonic acid is removed from blood (e.g., by decreasing Pa_{CO_2}). The line, BAC, defines the *buffer line* for arterial blood. (The slope of the buffer line for whole blood is actually greater than that for plasma, reflecting a smaller change in pH for a given change in P_{CO_2}. The difference arises because

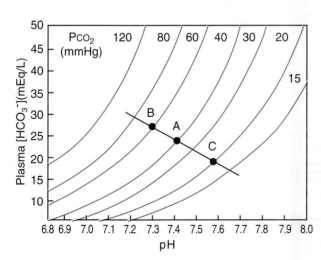

Figure 10-8. Davenport diagram, illustrating relationships among pH, P_{CO_2}, and bicarbonate concentration. Point A represents normal plasma. BAC is the buffer line created as carbonic acid is added or removed from whole blood. Changes in carbonic acid concentration are achieved through changes in P_{CO_2} (noted as P_{CO_2} isobars).

whole blood contains additional buffering systems, e.g., hemoglobin, that are absent in plasma.)

Alkalemia, or alkaline blood pH ($pH \geq 7.44$), arises when the plasma bicarbonate concentration is constant and Pa_{CO_2} is reduced (shift from point A to a P_{CO_2} isobar to the right of point A). Conversely, *acidemia,* or acidic blood pH ($pH \leq 7.36$), arises when the plasma bicarbonate concentration is constant and Pa_{CO_2} is increased (shift from point A to a P_{CO_2} isobar to the left of point A). Alkalemia or acidemia may also develop if the Pa_{CO_2} is constant and the bicarbonate concentration increases or decreases, respectively (i.e., bicarbonate concentration increases or decreases from point A along the same Pa_{CO_2} isobar).

Note that changes in pH accompanying changes in Pa_{CO_2} or bicarbonate concentration can be reduced by a concomitant alteration in the other variable. The degree of alkalemia or acidemia produced by a given increment or decrement, respectively, in bicarbonate concentration is reduced if Pa_{CO_2} rises or falls, respectively. Similarly, the degree of acidemia or alkalemia produced by a given increment or decrement, respectively, in Pa_{CO_2} is reduced if bicarbonate concentration rises or falls, respectively. These *compensatory* changes in Pa_{CO_2} and bicarbonate concentration are important homeostatic mechanisms for coping with *primary acid–base disturbances.*

PRIMARY ACID–BASE DISORDERS

There are four primary acid–base disorders: (1) respiratory acidosis, (2) respiratory alkalosis, (3) metabolic acidosis, and (4) metabolic alkalosis (Figs. 10-9 and 10-10). In addition, "mixed" acid–base disorders are not uncommonly observed in clinical practice (Fig. 10-11).

RESPIRATORY ACIDOSIS

When hypercapnia ($Pa_{CO_2} \geq 44$ mmHg) arises due to alveolar hypoventilation or significant ventilation–perfusion mismatching (see Chap. 13), *respiratory acidosis* develops. According to equation [10-18], a rise in Pa_{CO_2} that is unattended by a rise in $[HCO_3^-]$ produces a fall in pH. Examination of Figure 10-9A reveals that as Pa_{CO_2} rises, $[HCO_3^-]$ does increase a little, as a result of the dissociation of the H_2CO_3 produced into H^+ and HCO_3^-. However, the ratio of $[HCO_3^-]$ to ($\propto \cdot Pa_{CO_2}$) falls, producing the decline in pH. In Figure 10-9A, respiratory acidosis is denoted by movement from point A to point B.

A persistent increase in Pa_{CO_2} stimulates the renal tubular cells to secrete more hydrogen ion and to retain bicarbonate. As a consequence, serum bicarbonate concentration rises, tending to restore the ratio of $[HCO_3^-]$ to ($\propto \cdot Pa_{CO_2}$) toward normal. The pH is not completely restored to 7.40, however, and the process is referred to as a *compensated respiratory acidosis.* Analysis of Figure 10-9A indicates a shift to a new buffer line, which reflects the elevated $[HCO_3^-]$, less depressed pH, and increased Pa_{CO_2} (point C). The increase in $[HCO_3^-]$ from renal compensation is represented by the vertical difference between points A and C and constitutes the *base excess.*

RESPIRATORY ALKALOSIS

When hypocapnia ($Pa_{CO_2} \leq 36$ mmHg) arises due to alveolar hyperventilation, *respiratory alkalosis* develops. Although bicarbonate concentration falls

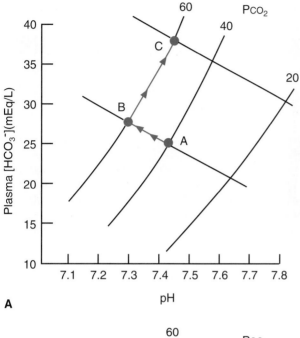

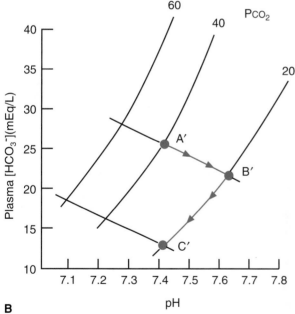

Figure 10-9. Davenport diagrams depicting primary respiratory acid–base disturbances. **(A)** Respiratory acidosis. Hypoventilation increases P_{CO_2} (point A to point B). Renal compensation increases $[HCO_3^-]$ (point C). **(B)** Respiratory alkalosis. Hyperventilation reduces P_{CO_2} (point A′ to point B′). Renal compensation decreases $[HCO_3^-]$ (point C′). See text for details.

slightly because of the equilibrium between CO_2 and H_2CO_3 (see equation [10-14]), the ratio of $[HCO_3^-]$ to $(\propto \cdot Pa_{CO_2})$ increases; therefore, pH rises (see equation [10-18]). In Figure 10-9B, a respiratory alkalosis is denoted by movement from point A′ to point B′.

With persistent hypocapnia, renal tubular cells excrete additional bicarbonate, restoring to ratio of $[HCO_3^-]$ to $(\propto \cdot Pa_{CO_2})$ toward normal. Restoration of pH may be nearly complete, and the process is referred to as a *compensated respiratory alkalosis*. The relationship among pH, Pa_{CO_2}, and bicarbonate concen-

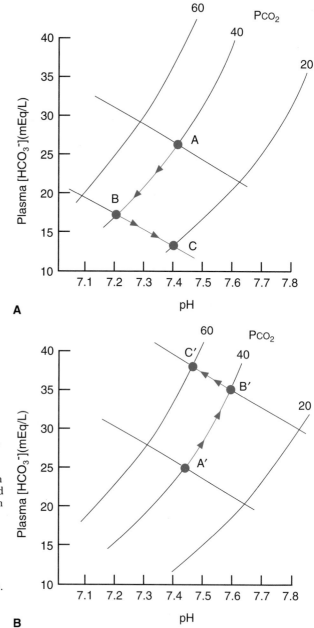

Figure 10-10. Davenport diagrams depicting primary metabolic acid–base disturbances. **(A)** Metabolic acidosis. Ingestion of excess fixed acid, or increased production or reduced excretion of fixed acid, lowers [HCO_3^-] (point A to point B). Respiratory compensation (increased $\dot{V}E$) reduces PCO_2 (point C). **(B)** Metabolic alkalosis. Excess HCO_3^- ingestion or retention raises [HCO_3^-] (point A′ to B′). Respiratory compensation (decreased $\dot{V}E$) raises PCO_2 (point C′). See text for details.

tration in a compensated respiratory alkalosis is shown at point C′ in Figure 10-9B. The vertical distance between points A′ and C′ represents the *base deficit* (or "negative base excess").

METABOLIC ACIDOSIS

When excess fixed acids are ingested (e.g., aspirin overdose) or metabolically produced (e.g., diabetic ketoacidosis, lactic acidosis, or renal failure), the ratio of [HCO_3^-] to ($\propto \cdot PaCO_2$) falls, as does the pH (see equation [10-18]). An

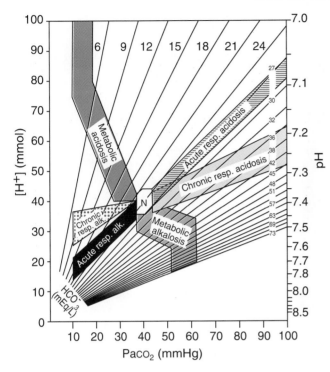

Figure 10-11. Nomogram for evaluating acid–base disturbances. Each band depicts the relationship among pH, $Paco_2$, and bicarbonate concentration in simple acid–base disturbances. Points falling between bands indicate mixed disturbances. N indicates the normal range. (From Goldberg M, Green SB, Moss ML, et al. Computer-based instruction and diagnosis of acid base disorders: A systemic approach. *JAMA* 223:269–275, 1973.)

example of the resulting *metabolic acidosis* is shown at point B in Figure 10-10A. The drop in pH stimulates peripheral chemoreceptors (see Chap. 16) which, in turn, stimulate a rise in minute ventilation. Hence, respiratory compensation for the metabolic acidosis occurs, resulting in hypocapnia. In Figure 10-10A, point C represents a *compensated metabolic acidosis*. The low $[HCO_3^-]$ reflects the base deficit (the difference in bicarbonate concentration between points A and C).

METABOLIC ALKALOSIS

A loss of acidic body fluids (e.g., through vomiting of gastric secretions), ingestion of alkali (e.g., excessive intake of antacids), or excessive renal retention of bicarbonate results in a rise in $[HCO_3^-]$ relative to ($\propto \cdot Paco_2$) (see equation [10-18]). A *metabolic alkalosis* develops, an example of which is shown at point B′ in Figure 10-10B. Respiratory compensation occurs through alveolar hypoventilation, resulting in hypercapnia. This *compensated metabolic alkalosis* is shown as point C′ in Figure 10-10B. The increased $[HCO_3^-]$ reflects the base excess (the difference in bicarbonate concentration between points A′ and C′). The magnitude of respiratory compensation in metabolic alkalosis is limited; in general, the $Paco_2$ does not rise above 55 mmHg.

MIXED ACID–BASE DISORDERS

As noted, the terms "acidemia" and "alkalemia" refer to acidic and alkaline blood pH, respectively. Although acidemia or alkalemia may arise from a single acid- or base-generating disturbance—that is, an acid*osis* or alkal*osis*, either respiratory or metabolic—in clinical practice, *mixed acid–base disorders* are not uncommon.

A detailed discussion of mixed acid–base disorders is beyond the scope of this chapter. The relationship among these respiratory and metabolic derangements, however, can be appreciated by considering the nomogram shown in Figure 10-11. The shaded areas indicate the expected values for pH, [HCO_3^-], and $Paco_2$ in "pure" disturbances; that is, the bands define the ranges of respiratory or metabolic compensation expected in each primary disturbance. Points falling between the bands constitute mixed disturbances; adjacent bands define the type of mixed disorder.

SELECTED READING

Effros RM. Acid–base balance. In: Murray JF, Nadel JA, eds. Textbook of Respiratory Medicine. Philadelphia: WB Saunders, 1988:129–148.

Goldberg M, Green SB, Moss ML, et al. Computer-based instruction and diagnosis of acid base disorders: A systemic approach. *JAMA* 223:269–275, 1973.

Murray JF. Acid–base equilibrium. In: The Normal Lung. 2nd ed. Philadelphia: WB Saunders, 1986:211–231.

Murray JF. Gas exchange and oxygen transport. In: The Normal Lung. 2nd ed. Philadelphia: WB Saunders, 1986:183–210.

Narins RG, Emmett M. Simple and mixed acid–base disorders: A practical approach. *Medicine* 58:161–187, 1980.

West JB. Gas transport to the periphery. In: Respiratory Physiology: The Essentials. 4th ed. Baltimore: Williams & Wilkins, 1990:69–85.

West JB. Ventilation, blood flow and gas exchange. In: Murray JF, Nadel JA, eds. Textbook of Respiratory Medicine. Philadelphia: WB Saunders, 1988:47–84.

Lippincott's Pathophysiology Series: Pulmonary Pathophysiology, edited by Michael A. Grippi. J. B. Lippincott Company, Philadelphia © 1995.

CHAPTER

11

Clinical Presentations: Gas Exchange and Transport

Michael A. Grippi

The following cases highlight the pathophysiology of a number of common clinical disorders characterized by abnormalities of oxygen or carbon dioxide exchange. The underlying principles are discussed in Chapters 9 and 10.

CASE 1

The patient is a 23-year-old man with a 9-month history of cough productive of one-quarter cup of purulent sputum daily, malaise, 30-pound weight loss, and progressive dyspnea on exertion. One day before admission to the hospital, he noted chills, fever, and hemoptysis consisting of two to three tablespoons of dark red clots mixed with purulent sputum. He has no history of cardiovascular or pulmonary disease. He has an 8-pack-year history of cigarette smoking.

The patient is a young man with a history of chronic purulent sputum production and systemic symptoms of weight loss, chills, and fever, in whom hemoptysis recently developed. The fever, chills, and purulent sputum suggest an acute infection, perhaps bacterial in etiology. The 9-month history, however, indicates an underlying, more indolent process. Neoplasm, a chronic inflammatory disorder, or chronic infection (e.g., tuberculosis) are among the primary considerations.

171

The patient's blood pressure is 130/76 mmHg, his pulse is 96 beats per minute, and his respiratory rate is 30 breaths per minute; his temperature is 101°F. He is in acute respiratory distress. There are fine, bibasilar, inspiratory rales throughout both lungs. No cardiac murmurs or gallops are noted. Cyanosis, clubbing, and edema of the extremities are absent.

The patient is febrile, tachypnic, and in respiratory distress. Diffuse rales suggest fluid within the lung parenchyma, due to either an inflammatory exudate or edema. Alternatively, the rales may be caused by a chronic process, such as pulmonary fibrosis.

Laboratory evaluation reveals a hemoglobin of 18.1 g/dl and a white blood cell count of 14,800/mm^3 with 71% polymorphonuclear leukocytes, 6% bands, 15% lymphocytes, and 8% monocytes. A Gram stain of sputum shows many polymorphonuclear leukocytes and gram-positive and gram-negative cocci in chains. Normal oropharyngeal flora are cultured from the sputum. Microscopic examination of three sputum specimens is negative for acid-fast bacilli. Chest radiography shows bilateral hilar lymphadenopathy and no parenchymal abnormalities.

The hemoglobin is elevated, perhaps because of dehydration and hemoconcentration. However, polycythemia secondary to chronic hypoxemia should also be considered, along with polycythemia vera. A leukocytosis is present, and the differential white blood cell count is "left shifted," suggesting acute bacterial infection. The sputum Gram stain is nonspecific, revealing mixed flora from the oropharynx, a finding suggested by the sputum culture. The fact that three sputum specimens are smear-negative for acid-fast bacilli argues against the diagnosis of tuberculosis but does not exclude it completely. Perhaps somewhat surprising is the fact that the chest radiograph shows no parenchymal infiltrates, as would be expected in acute pneumonia. The bilateral hilar lymphadenopathy is an abnormal finding, however.

The patient is treated with antibiotics for acute tracheobronchitis and improves within 72 hours. The white blood cell count decreases to 10,000/mm^3 with a normal differential count. The sputum becomes clear and thin. The bilateral hilar lymphadenopathy noted on chest radiography persists. Pulmonary function tests are performed, and the following results are obtained:

FVC	= 61% predicted
RV	= 99% predicted
FRC	= 78% predicted
TLC	= 71% predicted
D_{LCO}	= 49% predicted
FEV_1/FVC%	= 76

Arterial blood gas specimens, obtained while the patient was breathing room air at rest and during exercise, are as follows:

	Rest, Room Air	Exercise, Room Air
Pa_{O_2} (mmHg)	88	78
Pa_{CO_2} (mmHg)	44	28
pH	7.42	7.36
$[HCO_3^-]$ (mEq/L)	28	21

The patient's clinical improvement, clearing of the sputum, and decrease in white blood cell count indicate that the acute bacterial tracheobronchitis has responded to antibiotic treatment. The pulmonary function studies demonstrate a restrictive disorder, with a decreased FVC, normal FEV_1/FVC%, and reduced FRC and TLC (see Chap. 4). The reduced $D_{L_{CO}}$ represents a moderate impairment of gas transfer. Although resting oxygen saturation is normal, arterial desaturation occurs during exercise. At rest, the alveolar–arterial oxygen gradient is 9.2 mmHg (150 − 1.2[44] − 88 = 9.2). During exercise, the alveolar–arterial oxygen gradient is 38.4 mmHg (150 − 1.2[28] − 78 = 38.4).

A lung biopsy is performed (Fig. 11-1). The patient is discharged on an oral corticosteroid (prednisone). Repeat pulmonary function testing 3 months later reveals the following:

$$
\begin{aligned}
FVC &= 74\% \text{ predicted} \\
RV &= 92\% \text{ predicted} \\
FRC &= 75\% \text{ predicted} \\
TLC &= 79\% \text{ predicted} \\
D_{L_{CO}} &= 84\% \text{ predicted}
\end{aligned}
$$

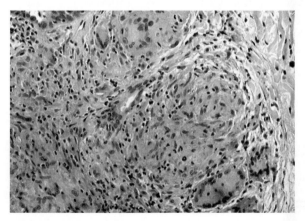

Figure 11-1. Case 1: open lung biopsy (Hematoxylin and eosin, original magnification × 200).

Repeat arterial blood gas results are as follows:

	Rest, Room Air	Exercise, Room Air
Pa_{O_2} (mmHg)	85	84
Pa_{CO_2} (mmHg)	38	41
pH	7.43	7.40
[HCO_3^-](mEq/L)	24	24

The lung biopsy shows noncaseating granulomas, consistent with the diagnosis of sarcoidosis. Sarcoidosis is a multisystem inflammatory disease that commonly affects the lungs. Granulomatous infiltration may be seen in virtually every organ, including the liver, skin, eyes, heart, central nervous system, bone marrow, and kidneys. After treatment with prednisone, the D_{LCO} and FVC are improved. Arterial O_2 desaturation with exercise no longer occurs.

Serial pulmonary function studies often provide a quantitative way to follow the response to therapy. Unfortunately, some patients do not improve with treatment, perhaps because the disease has already progressed to pulmonary fibrosis.

CASE 2

The patient is a 65-year-old man admitted to the hospital with a chief complaint of increasing shortness of breath and cough. He was in good health until approximately 8 years ago, when he began experiencing dyspnea on exertion that has progressed steadily. His appetite has decreased during the past year and he has lost approximately 20 pounds. The patient has smoked three packs of cigarettes daily for more than 20 years. He has had a chronic productive cough that is worse in the morning. During the week before admission, the patient incurred an upper respiratory tract infection. He has had constant swelling of his ankles during the past year. He sleeps on two pillows and frequently gets up during the night because lying flat aggravates his shortness of breath.

The patient has a long-standing smoking history, a cough that is productive of sputum, especially in the morning, and an 8-year history of dyspnea. The history strongly suggests chronic obstructive pulmonary disease (COPD) and, in particular, chronic bronchitis (see Chap. 6). The ankle swelling suggests right-sided heart failure (cor pulmonale) as a complication of COPD. The change in sputum color is consistent with an acute respiratory infection—a common precipitating factor for an exacerbation of COPD.

The patient's blood pressure is 160/60 mmHg; his pulse is 110 beats per minute, and his respiratory rate is 25 breaths per minute. Muscle wasting and plethora are noted. Chest examination shows an increased anteroposterior diameter, hyperresonant lungs, a prolonged expiratory

phase, diffuse wheezes, and no rales or rhonchi. The cardiac examination is notable for distant heart sounds and no murmurs or gallops. The liver is palpable 4 cm below the right costal margin. Cyanosis of the nailbeds and moderate pitting edema of the legs are present.

The hemoglobin is 19.2 g/dl and the white blood cell count is normal. The electrocardiogram shows low voltage and marked clockwise rotation, consistent with chronic lung disease.

The physical findings are consistent with COPD, showing hyperinflation (increased anteroposterior diameter, hyperresonance, distant heart sounds, and downward displacement of the liver) and airway obstruction (prolonged expiratory phase and wheezing). Plethora suggests an elevated hematocrit due to hypoxemia; nailbed cyanosis supports this consideration. Indeed, the hemoglobin is elevated at 19.2 g/dl. Muscle wasting indicates far advanced disease.

Pulmonary function tests are performed. The FVC is markedly decreased; the RV, FRC, and TLC are elevated. All expiratory airflow rates are reduced. The chest radiograph shows hyperinflation, but no infiltrates.

Diagnoses of COPD and acute tracheobronchitis are made. The following arterial blood gas results are obtained during the patient's hospitalization:

	Day 1	Day 2	Day 3	Day 4	Day 10	Day 15
F_{IO_2}	0.21	0.24	0.28	0.28	0.24	0.21
Pa_{O_2} (mmHg)	52	56	78	83	80	76
O_2 saturation (%)	80	84	94	95	95	93
Pa_{CO_2} (mmHg)	67	72	78	73	54	45
pH	7.31	7.29	7.29	7.32	7.38	7.34
$[HCO_3^-]$ (mEq/L)	33	36	38	38	30	23

The patient is treated with supplemental O_2, intravenous corticosteroids, and an inhaled β-agonist. He improves markedly.

The patient's respiratory failure is both acute and chronic. The high bicarbonate concentration represents renal compensation for chronic respiratory failure, and the low pH indicates a superimposed acute respiratory acidosis (see Chap. 10). The inspired Po_2 increased from 150 mmHg on room air (Day 1) to 171 mmHg on 24% O_2 (Day 2), whereas the arterial Po_2 increased from 52 mmHg (Day 1) to 56 mmHg (Day 2). The alveolar–arterial oxygen gradient, however, increased from 18 to 29 mmHg. Even in subjects with healthy lungs, the alveolar–arterial oxygen gradient widens slightly with administration of supplemental O_2, presumably due to worsening of ventilation–perfusion mismatching from relief of hypoxic pulmonary vasoconstriction (see Chaps. 12 and 13).

The decrease in pH on Day 2 was the result of worsening CO_2 retention. Although the precise reason that patients with flares of COPD experience hypercapnia on administration of supplemental O_2 remains unknown, several contributing mechanisms have been proposed: (1) improved oxygenation suppressing hypoxic ventilatory drive (see Chap. 16); (2) decreases in tidal volume or increases in physiologic dead space with resultant worsening in V_D/V_T and gas exchange (see Chaps. 3 and 13); and (3) increases in hemoglobin saturation, shifting bound CO_2 to the dissolved form and elevating $Paco_2$—the Haldane effect (see Chap. 10).

The arterial blood gas results during the first 3 days demonstrate worsening respiratory failure. Had the patient not improved, he would need to be intubated and mechanically ventilated to ensure adequate oxygenation without causing severe respiratory acidosis (see Chap. 18). In this setting of persistent hypoxemia, it would be inappropriate to decrease the Fio_2, which is contributing to the worsening hypercapnic respiratory failure by the mechanisms already described.

Finally, although the Pao_2 on Day 15 is higher than on Day 1, the alveolar–arterial oxygen gradient is slightly larger on Day 15 (18 mmHg on Day 1 and 20 mmHg on Day 15). Therefore, although the patient's respiratory status on Day 15 is improved with regard to oxygenation and ventilation, the magnitude of the physiologic defect in gas exchange is unchanged.

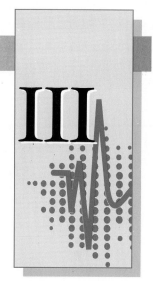

THE PULMONARY CIRCULATION AND ITS RELATIONSHIP TO VENTILATION

Lippincott's Pathophysiology Series: Pulmonary
Pathophysiology, edited by Michael A. Grippi.
J. B. Lippincott Company, Philadelphia © 1995.

CHAPTER

12

Pulmonary Circulation

Harold I. Palevsky

The pulmonary circulation is a high-capacity, low-resistance circuit "functionally" positioned between the right and left sides of the heart. Unlike the circulation to any other organ, the pulmonary circulation must accommodate the entire cardiac output, both at rest and during exertion. At rest, blood flow through the lungs is not uniform; most is through the lower, dependent regions (see Chap. 13). With exertion, blood vessel distention and "recruitment" (see section on Pulmonary Artery Pressure, later) permit the pulmonary vascular bed to accommodate a large increase in cardiac output with only a slight increment in pulmonary artery pressure (Table 12-1).

The pulmonary circulation differs from the systemic in that it is largely a "passive" vascular bed, lacking elaborate mechanisms for autoregulation of blood pressure. Although normal pulmonary blood flow is equal to systemic, the relatively small pulmonary vascular resistance allows for a low pulmonary artery pressure. At sea level, pulmonary blood flow is accomplished with an average mean pressure drop between the pulmonary artery and left atrium of only 5 to 10 mmHg (see Table 12-1). Even with significant increases in cardiac output during exercise, mean pulmonary artery pressure normally remains below 30 mmHg. In well trained athletes, who can achieve cardiac outputs greater than 20 L/minute, mean pulmonary artery pressure during peak exercise may be somewhat higher.

THE FETAL CIRCULATION AND CHANGES AT BIRTH

The normal adult and fetal pulmonary circulations are very different. Structural and functional changes in the pulmonary circulation begin with the newborn's first breath and continue during the first several weeks of life (Fig. 12-1).

TABLE 12-1. *NORMAL ADULT HEMODYNAMICS AT REST AND DURING EXERCISE*

	REST	EXERCISE
Cardiac output (L/min)	6	16*
Heart rate (beats/min)	80	130*
Pulmonary artery pressures (mmHg)		
Systolic	20–25	30–35
Diastolic	10–12	11–14
Mean	14–18	20–25
Pulmonary artery occlusion (wedge) pressure (mmHg)	6–9	10–12
Right atrial pressure (mmHg)	4–6	6–8
Systemic arterial pressure (mmHg)	120/80	150/95
Mean	90–100	110–120
Pulmonary vascular resistance (Wood units)	0.70–0.95	0.60–0.90

Representative values. Actual values vary with the subject and level of training.

In the fetus, oxygenated blood from the placenta flows through the *ductus venosus* into the inferior vena cava. On entering the right atrium, this portion of the venous return is shunted through the *foramen ovale* into the left atrium before entering the systemic circulation. Venous return from the superior vena cava passes through the right atrium and right ventricle into the main pulmonary artery, where it is diverted through the *ductus arteriosus* into the aorta. This flow pattern is maintained by intense vasoconstriction of small pulmonary arteries and high pulmonary vascular resistance.

At birth, dramatic changes in the fetal circulation accompany the first breath. Ventilation of the lungs results in a marked fall in pulmonary vascular resistance—a consequence of both the mechanical effects of alveolar expansion and relief of alveolar hypoxia (see section on Hypoxic Pulmonary Vasoconstriction, later). Within 24 hours of birth, pulmonary artery pressure falls to 50% of systemic levels. By the fourth week of life, pulmonary artery pressure approaches normal adult values, and the ductus arteriosus closes. With the decline in pulmonary vascular resistance and pulmonary artery pressure, structural remodeling of the pulmonary arteries and right ventricle occurs. Rarely, this sequence of events does not take place, resulting in the syndrome of persistent pulmonary hypertension of the newborn.

PULMONARY ARTERY PRESSURE

At sea level, the resting mean pulmonary artery pressure in a healthy adult is approximately 9 to 15 mmHg, one eighth that of the systemic circulation. Pulmonary artery systolic and diastolic pressures are 15 to 25 mmHg and 5 to 10 mmHg, respectively (see Table 12-1). With aging, pulmonary artery pressure increases, largely as a consequence of an elevation in left heart pressures, that is, an increase in "outflow" resistance (see section on Pulmonary Vascular Resistance, later).

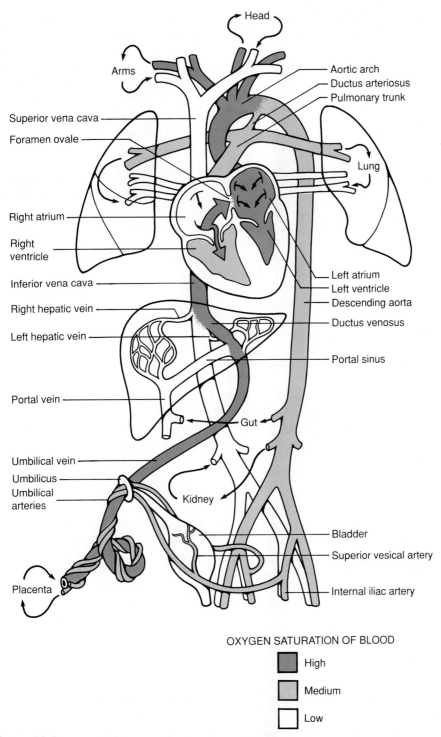

Figure 12-1. The fetal circulation. See text for details. (From Moore KL. The Developing Human: Clinically Oriented Embryology. 5th ed. Philadelphia: WB Saunders, 1993.)

A single, main pulmonary artery arising from the right ventricle divides sequentially into left and right pulmonary arteries, small muscular arteries, arterioles, and, ultimately, alveolar capillaries which interface with 70 m^2 of lung gas exchange surface. With progressive pulmonary vessel branching, the cross-sectional area at each successive level increases, and blood flow velocity decreases. The reverse is observed with confluence of the pulmonary veins leading to the left atrium.

Most pulmonary veins have thin walls, are collapsible and distensible, and are subject to the effects of both intravascular and extravascular pressures. As pulmonary blood flow increases, such as during exercise, distention of vessels and recruitment of additional vessels not normally perfused at rest result in an increase in vascular cross-sectional area. The recruited vessels include pulmonary capillaries that are not in close proximity to alveoli—so-called "extraalveolar" or "corner" vessels. The net result is blunting of the expected increase in pulmonary artery pressure. Unfortunately, increased flow through extraalveolar vessels contributes to intrapulmonary shunting and arterial hypoxemia (see Chap. 13), factors that may be clinically significant in patients with underlying pulmonary vascular disease.

PULMONARY VASCULAR RESISTANCE

Vascular resistance is a measure of a vessel's impediment to blood flow. In the normal pulmonary circulation, vascular resistance is not constant. An increase in cardiac output or in pulmonary artery pressure is accompanied by a decrease in the calculated pulmonary vascular resistance. Furthermore, the decrease is not linear; the pattern of change depends on the vasomotor tone that exists before cardiac output rises and on the levels of pulmonary artery pressure and blood flow achieved.

Analogous to calculation of electrical resistance using Ohm's law, *pulmonary vascular resistance* (PVR) is calculated as the driving pressure for blood flow across the circulation—that is, the difference between mean pulmonary artery pressure ($\overline{PAP}$) and left atrial pressure (LAP)—divided by pulmonary blood flow (cardiac output, C.O.):

$$PVR = \left(\frac{\overline{PAP} - LAP}{C.O.} \right)$$ [12-1]

As described later, left atrial pressure is approximated clinically by measurement of the *pulmonary artery occlusion pressure* (PAOP) or *pulmonary capillary wedge pressure* (PCWP).

When $\overline{PAP}$ and LAP are expressed in mmHg, and C.O. in L/minute, normal PVR is slightly less than 1.0 unit ("Wood" unit). Resistance may also be expressed in dyne · sec · cm^{-5} by multiplying the numerator of equation [12-1] by the conversion factor, 79.9. Expressed in this way, normal PVR is approximately 100 dyne · sec · cm^{-5}.

Equation [12-1] is based on an adaptation of Poiseuille's law, which applies to laminar flow of a Newtonian fluid through a rigid tube. Such conditions hardly apply to the pulmonary circulation, however, because pulmonary vessels are elastic and change in caliber with alterations in blood volume, blood flow, and pulmonary artery pressure. In addition, pulmonary blood flow is pulsatile and turbulent, not laminar. Finally, pulmonary blood volume is altered by changes in blood flow, transthoracic pressure, and body position. These factors complicate interpretation of calculated values for PVR, especially in evaluating therapy of pulmonary vascular disorders.

Because the relationship between pressure and flow in the normal pulmonary circulation is not linear, resistance is not constant; it varies with flow rate, the pressure drop across the pulmonary circulation, and other factors (Table 12-2). Hence, a change in resistance with a change in flow or pressure does not necessarily indicate that an "active" change in vascular tone (vasoconstriction or vasodilation) has occurred. Testing for active changes in pulmonary vascular resistance is always complicated by the possibility of concurrent passive changes. Among these passive changes, three warrant special mention: blood vessel recruitment or distention, lung volume, and alveolar pressure.

An increase in pulmonary arterial or pulmonary venous pressure automatically causes resistance to fall, either by opening segments of the pulmonary microcirculation previously closed (recruitment), or by distending resistance vessels already open (Fig. 12-2).

Lung volumes also passively affect pulmonary vascular resistance. Pulmonary vascular resistance is lowest at end-expiration (FRC); it increases as lung volume decreases toward residual volume or increases toward total lung capacity (Fig. 12-3).

Finally, unless left atrial pressure exceeds alveolar pressure in the portion of the pulmonary vascular bed under consideration, conventional calculation of pulmonary vascular resistance as noted in equation [12-1] is meaningless, because alveolar, rather than left atrial, pressure is the "outflow" pressure (see following section, Lung Zones).

TABLE 12-2. *FACTORS AFFECTING PULMONARY VASCULAR RESISTANCE (PVR)*

Passive Factors

Left atrial pressure (increase causes decrease in calculated PVR)

Pulmonary artery pressure (increase [when not caused by increase in left atrial pressure] causes decrease in calculated PVR)

Transpulmonary pressure (increase or decrease from value at FRC causes increase in PVR)

Pulmonary blood volume (shift of blood from systemic to pulmonary circulation causes decrease in PVR)

Blood viscosity (increase causes increase in PVR)

Active Factors

Alveolar hypoxia (increases PVR)

Acidemia (increases PVR)

Alveolar hypercarbia (increases PVR)

Humoral substances (catecholamines, F-series prostaglandins, endothelins, and angiotensin increase PVR; acetylcholine, bradykinin, E-series prostaglandins, prostacyclin, and nitric oxide decrease PVR)

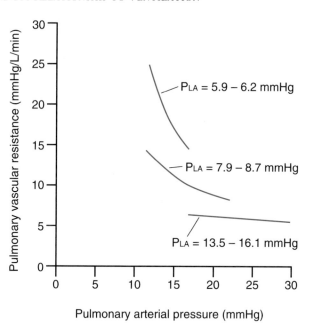

Figure 12-2. Effects of changes in pulmonary arterial pressure on pulmonary vascular resistance in three different ranges of left atrial pressure (P_{LA}). As pulmonary arterial pressure increases, pulmonary vascular resistance decreases, but the magnitude of effect progressively declines as left atrial pressure rises. At a constant pulmonary arterial pressure, a rise in left atrial pressure is accompanied by a decline in pulmonary vascular resistance. (From Murray JF. Circulation. In: *The Normal Lung.* 2nd ed. Philadelphia: WB Saunders, 1986:156.)

LUNG ZONES

Recognition of the effects of alveolar pressure on pressure and flow in the pulmonary circulation has led to the concept of four functional lung "zones." These zones are defined by the relationship among pulmonary arterial, pulmonary venous, and alveolar pressures (Fig. 12-4).

ZONE 1

Zone 1 of the upright lung is defined as the region where alveolar pressure (Palv) exceeds pulmonary arterial pressure (Ppa), which, in turn, exceeds pul-

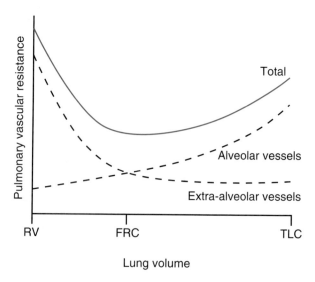

Figure 12-3. Lung volume and pulmonary vascular resistance. With inflation from residual volume (RV) to total lung capacity (TLC), resistance to flow through alveolar vessels increases, whereas resistance in extraalveolar vessels decreases. The net result is a U-shaped curve with the nadir at functional residual capacity (FRC). (From Murray JF. Circulation. In: *The Normal Lung.* 2nd ed. Philadelphia: WB Saunders, 1986:157.)

Pressure relationships

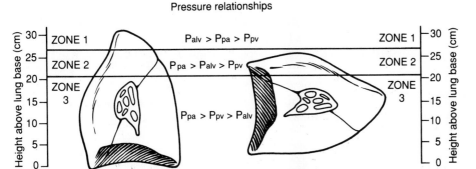

Figure 12-4. Functional lung zones in supine and upright positions. The relationship among pulmonary arterial pressure (Ppa), alveolar pressure (Palv), and pulmonary venous pressure (Ppv) determines the location of the zones. In the supine position, zone 1 is absent. See text for details. (From Fishman AP. The normal pulmonary circulation. In: *Pulmonary Diseases and Disorders*. 2nd ed. New York: McGraw-Hill, 1988:992.)

monary venous pressure (Ppv); that is, Palv > Ppa > Ppv. The pulmonary microvasculature is compressed to closure by the surrounding alveolar pressure, and blood flow in zone 1 is minimal. In fact, the apex of the upright lung would receive no flow were it not for the fact that pulmonary artery blood flow is pulsatile. During systole, the transient elevation in pulmonary artery pressure results in apical blood flow, despite a mean pressure that is too low to sustain the flow.

ZONE 2

In *zone 2*, pulmonary arterial pressure exceeds alveolar pressure, which, in turn, exceeds pulmonary venous pressure (Ppa > Palv > Ppv). As a consequence, blood flow is not determined by the usual gradient between mean pulmonary artery and left atrial pressures. Instead, the outflow pressure is alveolar pressure, and the driving gradient for flow is the pulmonary arterial–alveolar pressure difference.

Under the influence of gravity, pulmonary artery pressure increases about 1 cm H_2O per centimeter of vertical distance from the lung apex. On the other hand, alveolar pressure is homogeneous throughout the zone. Therefore, the driving pressure and, hence, blood flow, increase from apex to base (see Chap. 13). Changing relationships between alveolar and vascular pressures alternately shift the outflow pressure between alveolar and pulmonary venous, creating a so-called *Starling resistor*. Consequently, flow through zone 2 capillaries is pictured as intermittent, through channels that are open when pulmonary venous pressure exceeds alveolar pressure, and that are closed when alveolar pressure exceeds pulmonary venous pressure.

ZONE 3

In *zone 3*, pulmonary arterial pressure is greater than pulmonary venous pressure, which, in turn, is greater than alveolar pressure (Ppa > Ppv > Palv). As a result, blood flow is determined by the pulmonary arterial–pulmonary venous pressure difference (because both exceed alveolar pressure), and conventional calculations of pulmonary vascular resistance are valid. Resistance to blood flow in zone 3 is less than in zone 2, because the driving pressure for flow remains constant throughout both lung zones, while gravity causes arterial and venous pressures to increase equally per centimeter of vertical distance from the lung apex. Consequently, flow is higher at the lung base, where resistance is reduced. In contrast to zone 2, where the increase in blood flow from top to bottom of the zone is predominantly the result of recruitment of vessels previously closed, an increase in blood flow in zone 3 is effected largely by distention of already patent capillaries.

ZONE 4

In the most dependent portion of the erect lung are regions of decreased pulmonary blood flow that constitute *zone 4*. The paradox of high vascular pressures (due to gravitational effects, as described) and low blood flow cannot be explained in terms of a three-zone model, which considers only the effects of pulmonary arterial, pulmonary venous, and alveolar pressures. In zone 4, resistance to blood flow is believed to reside in the extraalveolar, rather than alveolar, vessels. Zone 4 disappears with deep inspiration, presumably because distortion of these vessels, which contributes to the increased resistance, is relieved as the lung is inflated (see Fig. 12-3).

The zones described are functional constructs, not discrete anatomic areas. The interfaces between zones are not fixed topographically, but vary in the vertical dimension according to shifts in the relationship among pulmonary arterial, pulmonary venous, and alveolar pressures. For example, institution of mechanical ventilation (positive pressure breathing, which increases alveolar pressure) or diuresis (which decreases vascular pressures) enlarges zone 2 while it diminishes zone 3, and enlarges zone 1 while it diminishes zone 2. Awareness of the functional nature of these relationships affects the interpretation of changes in calculated PVR. For vessels in zone 2, where alveolar, rather than pulmonary venous, pressure is the outflow pressure, the conventional calculation of pulmonary vascular resistance is meaningless. Only for hemodynamic measurements made in zone 3, where pulmonary venous, rather than alveolar, pressure determines blood flow, is the calculation of PVR useful.

HYPOXIC PULMONARY VASOCONSTRICTION

Although many factors induce pulmonary vasoconstriction, hypoxia is the most potent. *Hypoxic pulmonary vasoconstriction* (HPV), a response to alveolar hypoxia, results in marked narrowing of adjacent, precapillary muscular pulmonary arteries and arterioles. When alveolar hypoxia is localized, such as in pneumonia or regional atelectasis, pulmonary vasoconstriction is also localized, diverting blood flow away from the hypoxic region. The degree of ventilation–perfusion mismatching is thereby minimized (see Chap. 13). When alveolar hypoxia is diffuse, however, the resulting pulmonary vasoconstriction affects the entire lung. In the fetus, diffuse HPV is desirable, since it increases PVR and increases the proportion of placental blood flow shunted through the foramen ovale. In adults, the increased PVR seen at high altitude is a consequence of HPV, as is a component of the increased pulmonary vascular resistance seen in chronic obstructive pulmonary disease.

PATHOGENESIS OF PULMONARY HYPERTENSION

Although changes in pressure in the left side of the heart (left heart "filling" pressure), cardiac output, heart rate, hematocrit, and blood volume may contribute to development of pulmonary hypertension, the most important pathophysiologic factor is an elevation in pulmonary vascular resistance, localized primarily to the precapillary arteries and arterioles. The increase may be on an anatomic basis (from narrowing or occlusion of the microcirculation) or caused by vasoconstriction; often both mechanisms may be operative.

Regardless of etiology, when vascular reserve is compromised by a progressive reduction in the extent or distensibility of the pulmonary vascular bed, increases in cardiac output result in pulmonary hypertension. Over time, smaller increments in cardiac output result in an elevation of pulmonary artery pressure. A number of physiologic parameters affect pulmonary artery pressure.

OXYGEN AND CARBON DIOXIDE TENSIONS

As noted, the most potent stimulus for pulmonary vasoconstriction is alveolar hypoxia, which acts on adjacent small pulmonary arteries and arterioles. The mediators involved in HPV have not yet been identified. Systemic arterial hypoxemia augments the local effects of alveolar hypoxia indirectly through sympathetic neural reflexes. In chronic hypoxemia, the effects of pulmonary vasoconstrictor stimuli are often augmented by increased blood viscosity due to secondary polycythemia. Episodic exacerbations of hypoxemia result in progressive pulmonary vascular remodeling and may progress to sustained pulmonary hypertension, even though early episodes are completely reversible.

Unlike hypoxia, hypercapnia appears to contribute to pulmonary hypertension by producing acidemia, rather than by direct vasoconstriction. Carbon dioxide retention may be self-perpetuating; hypercapnia blunts the responsiveness of respiratory centers to CO_2 (see Chap. 16) and promotes retention of bicarbonate by the kidney (see Chap. 10). The hypercapnia due to disorders of the lungs or ventilatory pump, and that arising as compensation for metabolic alkalosis, each result in ventilatory depression, worsening of the hypercapnia, hypoxia, and pulmonary vasoconstriction.

ACID–BASE STATUS

Significant acidemia (blood pH < 7.2) causes pulmonary vasoconstriction. In humans, acidemia acts synergistically with hypoxia. Significant alkalemia (blood pH > 7.5) diminishes the vasoconstrictive response to hypoxia. The biologic basis for these responses and the mediators involved are unknown.

MEDIATORS REGULATING PULMONARY VASCULAR TONE

The pulmonary endothelium comes in contact with the entire cardiac output and is in a unique position to regulate levels and activity of vasoactive substances. Circulating compounds can be processed, activated, or cleared from the blood. The endothelium also serves an endocrine function, releasing growth factors and potent mediators of vasodilation or vasoconstriction.

Among the endothelium-related compounds thus far described, *prostacyclin* (*prostaglandin I_2*), the predominant metabolite of arachidonic acid, appears to play an important role in the local modulation of vascular tone, serving as a potent vasodilator.

Endothelium-derived relaxing factor (EDRF) is a product of the intact vascular endothelium that vasodilates through effects on adjacent vascular smooth muscle. EDRF appears to be the free radical, nitric oxide (NO ·), which stimulates guanylate cyclase in vascular smooth muscle, thereby increasing cyclic guanosine monophosphate levels.

Endothelins, a family of peptides, are circulating hormones that stimulate smooth muscle contraction. These compounds are produced by pulmonary vascular endothelial cells and bronchiolar respiratory epithelial cells. In experimental preparations, endothelins cause both significant pulmonary vasoconstriction and airway smooth muscle contraction. Endothelins may be the mediators of HPV.

VASCULAR HISTOLOGIC CHANGES

Pulmonary vascular histologic changes that are primary or develop as a consequence of increased flow, pressure, or shear stress contribute to pulmonary vascular disease. Changes may be observed in the media, intima, or blood vessel lumen. Although microvascular changes may be reversible initially if the inciting mechanism is eliminated, they can become fixed over time.

In addition to proliferative histologic changes, in situ thrombosis increases vascular resistance. In situ thrombosis appears to be a consequence of: (1) alterations in endothelial function, which either reduce local fibrinolytic activity or the release of inhibitors of platelet activation (e.g., prostacyclin); and (2) endothelial injury, which predisposes to platelet activation and deposition and initiation of thrombosis.

CAUSES OF PULMONARY HYPERTENSION

Pulmonary hypertension due to an identifiable disease is far more common than primary or "idiopathic" pulmonary hypertension (Table 12-3). The mechanisms by which these underlying conditions result in pulmonary hypertension are variable. Right heart catheterization is often necessary to establish the diagnosis and to determine the etiology. Although a number of clinical disorders associated with pulmonary hypertension are described elsewhere in this book, one deserves special mention here—pulmonary embolism.

PULMONARY EMBOLISM

Pulmonary hypertension may arise from acute emboli or chronic occlusion of pulmonary vessels by unresolved, "organized" clots.

After an acute pulmonary embolism, the patient's physiologic (and clinical) status depends primarily on three factors: (1) preexisting cardiac and pulmonary function; (2) size of the embolism and extent of vascular obstruction; and (3) pathophysiologic effects of released humoral mediators.

Only relatively recently has the important role of humoral mediators in determining the physiologic consequences of pulmonary emboli been appreciated. This role is based on the observation that changes in hemodynamics and

TABLE 12-3. *PULMONARY HYPERTENSION: PATHOPHYSIOLOGIC CATEGORIES AND DISORDERS*

Hyperkinetic

Intracardiac shunts (e.g., atrial septal defect, ventricular septal defect)

Pulmonary arteriovenous fistulas

Passive

Elevated left ventricular end-diastolic pressure (e.g., coronary artery disease, cardiomyopathy, aortic valve disease, constrictive pericarditis)

Mitral valve stenosis or obstruction

Left atrial obstruction (e.g., neoplasm, thrombus)

Pulmonary venous obstruction (e.g., lymphadenopathy, neoplasm, fibrosing mediastinitis)

Obliterative

Pulmonary parenchymal disease (e.g., obstructive and restrictive lung diseases)

Pulmonary arteritis (e.g., collagen vascular diseases, schistosomiasis)

Obstructive

Pulmonary embolism, acute and chronic (e.g., venous thromboemboli, tumor emboli)

Pulmonary arterial thrombosis (e.g., sickle cell disease)

Vasoconstrictive

Hypoxemia (e.g., sleep apnea syndrome, neuromuscular disorders)

High altitude

Idiopathic

Primary pulmonary hypertension, including pulmonary veno-occlusive disease

Dietary pulmonary hypertension (e.g., Aminorex ingestion, toxic oil syndrome)

Coexistent portal and pulmonary hypertension

Human immunodeficiency virus-associated pulmonary hypertension

Persistent fetal circulation

---

gas exchange often exceed what is expected from the extent of vascular occlusion. In contrast to the usually well tolerated consequences of clamping a pulmonary artery during surgical removal of a lobe or whole lung, a pulmonary embolism obstructing a lobar or main pulmonary artery can be life threatening.

Other observations support an important role for humoral mediators in determining the consequences of pulmonary emboli. For example, in experimental models, serotonin antagonists block many of the acute hemodynamic and airway responses. In addition, bronchoconstriction, either localized or diffuse, sometimes occurs after acute pulmonary embolism, suggesting that mediator release from the pulmonary vasculature may be responsible.

Pulmonary embolism is associated with release of other potentially important mediators as well. Among these are both pulmonary vasoconstrictors and vasodilators. Arachidonic acid metabolites, peptidoleukotrienes, platelet-activating factor, and platelet-derived growth factor, released from formed blood elements, promote vasoconstriction. In contrast, prostacyclin and EDRF, released from pulmonary vascular endothelium, promote pulmonary vasodilation.

Finally, neurohumoral reflexes triggered by receptors in the pulmonary vasculature, particularly at points of vessel bifurcation, may also participate in the pulmonary vascular response to thromboembolism.

PULMONARY ARTERY CATHETERIZATION

Measurement of the pulmonary hemodynamics described previously has become standard practice in the management of critically ill patients, including those suspected of having pulmonary vascular disease. A brief description of the catheter, primary measurements, and derived calculations follows.

THE PULMONARY ARTERY CATHETER AND ITS INSERTION

The catheter used clinically for measuring pulmonary hemodynamics is known as the *balloon flotation catheter* or *Swan-Ganz catheter* (Fig. 12-5). The standard catheter has three inner lumens and is 110 cm in length. One lumen opens at the catheter tip, another opens at a point 30 cm proximal to the tip, and the third communicates with a balloon near the tip. The balloon engulfs the tip when inflated, allowing the catheter to "float" in the blood stream as it is passed through the heart and pulmonary vessels.

When the catheter, with balloon inflated, is placed in a branch of the pul-

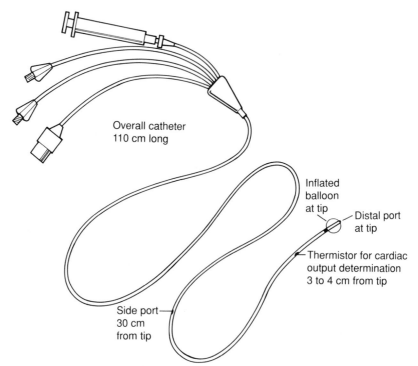

Overall catheter
110 cm long

Inflated
balloon
at tip

Distal port
at tip

Thermistor for cardiac
output determination
3 to 4 cm from tip

Side port—
30 cm
from tip

Figure 12-5. Pulmonary artery flotation (Swan-Ganz) catheter. See text for description.

monary artery, the vessel is occluded, enabling measurement of the PAOP or PCWP, as described below. In addition, a thermistor lead located 3 to 4 cm from the tip permits measurement of cardiac output, also detailed later.

The pulmonary artery catheter is introduced percutaneously through the internal jugular, external jugular, subclavian, femoral, or antecubital veins; during insertion, the electrocardiogram is monitored continuously and vascular pressure is measured at the tip.

ROUTINE HEMODYNAMIC MEASUREMENTS

Table 12-4 summarizes measurements commonly made using the balloon flotation catheter. Of particular note is the fact that such a catheter placed through the *right* side of the heart can provide information about *left* heart hemodynamics.

Occlusion of a pulmonary artery segment with balloon inflation interrupts flow distally; consequently, the pressure recorded at the catheter tip (PAOP) reflects the pressure in patent pulmonary veins carrying blood to the left atrium. In healthy subjects, PAOP approximates pulmonary venous pressure. Furthermore, because the normal pressure drop between pulmonary veins and left atrium is small, the measurement also approximates left atrial and left ventricular end-diastolic pressures (see equation [12-1]).

Even in a normal lung, PAOP provides a meaningful measure of left atrial pressure only under zone 3 conditions—that is, when the column of blood between the catheter tip and the left heart is uninterrupted (see section on Lung Zones, earlier). As a rule, the balloon flotation catheter floats into an area that satisfies the hemodynamic criteria for zone 3.

When these measurements are combined with hemodynamic and blood gas determinations obtained using an indwelling arterial catheter, basic physiologic parameters of cardiovascular function can be calculated (Table 12-5).

TABLE 12-4. *MEASUREMENTS OBTAINED USING A PULMONARY ARTERY CATHETER*

Pressures
  Right atrial
  Right ventricular
  Pulmonary artery (systolic, diastolic, mean)
  Pulmonary artery occlusion (wedge)
Flow
  Cardiac output
Blood Samples
  Mixed venous blood
  Pulmonary capillary blood
Oxygen Saturation
  Right atrial
  Right ventricular
  Pulmonary artery

TABLE 12-5. *CLINICALLY USEFUL CALCULATIONS BASED ON MEASUREMENTS MADE USING A PULMONARY ARTERY CATHETER*

Cardiac Index (L/min/m²)

$$CI = \frac{\dot{Q}_T}{BSA}$$

where $\dot{Q}_T$ is cardiac output in L/min and BSA is body surface area in m².

Pulmonary Vascular Resistance (dynes · sec · cm⁻⁵)

$$PVR = \frac{\overline{Ppa} - \overline{Pw}}{\dot{Q}_T} \cdot 79.9$$

where $\overline{Ppa}$ is mean pulmonary arterial pressure in mmHg, $\overline{Pw}$ is mean pulmonary wedge pressure in mmHg, $\dot{Q}_T$ is cardiac output in L/min, and 79.9 is a conversion factor for adjusting to the unit, dynes · sec · cm⁻⁵.

Systemic Vascular Resistance (dynes · sec · cm⁻⁵)

$$SVR = \frac{\overline{Pa} - \overline{Pra}}{\dot{Q}_T} \cdot 79.9$$

where $\overline{Pa}$ is mean systemic arterial pressure in mmHg, $\overline{Pra}$ is mean right atrial pressure in mmHg, $\dot{Q}_T$ is cardiac output in L/min, and 79.9 is a conversion factor for adjusting to the unit, dynes · sec · cm⁻⁵.

Stroke Volume Index (ml/beat/m²)

$$SVI = \frac{\dot{Q}_T/HR}{BSA}$$

where $\dot{Q}_T$ is cardiac output in ml/min, HR is heart rate in beats per minute, and BSA is body surface area in m².

Right Ventricular Stroke Work Index (g · m/m²)

$$RVSWI = SVI \cdot (\overline{Ppa} - \overline{Pw}) \cdot 0.0136$$

where SVI is stroke volume index in ml/beats/m², $\overline{Ppa}$ is mean pulmonary arterial pressure in mmHg, $\overline{Pw}$ is mean pulmonary wedge pressure in mmHg, and 0.0136 is a conversion factor for adjusting to the unit, g · m/m².

Left Ventricular Stroke Work Index (g · m/m²)

$$LVSWI = SVI \cdot (\overline{Pa} - \overline{Pra}) \cdot 0.0136$$

where SVI is stroke volume index in ml/beat/m², $\overline{Pa}$ is mean systemic arterial pressure in mmHg, $\overline{Pra}$ is mean right atrial pressure in mmHg, and 0.0136 is a conversion factor for adjusting to the unit, g · m/m².

Arteriovenous Difference in O₂ Content (Vols %)

$$(a-v)\,DO_2 = CaO_2 - C\bar{v}O_2$$

where O_2 content = $([Hb] \cdot 1.34 \cdot \%\ saturation) + (0.0031 \cdot PaO_2)$ for both arterial (CaO_2) and mixed venous ($C\bar{v}O_2$) specimens.

TABLE 12-5 *(Continued)*

Shunt Fraction (%)

$$\frac{\dot{Q}s}{\dot{Q}_T} = \frac{Cc_{O_2} - Ca_{O_2}}{Cc_{O_2} - C\bar{v}_{O_2}}$$

where Cc_{O_2} is pulmonary capillary O_2 content, Ca_{O_2} is systemic arterial O_2 content, and $C\bar{v}_{O_2}$ is mixed venous O_2 content.

Fick Equation for Cardiac Output (L/min)*

$$\text{Systemic Blood Flow} = \frac{\dot{V}_{O_2}}{Ca_{O_2} - C\bar{v}_{O_2}}$$

where $\dot{V}_{O_2}$ is oxygen consumption in ml/min, Ca_{O_2} is systemic arterial O_2 content in ml/L, and $C\bar{v}_{O_2}$ is mixed venous O_2 content in ml/L.

$$\text{Pulmonary Blood Flow} = \frac{\dot{V}_{O_2}}{Cpv_{O_2} - Cpa_{O_2}}$$

where $\dot{V}_{O_2}$ is oxygen consumption in ml/min, Cpv_{O_2} is pulmonary venous O_2 content in ml/L, and Cpa_{O_2} is pulmonary arterial O_2 content in ml/L.

*If measured O_2 consumption is used in the calculation, this is a Fick determination of cardiac output. If O_2 consumption is estimated, then the calculation provides an "estimated" determination of cardiac output using the Fick principle. The difference between pulmonary blood flow and systemic blood flow can be used to detect the presence of a left-to-right intracardiac shunt.

CARDIAC OUTPUT MEASUREMENTS USING THE THERMODILUTION METHOD

Cardiac output can be determined using the balloon flotation catheter by application of the indicator–dilution technique; less often, cardiac output is determined using the *Fick principle*, described in Chapter 10 (also see Table 12-5).

The most common application of the indicator–dilution technique is the *thermodilution method*. An aliquot of saline, at known temperature, is injected through the lumen leading to the proximal port. Downstream, at the catheter tip, a thermistor measures the temperature of the flowing fluid. The magnitude of the change in temperature of the injected fluid allows calculation of flow (cardiac output) using a table-top computer. The thermodilution method may be inaccurate when the cardiac output is low or when tricuspid regurgitation, pulmonic regurgitation, or shunts (see Chap. 13) are present.

EFFECT OF CHANGES IN INTRATHORACIC PRESSURE ON HEMODYNAMIC MEASUREMENTS

Changes in intrathoracic pressure may distort pulmonary hemodynamic measurements—measurements that are made relative to atmospheric pressure, rather than intrathoracic. In all patients, including those on mechanical ventilation, pleural pressures most closely approximate atmospheric pressure at end-expiration. Therefore, vascular pressure measurements should be made at end-expiration. *Trends* in measured hemodynamic parameters are more useful than is any single determination in following a patient's course and in evaluating the effects of therapeutic interventions.

SELECTED READING

Fishman AP. The normal pulmonary circulation. In: Fishman AP, ed. Pulmonary Diseases and Disorders, 2nd ed. New York: McGraw-Hill, 1988:975–994.

Fishman AP, ed. The Pulmonary Circulation: Normal and Abnormal. Philadelphia: The University of Pennsylvania Press, 1990.

Harris P, Heath D. The Human Pulmonary Circulation: Its Form and Function in Health and Disease. New York: Churchill-Livingstone, 1986.

Palevsky HI. Exercise and the pulmonary circulation. In: Leff A, ed. Cardiopulmonary Exercise Testing. Orlando, FL: Grune & Stratton, 1986:89–106.

Palevsky HI. Pulmonary hypertension and right heart failure. In: Carlson RW, Geheb MA, eds. The Principles and Practice of Medical Intensive Care. Philadelphia: WB Saunders, 1993:838–849.

Weir EK, Reeves JT, eds. Pulmonary Vascular Physiology and Pathophysiology. New York: Marcel Dekker, 1989.

Lippincott's Pathophysiology Series: Pulmonary Pathophysiology, edited by Michael A. Grippi. J. B. Lippincott Company, Philadelphia © 1995.

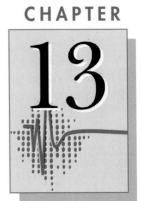
Ventilation–Perfusion Relationships

Paul N. Lanken

In Chapter 9, the concept that gas exchange is critically dependent on events occurring at the alveolar–capillary membrane is emphasized. In this chapter, the importance of the physiologic *coupling* between ventilation and perfusion in individual alveoli, and throughout the lung as a whole, is highlighted.

First, the role of ventilation–perfusion relationships in determining alveolar P_{CO_2} and P_{O_2} is described. Next, ventilation and perfusion *gradients* through the lung are detailed, and changes in the relationship between the two are outlined. The effects of these gradients on gas exchange are summarized before a final, brief description of ventilation–perfusion relationships in disease states is given.

THE CONCEPT OF VENTILATION–PERFUSION MATCHING

In most patients with obstructive lung diseases, such as asthma (see Chap. 5) or chronic obstructive pulmonary disease (see Chap. 6), as well as those with various interstitial lung diseases (see Chap. 7), a disturbance in the coupling between ventilation and perfusion results in serious alterations in gas exchange that, if progressive, lead to respiratory failure (see Chap. 18). The quantitative relationship between ventilation and perfusion is expressed as the *ventilation–perfusion ratio* ($\dot{V}/\dot{Q}$).

The magnitude of pathophysiologic effects on arterial oxygenation due to abnormal ventilation–perfusion ratios far exceeds those secondary to other basic mechanisms of hypoxemia, including hypoventilation (see Chaps. 17 and 18), diffusion block (see Chap. 9), and shunt (see Chaps. 3 and 12). In healthy subjects, less than perfect matching between ventilation and perfusion is also the major reason for the small difference between alveolar and arterial oxygen tensions, the *alveolar–arterial oxygen difference* or *alveolar–arterial oxygen gradient*, (A − a) Po_2, discussed in Chapter 3 (Fig. 13-1).

In Chapters 3 and 9, the lung is considered a single gas exchanging unit that has a *single* mean alveolar Po_2, determined by the alveolar gas equation. This value for Po_2 is regarded as an *ideal* mean value that, although valid for this model, must be contrasted with the real lung in which there is a *distribution* of values for alveolar Po_2 among 300 million alveoli. The Po_2 in any one of these alveoli is determined by the relationship between ventilation and perfusion in the alveolus—the $\dot{V}/\dot{Q}$. We can now consider a more complex, but more realistic, model of the lung: a network of gas-exchanging units organized in parallel, with a distribution of $\dot{V}/\dot{Q}$'s and corresponding values for alveolar Po_2. Understanding this model is essential in appreciating the effects of $\dot{V}/\dot{Q}$ on gas exchange and ventilation in health and disease.

DETERMINATION OF ALVEOLAR Po_2 AND Pco_2

Once the barometric pressure and Fio_2 are specified (see Chap. 9), the critical element in determining gas tensions in an individual alveolus is the $\dot{V}/\dot{Q}$ of the alveolus (Fig. 13-2). For example, with an Fio_2 of 0.21 at sea level, an alveolus with one unit of ventilation and one unit of perfusion, that is, a $\dot{V}/\dot{Q}$ of 1.0, has a Pao_2 of 100 mmHg and a $Paco_2$ of 40 mmHg (see Fig. 13-2A).

In one extreme of ventilation–perfusion mismatch, an alveolus is perfused,

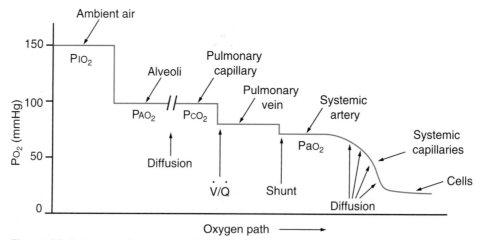

Figure 13-1. Physiologic decrements in Po_2 from atmosphere to cell. The drop in Po_2 from inspired air to alveolus is caused by the "dilutional" effect of alveolar Pco_2, as described by the alveolar gas equation. Subsequent decrements are caused by the mechanisms indicated in the figure (diffusion impairment, ventilation–perfusion inequalities, and right-to-left shunts across the lungs and heart). Pio_2, oxygen tension in inspired gas; Pao_2, alveolar Po_2; Pco_2, pulmonary capillary Po_2; Pao_2, arterial Po_2. Normally, there is no decrement in Po_2 from alveolus to pulmonary capillaries. The alveolar–capillary membrane is denoted by the parallel vertical lines. (Modified from West JB. Ventilation–perfusion relationships. In: Respiratory Physiology: The Essentials. 4th ed. Baltimore: Williams & Wilkins, 1990:52.)

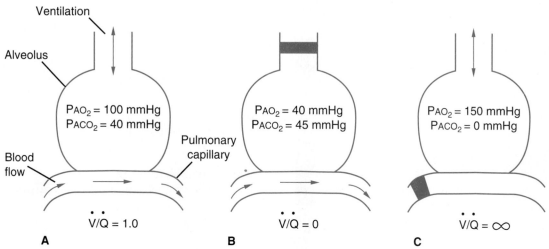

Figure 13-2. Three-compartment model for analysis of effects of differing $\dot{V}/\dot{Q}$ on P_{AO_2} and P_{ACO_2}. Assumptions include an inspired P_{O_2} of 150 mmHg, a mixed venous P_{O_2} of 40 mmHg, and a P_{ACO_2} of 45 mmHg (and, therefore, a P_{aCO_2} of 45 mmHg). **(A)** $\dot{V}/\dot{Q}$ = 1.0. The unit's ventilation and perfusion are perfectly matched. P_{AO_2} is 100 mmHg and P_{ACO_2} is 40 mmHg, as predicted by the alveolar gas equation. **(B)** $\dot{V}/\dot{Q}$ = 0. The unit is perfused but not ventilated. Alveolar gas tensions equal those of mixed venous blood. **(C)** $\dot{V}/\dot{Q}$ = ∞. The unit is ventilated but not perfused. Alveolar gas tensions equal those of inspired gas.

but not ventilated; that is, $\dot{V}/\dot{Q}$ = 0 (see Fig. 13-2B). The alveolar gas tensions equal those in alveolar capillary blood, which, under these circumstances, is equivalent to mixed venous blood (see Chaps. 9 and 12).

In another extreme of ventilation–perfusion mismatch, an alveolus is ventilated, but not perfused; that is, $\dot{V}/\dot{Q}$ = ∞ (see Fig. 13-2C). The alveolar gas tensions equal those in inspired gas.

An assumption underlying these considerations of the effects of $\dot{V}/\dot{Q}$ on P_{O_2} and P_{CO_2} is that full equilibration has occurred between alveolar and end-capillary gas tensions; in other words, there is no diffusion limitation across the alveolar–capillary membrane. Although this assumption is valid under the circumstances described in this chapter, there are clinically important disorders in which the deleterious effects of $\dot{V}/\dot{Q}$ mismatch in causing hypoxemia are made worse by a concomitant limitation in diffusion (see Chap. 9).

RELATIONSHIP BETWEEN $\dot{V}/\dot{Q}$ AND P_{ACO_2}

Analysis of the relationship between $\dot{V}/\dot{Q}$ and alveolar gas tensions begins with consideration of the determinants of alveolar P_{CO_2} (P_{ACO_2}).

Inspired gas contains no CO_2. Therefore, all CO_2 exhaled from the lungs arises from metabolic production and is calculated according to the following equation:

$$\dot{V}_{CO_2} = P_{ACO_2} \cdot \dot{V}_A / K \qquad [13\text{-}1]$$

where

$\dot{V}_{CO_2}$ = minute CO_2 production
$\dot{V}_A$ = alveolar ventilation
K = a constant

(Equation [13-1] is a rearrangement of equation [3-10] in Chap. 3). Furthermore, CO_2 cleared from the circulation by the lungs is described by application of the Fick equation for CO_2 production:

$$\dot{V}_{CO_2} = \dot{Q} \cdot (C\bar{v}_{CO_2} - Cc_{CO_2}) \qquad [13\text{-}2]$$

where

$\dot{Q}$ = cardiac output
$C\bar{v}_{CO_2}$ = CO_2 content of mixed venous blood
Cc_{CO_2} = CO_2 content of pulmonary end-capillary blood

In a steady state, the total CO_2 expired equals the CO_2 cleared from the circulation by the lungs. Therefore, the right side of equation [13-1] equals the right side of equation [13-2]:

$$P_{ACO_2} \cdot \dot{V}_A / K = \dot{Q} \cdot (C\bar{v}_{CO_2} - Cc_{CO_2}) \qquad [13\text{-}3]$$

Rearrangement of equation [13-3] yields the following:

$$\frac{\dot{V}_A}{\dot{Q}} = \frac{(C\bar{v}_{CO_2} - Cc_{CO_2})}{(P_{ACO_2}/K)} \qquad [13\text{-}4]$$

Equation [13-4] can be rearranged to provide the following expression for P_{ACO_2}:

$$P_{ACO_2} = \frac{(C\bar{v}_{CO_2} - Cc_{CO_2})}{(\dot{V}_A/\dot{Q})/K} \qquad [13\text{-}5]$$

Analysis of equation [13-5] reveals that an increase in $\dot{V}_A/\dot{Q}$ (or, as written generically, $\dot{V}/\dot{Q}$) lowers P_{ACO_2} and a decrease raises P_{ACO_2}. Note that at one extreme, when $\dot{V}/\dot{Q} = \infty$, $P_{ACO_2} = 0$ (see Fig. 13-2C). P_{ACO_2} as a function of $\dot{V}/\dot{Q}$ is shown graphically in Figure 13-3.

RELATIONSHIP BETWEEN $\dot{V}/\dot{Q}$ AND P_{AO_2}

As in the case for CO_2, the relationship between $\dot{V}/\dot{Q}$ and P_{AO_2} is derived by considering the mass balance of O_2 across the alveolar–capillary membrane. The analysis for O_2 is more complex than that for CO_2 because only a portion of the inspired O_2 is taken up across the alveolar–capillary membrane, and O_2 is present in alveoli throughout respiration. The same principles apply, however.

The quantity of O_2 diffusing from alveoli into the circulation is described by the Fick equation for O_2 consumption:

$$\dot{V}_{O_2} = \dot{Q} \cdot (Ca_{O_2} - Cc_{O_2}) \qquad [13\text{-}6]$$

where

$\dot{V}_{O_2}$ = minute O_2 consumption
Ca_{O_2} = O_2 content of arterial blood
Cc_{O_2} = O_2 content of pulmonary end-capillary blood

Under steady-state conditions, the difference between the O_2 contents of inspired and mixed expired gas equals the amount of O_2 diffusing across the lungs. The O_2 contents of inspired and expired gas are proportional to the

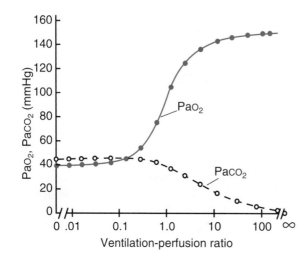

Figure 13-3. Graphical relationships between Pao_2 and $\dot{V}/\dot{Q}$, and $Paco_2$ and $\dot{V}/\dot{Q}$. Pao_2 and $Paco_2$ in regions with $\dot{V}/\dot{Q}$ of 1, 0, and ∞ are the same as those shown in Figure 13-2. (Modified from West JB. State of the Art: Ventilation–perfusion relationships. Am Rev Respir Dis 116:919–943, 1977.)

partial pressures of O_2 in inspired and mixed expired gas, respectively (see Chap. 9):

$$\dot{V}o_2 = [Pio_2 - P\bar{E}o_2] \cdot \dot{V}A \cdot K' \qquad [13\text{-}7]$$

where

$$Pio_2 = Po_2 \text{ of inspired gas}$$
$$P\bar{E}o_2 = Po_2 \text{ of mixed expired gas}$$
$$K' = \text{a constant}$$

Furthermore, under steady-state conditions, the amount of O_2 diffusing across the lungs equals that taken up by the circulation. Therefore, setting the right side of equation [13-6] equal to the right side of equation [13-7] yields the following expression:

$$\dot{Q} \cdot (Cao_2 - Cco_2) = [Pio_2 - P\bar{E}o_2] \cdot \dot{V}A \cdot K' \qquad [13\text{-}8]$$

Equation [13-8] can be rearranged as follows:

$$\frac{\dot{V}A}{\dot{Q}} = \frac{(Cao_2 - Cco_2)}{[Pio_2 - P\bar{E}o_2] \cdot K'} \qquad [13\text{-}9]$$

The algebraic solution of equation [13-9] for Pao_2 is more problematic than solution of equation [13-4] for $Paco_2$ because of the complex interrelationships among these variables. The graphical solution to equation [13-9] is shown in Figure 13-3.

$\dot{V}/\dot{Q}$ RELATIONSHIPS IN THE NORMAL LUNG

Thus far, the analysis has been based on consideration of the lung as a single, homogeneous entity. Ventilation and perfusion, however, are *not* homogeneously distributed throughout the lung. Gradients of ventilation and perfusion exist, resulting in slight mismatching of these variables, even in the healthy organ. An understanding of the factors that determine regional ventilation and perfusion is important in appreciating how the lung efficiently accomplishes gas exchange. The basic physiologic underpinnings are described in Chapter 2

(Respiratory Mechanics), Chapter 3 (Distribution of Ventilation), Chapter 9 (Gas Exchange in the Lung), and Chapter 12 (Pulmonary Circulation).

APICAL–BASAL GRADIENT OF VENTILATION

As described in Chapter 3, gravity has significant effects on the upright human lung and chest wall. An apical–basal gradient of pleural pressure exists, with pleural pressure decreasing (i.e., becoming less negative) from apex to base (see Fig. 3-6). As a result, alveoli in the apex and in the base have different *end-expiratory* volumes because the alveoli lie at different points on their individual static pressure–volume curves (Fig. 13-4A). Furthermore, because static lung compliance during inspiration is different for these two points, for the same change in pleural pressure, alveoli in the apex undergo smaller increases in volume than those in the base (Fig. 13-4B). As a result, a gradient of ventilation

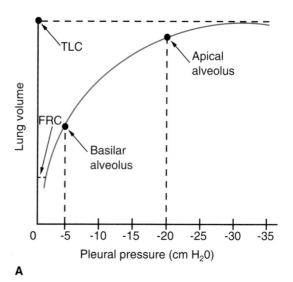

Figure 13-4. Apical–basal gradient of alveolar volume and lung compliance. **(A)** Normal static pressure–volume curve from functional residual capacity (FRC) to total lung capacity (TLC). The two points identified on the curve represent apical and basal alveoli. The apical alveolus lies on the flat part of the curve; that is, its compliance is less than the basal unit. **(B)** A change in pleural pressure of −5 cm H_2O expands both apical and basal units. The change in volume of each unit (for the same change in pleural pressure) is greater for the basal than apical alveolus. See text for discussion.

exists, with relatively more ventilation (per unit lung volume) to the base than the apex (Fig. 13-5A). Overall ventilation to the base is also greater because the lung base is larger than the apex.

APICAL–BASAL GRADIENT OF PERFUSION

An apical–basal gradient for lung perfusion also exists, with the lung base having greater perfusion per unit lung volume than the apex. Hence, the distribution gradient for ventilation is in the same direction as that for perfusion. As described in Chapter 12, the principal factor determining regional perfusion is the relationship among pulmonary arterial pressure, pulmonary venous pressure, and alveolar pressure—pressure relationships that determine zones 1, 2, 3, and 4 of the lung. The apical–basal gradient of lung perfusion is shown graphically in Figure 13-5B.

OVERALL $\dot{V}/\dot{Q}$ RELATIONSHIPS IN THE HEALTHY UPRIGHT LUNG

Although the apical–basal gradients for ventilation and perfusion are in the same direction, the magnitudes of the changes in ventilation and perfusion from apex to base are different. In particular, the increment in perfusion per centimeter of vertical distance from the apex is greater than that for ventilation; that is, the slope of the plot of perfusion versus distance from apex is steeper than that for ventilation (Fig. 13-6A). As a result, $\dot{V}/\dot{Q}$ decreases from top to bottom of the lung, and a corresponding *distribution* of alveolar P_{O_2} and P_{CO_2} is

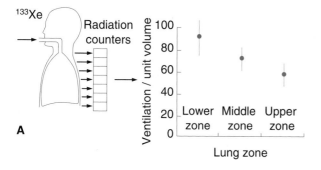

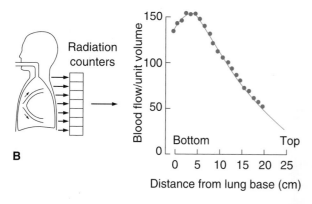

Figure 13-5. Measurement of regional lung ventilation and perfusion. **(A)** Apical–basal gradient of ventilation. Radioactive xenon is inhaled with a normal tidal volume breath by the upright subject. Radioactivity is measured using a panel of external radioactivity counters. The data are "normalized" for a smaller lung volume in the apex than in the base. **(B)** Apical–basal gradient of perfusion. By similar methodology, perfusion per unit lung volume is measured after intravenous injection of a radioisotope. See text for discussion. (From West JB. Blood flow and metabolism. In: Respiratory Physiology: The Essentials. 4th ed. Baltimore: Williams & Wilkins, 1990:40.)

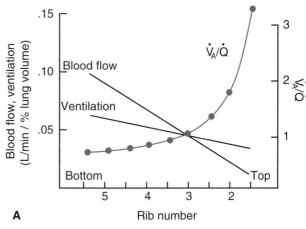

A

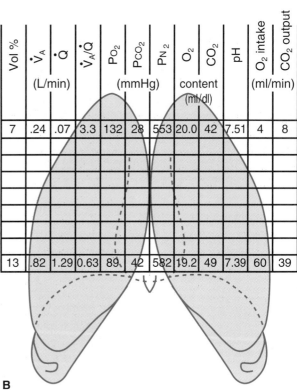

Figure 13-6. Regional variation in lung function. **(A)** Ventilation, perfusion, and V̇/Q̇ from lung apex to base. Ventilation and perfusion are greater at the base. The apical–basal difference for perfusion is greater than for ventilation, however, and V̇/Q̇ is lower at the base. **(B)** Apical–basal differences in multiple respiratory variables in the healthy, upright lung. The lung is conceptualized as multiple discrete levels from base to apex, each having a certain V̇/Q̇. The V̇/Q̇ of each level determines its corresponding alveolar PO_2 and PCO_2, as well as the O_2 and CO_2 contents of blood leaving the level. For purposes of simplification, only values for the top and bottom levels are shown. The range of V̇/Q̇ and corresponding PO_2 values is large, even in the normal lung—a finding attributable primarily to the relative lack of perfusion of the lung apex. (From West JB. Ventilation–perfusion relationships. In: Respiratory Physiology: The Essentials. 4th ed. Baltimore: Williams & Wilkins, 1990:61,63.)

B

| Vol % | $\dot{V}_A$ | $\dot{Q}$ | $\dot{V}_A/\dot{Q}$ | PO_2 | PCO_2 | PN_2 | O_2 | CO_2 | pH | O_2 intake | CO_2 output |
	(L/min)			(mmHg)			content (ml/dl)			(ml/min)	
7	.24	.07	3.3	132	28	553	20.0	42	7.51	4	8
13	.82	1.29	0.63	89	42	582	19.2	49	7.39	60	39

seen (Fig. 13-6B). These distributions of V̇/Q̇, Pao_2, and $Paco_2$ depend, of course, on lung position. The gradient is front-to-back in a supine subject and base-to-apex in a subject doing a handstand (or in a sleeping bat!).

EFFECTS OF THE V̇/Q̇ GRADIENT ON GAS EXCHANGE AND VENTILATION

From the previous discussion, it is apparent that ventilation–perfusion relationships in the healthy lung are rather intricate. The physiologic impact of the distribution of $\dot{V}/\dot{Q}$ is highlighted by considering its effect on normal gas exchange and ventilation. First, the major effect on arterial oxygenation of alveoli with $\dot{V}/\dot{Q}$ less than 1.0 is examined. Subsequently, a three-compartment model, including a compartment with $\dot{V}/\dot{Q}$ greater than 1.0, is described.

EFFECT ON Pa$_{O_2}$ OF ALVEOLI WITH VENTILATION–PERFUSION RATIOS LESS THAN ONE

Alveoli with $\dot{V}/\dot{Q}$ less than 1.0 contribute to the normal difference between ideal mean Pa$_{O_2}$ and Pa$_{O_2}$—that is, the alveolar–arterial oxygen difference [(a − a) P$_{O_2}$]. Normally, this difference (or gradient) is 5 to 10 mmHg in young subjects; it may increase to 20 mmHg in healthy elderly subjects. Two mechanisms are responsible for the alveolar–arterial oxygen difference: (1) relatively greater blood flow to the lung base, and (2) the curvilinear nature of the oxyhemoglobin dissociation curve. Each of these mechanisms is discussed in the following sections.

Effects of the Apical–Basal Blood Flow Gradient

Consider a hypothetical lung consisting of only two alveoli, one apical and one basal (Fig. 13-7A). Alveolar ventilation, perfusion, and Pa$_{O_2}$ for each unit are derived from the data for apical and basal lung regions illustrated in Figure 13-6B. In this initial analysis, we will assume that the oxyhemoglobin dissociation curve is *linear* (Fig. 13-7B).

According to the principle of conservation of mass, the total O_2 content of expired gas equals the sum of the O_2 contents of gas from the apex and the base. Furthermore, because in the gaseous phase O_2 content corresponds to P$_{O_2}$, the following expression can be derived:

$$\text{Pa}_{O_2} \cdot \dot{V}_A \text{ (total)} = [\text{Pa}_{O_2} \text{ (apex)} \cdot \dot{V}_A \text{ (apex)}] \quad \text{[13-10]}$$
$$+ [\text{Pa}_{O_2} \text{ (base)} \cdot \dot{V}_A \text{ (base)}]$$

where

Pa$_{O_2}$	= weighted mean alveolar P$_{O_2}$
$\dot{V}_A$ (total)	= total alveolar ventilation
Pa$_{O_2}$ (apex)	= alveolar P$_{O_2}$ in apical alveolus
$\dot{V}_A$ (apex)	= alveolar ventilation in apical alveolus
Pa$_{O_2}$ (base)	= alveolar P$_{O_2}$ in basal alveolus
$\dot{V}_A$ (base)	= alveolar ventilation in basal alveolus

By substituting into equation [13-10] the numerical values for the apical and basal regions of the lung illustrated in Figure 13-6B, and adding the apical and basal alveolar ventilation to derive total alveolar ventilation ($\dot{V}_A$ [total]), the following expression may be written:

$$\text{Pa}_{O_2} \cdot 1.06 \text{ L/min} = [(132 \text{ mmHg} \cdot 0.24 \text{ L/min})]$$
$$+ [(89 \text{ mmHg} \cdot 0.82 \text{ L/min})] \quad \text{[13-11]}$$

$$\text{Pa}_{O_2} = 98.7 \text{ mmHg} \quad \text{[13-12]}$$

This Pa$_{O_2}$ represents the overall P$_{O_2}$ of the exhaled gas derived from both apical and basal alveoli, that is, the lung's *mean alveolar P$_{O_2}$.*

Application of the principle of conservation of mass to O_2 content of the blood yields the following:

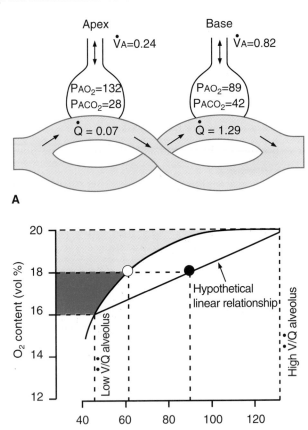

Figure 13-7. Lung model consisting of idealized apical and basal units. **(A)** Calculated values for PAO_2 and $PACO_2$ derived from data provided in Figure 13-6B. **(B)** Effect of curvilinear nature of oxyhemoglobin dissociation curve on PO_2 in presence of alveoli with low (<1) and high (>1) $\dot{V}/\dot{Q}$. If blood flow from an alveolus with low $\dot{V}/\dot{Q}$ (PO_2 of 46 mmHg and O_2 content of 16 ml/dl) mixes with an *equal* blood flow from an alveolus with high $\dot{V}/\dot{Q}$ (PO_2 of 132 mmHg and O_2 content of 20 ml/dl), the O_2 content of the resulting mixture (which is equivalent to arterial blood) is 18 ml/dl, as determined by equation [13-13] in the text. The PO_2 of this *mixed blood* varies markedly, however, depending on the nature of the oxyhemoglobin dissociation relationship. If the relationship were linear, the PO_2 would be 89 mmHg (solid circle); however, because it is curvilinear, the PO_2 is 62 mmHg (open circle).

$$Cao_2 \cdot \dot{Q} \text{ (total)} = [Cco_2 \text{ (apex)} \cdot \dot{Q} \text{ (apex)}] + [Cco_2 \text{ (base)} \cdot \dot{Q} \text{ (base)}] \qquad [13\text{-}13]$$

where

Cao_2	= weighted mean O_2 content of the blood leaving the lung (arterial blood)
$\dot{Q}$ (total)	= total blood flow through the lung (cardiac output)
Cco_2 (apex)	= O_2 content of end-capillary blood in apical alveolus
$\dot{Q}$ (apex)	= blood flow to apical alveolus
Cco_2 (base)	= O_2 content of end-capillary blood in basal alveolus
$\dot{Q}$ (base)	= blood flow to basal alveolus

Because we have assumed a *linear* oxyhemoglobin curve, we may substitute the term, $PO_2 \cdot K'$, where K' is a constant, for each corresponding term for O_2 content in equation [13-13] and then divide both sides of equation [13-13] by K':

$$Pao_2 \cdot \dot{Q} \text{ (total)} = [Pco_2 \text{ (apex)} \cdot \dot{Q} \text{ (apex)}] + [Pco_2 \text{ (base)} \cdot \dot{Q} \text{ (base)}] \qquad [13\text{-}14]$$

where

Pa_{O_2} = weighted mean P_{O_2} of blood leaving the lung (arterial blood)

Pc_{O_2} (apex) = P_{O_2} of end-capillary blood in apical alveolus

Pc_{O_2} (base) = P_{O_2} of end-capillary blood in basal alveolus

Substitution of numerical values from Figure 13-6B into equation [13-14] yields the following:

$$Pa_{O_2} \cdot 1.36 \, L/min = [(132 \, mmHg \cdot 0.07 \, L/min)] \qquad [13\text{-}15]$$
$$+ \, [(89 \, mmHg \cdot 1.29 \, L/min)]$$

$$Pa_{O_2} = 91.2 \, mmHg \qquad [13\text{-}16]$$

From equations [13-12] and [13-16], the alveolar—arterial oxygen gradient can be calculated:

$$P_{A_{O_2}} - Pa_{O_2} = 98.7 \, mmHg - 91.2 \, mmHg = 7.5 \, mmHg$$
$$[13\text{-}17]$$

Hence, this portion of the alveolar—arterial oxygen gradient is the result of the apical—basal perfusion gradient and resultant effects on regional values for alveolar and arterial P_{O_2}.

Effects of the Curvilinear Oxyhemoglobin Dissociation Curve

We must now consider the physiologic contribution to the alveolar—arterial oxygen difference of the *nonlinearity* of the oxyhemoglobin dissociation curve. Once again, the model depicted in Figure 13-7A is useful in the analysis.

The calculations for $P_{A_{O_2}}$ are identical to those performed previously. The mean $P_{A_{O_2}}$ is 98.7 mmHg (equations [13-11] and [13-12]). Because the oxyhemoglobin dissociation curve is nonlinear, we cannot use equation [13-10]; rather we must solve equation [13-13] for Ca_{O_2}. If we assume a hemoglobin of 15.0 g/dl, the following equation may be written:

$$Ca_{O_2} \cdot 1.36 \, L/min = [(20.0 \, ml/dl \cdot 0.07 \, L/min)] \qquad [13\text{-}18]$$
$$+ \, [(19.2 \, ml/dl \cdot 1.29 \, L/min)]$$

$$Ca_{O_2} = 19.24 \, ml/dl \qquad [13\text{-}19]$$

An arterial O_2 content of 19.24 ml/dl corresponds to a Pa_{O_2} of 89.2 mmHg (based on a normal oxyhemoglobin dissociation curve, as depicted in Chap. 10, Fig. 10-2). Substitution of this value into equation [13-17] yields an alveolar—arterial oxygen gradient of 9.5 mmHg ($P_{A_{O_2}} - Pa_{O_2} = 98.7 \, mmHg - 89.2 \, mmHg = 9.5 \, mmHg$). Hence, an additional 2.0 mmHg of the normal alveolar—arterial oxygen difference is the result of the nonlinearity of the oxyhemoglobin dissociation curve.

THREE-COMPARTMENT LUNG MODEL

A convenient way of analyzing the effects of having a distribution of ventilation—perfusion ratios in the lung is based on the three-compartment model described in Figure 13-2. The three idealized compartments include: (1) a "normal" compartment having $\dot{V}/\dot{Q} = 1$; (2) a second compartment, denoting *physiologic shunt*, having $\dot{V}/\dot{Q} = 0$; and (3) a third compartment, denoting *physiologic dead space*, having $\dot{V}/\dot{Q} = \infty$.

Physiologic Shunt

From a conceptual standpoint, the effect of lung units having $\dot{V}/\dot{Q}$ less than 1, but not zero, can be described *as if* the units were the *functional equivalent* of a right-to-left shunt across the lungs (see Chap. 12). When a subject breathes gas having a fractional inspired oxygen concentration of less than 1.0, *both true right-to-left shunts and units with low $\dot{V}/\dot{Q}$ contribute to lowering of Pa_{O_2} relative to PA_{O_2}.* (In this model, hypoventilation and diffusion block are ignored as possible contributing causes of hypoxemia.)

Physiologic shunt is the term used to describe, quantitatively, the effects of both true shunt (anatomic shunt) and regions with low $\dot{V}/\dot{Q}$. Physiologic shunt is calculated using the shunt equation (see Chap. 12, Table 12-5), in which the term, $\dot{Q}_{PS}$ (physiologic shunt), is substituted for $\dot{Q}_S$ (shunt). Normally, physiologic shunt is less than 5% of cardiac output. The similar physiologic effects of alveoli with very low ventilation–perfusion ratios and true shunt are illustrated in Figure 13-8.

Physiologic Dead Space

Conceptually, the physiologic effect of alveoli having $\dot{V}/\dot{Q}$ greater than 1, but not infinity, can be described *as if* the units were the *functional equivalent* of extra dead space, that is, "alveolar dead space." Total dead space, referred to as *physiologic dead space*, comprises two components, anatomic and alveolar. The effect of units having high $\dot{V}/\dot{Q}$ is calculated using the Bohr equation (see Chap. 3):

$$\frac{V_{D_{phys}}}{V_T} = \frac{Pa_{CO_2} - P\bar{E}_{CO_2}}{Pa_{CO_2}} \qquad [13\text{-}20]$$

where

$$\begin{aligned}
V_{D_{phys}} &= \text{physiologic dead space} \\
V_T &= \text{tidal volume} \\
P\bar{E}_{CO_2} &= P_{CO_2} \text{ in mixed expired gas}
\end{aligned}$$

Pa_{CO_2} is assumed to equal PA_{CO_2}.

Although alveolar units with low $\dot{V}/\dot{Q}$ usually produce a decrease in Pa_{O_2}, as described previously, it is uncommon for alveolar units with low $\dot{V}/\dot{Q}$ to produce an elevation in Pa_{CO_2}. This finding is *not* related to the greater solubility of CO_2 than O_2, because, normally, a diffusion limitation for O_2 uptake does not exist. Rather, subjects with modest increases in the fraction of alveoli with high $\dot{V}/\dot{Q}$ can readily increase their *total* ventilation ($\dot{V}_E$); they excrete more CO_2 from other lung units and compensate for the additional dead space. This effect is possible because of the relatively linear CO_2–hemoglobin dissociation curve; that is, the CO_2 content of blood is linearly related to Pa_{CO_2} (see Chap. 10).

A similar compensatory effect in response to hypoxemia arising from units with low $\dot{V}/\dot{Q}$ does not exist. Although an increase in total ventilation increases PA_{O_2} in alveoli with $\dot{V}/\dot{Q}$ greater than 1, the increment in *O_2 content* in end-

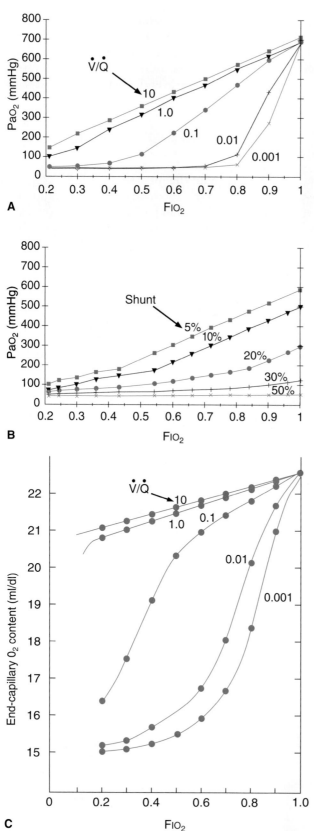

Figure 13-8. $\dot{V}/\dot{Q}$ and arterial oxygenation. **(A)** Effects of increasing and decreasing $\dot{V}/\dot{Q}$ on Pa_{O_2} as inspired O_2 concentration is increased. A high FI_{O_2} is necessary to raise Pa_{O_2} in regions with low $\dot{V}/\dot{Q}$. **(B)** Effect of increasing FI_{O_2} on Pa_{O_2} at differing levels of true right-to-left shunt. With a large shunt (e.g., 50%), even inspiration of pure oxygen ($FI_{O_2} = 1.0$) cannot raise Pa_{O_2} to 100 mmHg. **(C)** Effects of increasing and decreasing $\dot{V}/\dot{Q}$ on end-capillary O_2 content as inspired O_2 concentration is increased. For alveoli with very low $\dot{V}/\dot{Q}$ (e.g., 0.001), FI_{O_2} must be increased markedly to raise end-capillary O_2 content. A 10-fold increase in $\dot{V}/\dot{Q}$ only minimally increases end-capillary O_2 content; however, the presence of low $\dot{V}/\dot{Q}$ regions results in profound lowering of end-capillary O_2 content. Hence, the presence of alveoli with high $\dot{V}/\dot{Q}$ cannot compensate for hypoxemia resulting from alveoli with low $\dot{V}/\dot{Q}$. (From West JB. State of the Art: Ventilation–perfusion relationships. Am Rev Respir Dis 116:919–943, 1977.)

capillary blood in minimal (Fig. 13-8C), and it is inadequate to offset the effect of desaturated blood coming from alveoli with low $\dot{V}/\dot{Q}$.

In general, hypercapnia develops only when the fraction of alveoli with high $\dot{V}/\dot{Q}$ is so great that physiologic dead space becomes significantly elevated and $\dot{V}E$ is unsustainable. Under these circumstances, ventilatory demand exceeds ventilatory supply, as described in Chapter 18.

DISTRIBUTION OF VENTILATION–PERFUSION RATIOS IN HEALTH AND DISEASE

The actual distribution of $\dot{V}/\dot{Q}$ throughout the lung is much more complicated than the simple, three-compartment model described earlier. A continuous spectrum of $\dot{V}/\dot{Q}$ exists in both healthy subjects and in patients with lung disease. Mathematical analysis of data generated experimentally using the so-called "multiple inert gas technique" (the principles of which will not be described here) has been used in addressing the topic of "dispersion of $\dot{V}/\dot{Q}$."

Findings from application of the multiple inert gas technique to study of the normal lung are illustrated in Figure 13-9. The range of $\dot{V}/\dot{Q}$ is shown on the abscissa in a log normal distribution. As noted in the figure, intrapulmonary shunts are absent in the healthy lung. (Normally occurring, nonpulmonary shunts, e.g., the Thebesian veins that drain into the left ventricle, are not detected by this technique.) In addition, the number of units with either very low or very high $\dot{V}/\dot{Q}$ is minimal.

The distribution of $\dot{V}/\dot{Q}$ in a variety of lung diseases has been studied. Two examples are illustrated in Figure 13-10.

In Figure 13-10A, a pattern typical for patients with asthma, a bimodal distribution of $\dot{V}/\dot{Q}$ is evident. A peak of low $\dot{V}/\dot{Q}$, comprising up to 20% of cardiac output, and the main distribution, with a normal range of $\dot{V}/\dot{Q}$, are present. The peak of low $\dot{V}/\dot{Q}$ signifies the presence of alveoli whose small peripheral airways are either occluded or narrowed by mucus or edema (see Chap. 5).

In Figure 13-10B, a pattern typical for patients with adult respiratory distress syndrome (ARDS; see Chap. 14), complex changes in the relationship between ventilation and perfusion are highlighted: (1) an increase in true right-to-

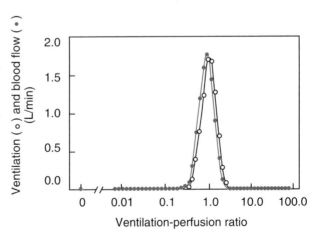

Figure 13-9. Multiple inert gas technique. Shown are ventilation (open circles) and perfusion (closed circles) relative to $\dot{V}/\dot{Q}$ (log normal scale) in the healthy, upright lung. The distribution of ratios is clustered around 1.0, and regions with either high or low ratios are absent. (From West JB, Wagner PD. Ventilation–perfusion relationships. In: Crystal RG, West JB, eds. The Lung: Scientific Foundations. vol. 2. New York: Raven Press, 1991:1299.)

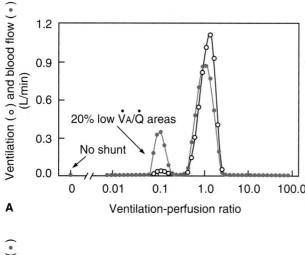

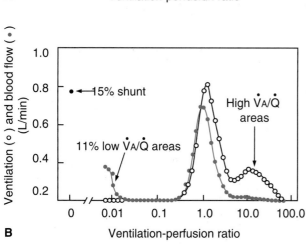

Figure 13-10. Changes in distribution of ventilation (open circles) and perfusion (closed circles) in patients with lung disease. (**A**) Distribution of $\dot{V}/\dot{Q}$ in chronic asthma. Compared with the normal distribution shown in Figure 13-9, a bimodal population of units is seen. A considerable fraction of perfusion goes to poorly ventilated regions centered around a $\dot{V}/\dot{Q}$ of 0.1. (From Wagner PD, Dantzker DR, Iacovoni VE, et al. Ventilation–perfusion inequality in asymptomatic asthma. Am Rev Respir Dis 118: 511–524, 1978.) (**B**) Distribution of $\dot{V}/\dot{Q}$ in ARDS. The predominant peak remains at a $\dot{V}/\dot{Q}$ of 1.0. However, three additional findings are of note: (1) a significant (15%) right-to-left shunt ($\dot{V}/\dot{Q} = 0$); (2) a region with very low $\dot{V}/\dot{Q}$; and (3) a region with increased $\dot{V}/\dot{Q}$. Shunt and regions of low $\dot{V}/\dot{Q}$ underlie the profound hypoxemia that characterizes this disorder. (From Dantzker DR, Brook LJ, Dehart P, et al. Ventilation–perfusion distributions in the ARDS. Am Rev Respir Dis 120:1039–1052, 1979.)

left shunt; (2) a compartment with very low $\dot{V}/\dot{Q}$; (3) a predominance of units with a normal range of $\dot{V}/\dot{Q}$; and (4) a compartment with high $\dot{V}/\dot{Q}$. Patients with ARDS characteristically demonstrate hypoxemia that is poorly responsive to increases in F_{IO_2}. This finding might be expected on the basis of increased right-to-left shunt and the shunt-like effects of regions with very low $\dot{V}/\dot{Q}$ (see Fig. 13-8).

SELECTED READING

Dantzker DR, Brook LJ, Dehart P, Lynch JP, Weg JG. Ventilation–perfusion distributions in the ARDS. Am Rev Respir Dis 120:1039–1052, 1979.

Rahn H, Fenn WO. A Graphical Analysis of the Respiratory Gas Exchange. Washington, DC: American Physiological Society, 1955.

Riley RL, Cournand A. "Ideal" alveolar air and the analysis of ventilation–perfusion relationships in the lungs. J Appl Physiol 1:825–847, 1949.

Wagner PD, Dantzker DR, Iacovoni VE, Tomlin WC, West JB. Ventilation–perfusion inequality in asymptomatic asthma. Am Rev Respir Dis 118:511–524, 1978.

West JB. State of the Art: Ventilation–perfusion relationships. Am Rev Respir Dis 116:919–943, 1977.

West JB. Ventilation/Blood Flow and Gas Exchange. 5th ed. Philadelphia: JB Lippincott, Oxford Blackwell Scientific Publications, 1990.

West JB. Ventilation–perfusion relationships. In: Respiratory Physiology: The Essentials. 4th ed. Baltimore: Williams & Wilkins, 1990:51–68.

West JB, Wagner PD. Ventilation–perfusion relationships. In: Crystal RG, West JB, eds. The Lung: Scientific Foundations. vol. 2. New York: Raven Press, 1991:1289–1305.

Lippincott's Pathophysiology Series: Pulmonary
Pathophysiology, edited by Michael A. Grippi.
J. B. Lippincott Company, Philadelphia © 1995.

CHAPTER

14

Cardiogenic and Noncardiogenic Pulmonary Edema

John Hansen-Flaschen

Pulmonary edema, defined as excess water in the extravascular spaces of the lung, is not a specific disease. It is a pathologic condition resulting from failure of physiologic compensatory mechanisms to maintain a balance between the amount of fluid entering and leaving the lung.

Pulmonary edema can be caused by acute injury to the lung itself (*permeability pulmonary edema*) or by severe dysfunction of the heart or kidneys (*hemodynamic pulmonary edema*); occasionally, both mechanisms operate in concert. Pulmonary edema may even occur in the absence of any organ dysfunction if a large quantity of fluid is administered intravenously at a rapid rate.

In its mildest form, pulmonary edema causes no symptoms and may be undetectable by physical examination or chest radiograph. On the other hand, acute, severe pulmonary edema is among the most dramatic clinical disorders of humans. The clinical recognition and treatment of pulmonary edema depend on a thorough understanding of the anatomic and physiologic basis of fluid balance in the lung in both health and disease.

The pathophysiologic consequences of pulmonary edema are directly related to a number of concepts discussed elsewhere in this book—most notably, diffusion (see Chap. 9), the pulmonary circulation (see Chap. 12), and ventilation–perfusion relationships (see Chap. 13).

ANATOMIC PATHWAY FOR FLUID MOVEMENT IN THE LUNG

In the healthy lung, a small amount of fluid continuously filters across the walls of small pulmonary blood vessels into the adjacent interstitium. Approximately one third of the filtered fluid moves into the interstitium across the surfaces of arterioles and venules. The rest of the fluid moves across alveolar capillary surfaces. Collectively, the fluid-exchanging arterioles, capillaries, and venules supplied by the pulmonary artery are referred to as the *pulmonary microcirculation*.

THE ALVEOLAR–CAPILLARY MEMBRANE

For a long time, physiologists wondered how fluid exchange could take place across the walls of alveolar capillaries without interfering with gas exchange. The development of the electron microscope provided the answer to this question (Fig. 14-1).

Practically all of the alveolar interstitial connective tissue lies on one side of the capillary, the so-called "thick side." On the other side, the endothelial basement membrane is fused directly to the epithelial basement membrane so that an exceedingly thin surface is formed, the "thin side." The thick side of the capillary contains collagen and elastin fibrils that provide the structural framework for the alveolar walls; the thick side also subserves the fluid exchanging function of the microcirculation. The thin side allows for rapid exchange of respired gases across the delicate, highly diffusable *alveolar–capillary membrane*.

Most of the fluid traversing the walls of the pulmonary microcirculation is thought to move through gaps in the junctions between endothelial cells (Fig. 14-2). Water, small solutes (e.g., glucose), and small plasma proteins (e.g., transferrin and albumin) move passively through these junctions by convection and diffusion. The pathway and mechanism for transendothelial movement of larger plasma proteins, such as gamma globulin, are debated.

Some evidence points to these larger molecules moving passively across the endothelium through intercellular channels formed by transient fusion of cell membrane invaginations and cytoplasmic vesicles. Other observations suggest that proteins are transported within vesicles that move from one surface of

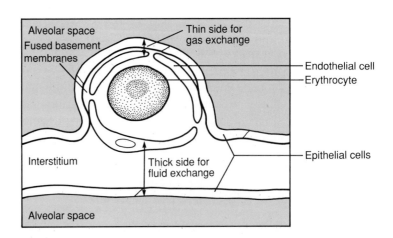

Figure 14-1. Functional anatomy of the alveolar–capillary membrane. Fluid enters the interstitial space on the "thick side" of the membrane. The "thin side" is ideally suited for gas exchange. See text for details.

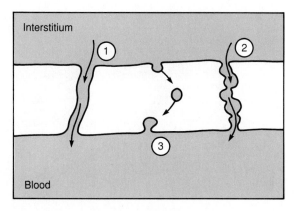

Figure 14-2. Likely pathways for movement of water and solutes across the pulmonary endothelium: (1) intercellular junctions, (2) vesicular channels, and (3) vesicular transcytosis.

pulmonary endothelial cells to the other. Ultrastructural studies have shown that the luminal surface of the pulmonary capillary endothelium is richly endowed with binding sites for various plasma constituents, including albumin and low-density plasma lipids. These binding sites may allow for selectivity and modulation in the transvesicular transport of macromolecules across the endothelium.

Junctions between alveolar epithelial cells are much "tighter" than those that separate pulmonary endothelial cells. Consequently, solutes larger than urea do not move passively from the alveolar interstitium into the air spaces of the normal lung. Instead, the microvascular filtrate moves from the alveolar walls, down a hydrostatic pressure gradient, into the interstitial spaces beneath the pleural surface and within the bronchovascular bundles.

THE PULMONARY LYMPHATICS

The terminal pouches of the pulmonary lymphatic system are located within the subpleural and peribronchial connective tissue spaces (Fig. 14-3). Fluid enters the lymphatic pouches through discontinuities in the lymphatic endothelium; it is pumped by peristaltic action past a series of one-way valves into the collecting lymphatics in the hila of the lungs. From there, the fluid moves through mediastinal lymphatic vessels and associated lymph nodes into the thoracic duct, where it rejoins the blood. This pathway is depicted schematically in Figure 14-4 (see also Chap. 1).

Fluid probably also moves from the subpleural interstitial tissue into the pleural space through gaps in the visceral pleura. Fluid that enters the pleural space is taken up in lymphatics that terminate on the parietal pleural surface. Like the pulmonary lymphatics, these chest wall lymph vessels drain through the mediastinal collecting system into the thoracic duct.

DEVELOPMENT OF PULMONARY EDEMA

Pulmonary edema occurs when fluid filters across the pulmonary microcirculation into the lungs faster than it is removed by the lymphatic system. Initially, the fluid collects within the interstitial spaces of the lungs (*interstitial edema*). The thick sides of the alveolar walls swell slightly; however, most of the edema fluid flows into the interstitial spaces beneath the pleura and around the bronchovascular bundles. These spaces are much more compliant than the spaces within

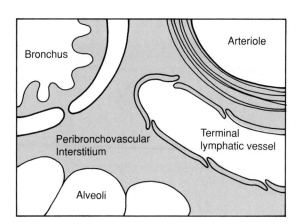

Figure 14-3. Terminal lymphatic vessel. Pulmonary lymphatic vessels terminate in peribronchovascular interstitial tissue. Fluid enters through gaps between lymphatic endothelial cells. Note the flap-like configuration of these intercellular gaps.

the alveolar walls. In effect, the subpleural and peribronchial connective tissue serves as a "sink" that draws excess fluid away from the alveolar membranes, thereby preserving the gas-exchanging function of the lung. The pleural spaces function as a second sink for promoting fluid movement away from the gas-exchanging surfaces.

If large quantities of fluid enter the pulmonary interstitium rapidly, or if the alveolar epithelium is damaged, fluid enters the air spaces and floods the alveoli (*alveolar edema*). The pathway for leakage of fluid into the air spaces is controversial. Some evidence indicates that leakage occurs between epithelial cells in the walls of alveolar ducts or other small airways. Other observations suggest that the tight junctions between alveolar epithelial cells open to allow passage of water and soluble proteins when the interstitial pressure exceeds a threshold value. As alveoli fill, frothy fluid backs up into the bronchi. At this stage, gas exchange is severely compromised by shunting of blood across fluid-filled alveoli (see Chap. 13). The compliance of the lungs is also markedly reduced (see Chap. 2).

Chronic hemodynamic edema is often accompanied by pleural effusions. Fluid accumulates in the pleural spaces when the rate of transudation exceeds the rate of removal of fluid by the parietal lymphatic vessels. If large, the pleural effusions compress adjacent lung and contribute to the gas exchange abnormality.

Figure 14-4. Anatomic pathway for lung fluid exchange. Fluid moves from the alveolar capillaries across the endothelium into the interstitium on the "thick" sides of the capillaries. From there, the fluid percolates through the interstitial space to the terminal lymphatics, which are located in the connective tissue surrounding blood vessels and bronchi.

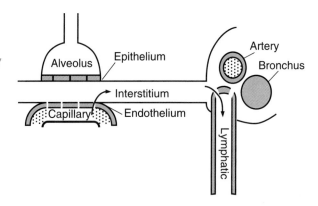

PHYSIOLOGIC BASIS OF FLUID EXCHANGE IN THE LUNG

The rate of movement of fluid across the microvascular endothelium into the interstitium is determined by the net hydrostatic and oncotic pressures acting across the microvascular walls. This relationship is described by the *Starling equation:*

$$Q_f = K_f[(P_{mv} - P_i) - \sigma(\Pi_{mv} - \Pi_i)] \qquad [14\text{-}1]$$

where

Q_f = fluid filtration rate
K_f = filtration coefficient
P_{mv} = microvascular hydrostatic pressure
P_i = interstitial space hydrostatic pressure
σ = osmotic reflection coefficient
Π_{mv} = microvascular oncotic pressure
Π_i = interstitial space oncotic pressure

Normal values for each of the terms in the Starling equation are given in Table 14-1.

The *hydrostatic pressure gradient* ($P_{mv} - P_i$) drives fluid from the pulmonary microcirculation into the interstitium. The hydrostatic pressure gradient is opposed by the *oncotic pressure gradient* ($\Pi_{mv} - \Pi_i$), which favors movement of fluid in the opposite direction.

The two constants in the Starling equation define the physical properties of the microvascular endothelium with respect to fluid exchange.

The *filtration coefficient* (K_f) determines the relationship between the net driving pressure and the rate of flow of fluid across the endothelium per 100 g of lung tissue. This relationship defines the permeability characteristics of the membrane. The *osmotic reflection coefficient* (σ) determines the relative contribution of the oncotic pressure gradient to the net driving pressure across the endothelial membrane. Values for σ range from 0 to 1.

TABLE 14-1. *THE STARLING EQUATION:*
$$Q_f = K_f[(P_{mv} - P_i) - \sigma(\Pi_{mv} - \Pi_i)]$$

TERM	SYMBOL	NORMAL MEAN VALUE
Fluid filtration rate	Q_f	—
Filtration coefficient	K_f	0.2 ml/min · 100 g · mmHg
Hydrostatic pressure in pulmonary microvessels	P_{mv}	9 mmHg
Hydrostatic pressure in perimicrovascular interstitial space	P_i	−4 mmHg
Osmotic reflection coefficient	σ	0.8
Oncotic pressure in pulmonary microvessels	Π_{mv}	24 mmHg
Oncotic pressure in perimicrovascular interstitial space	Π_i	14 mmHg

When σ is 0, the membrane allows unrestricted passage of protein; under these circumstances, the oncotic pressure gradient across the membrane makes no contribution to the net transmembrane driving pressure for fluid. When σ is 1, the membrane allows no passage of protein (i.e., all plasma proteins are "reflected back"), and the oncotic pressure gradient contributes maximally to the net transmembrane driving pressure.

Because the hydrostatic driving force ($P_{mv} - P_i$) exceeds the oncotic absorptive force [$\sigma(\Pi_{mv} - \Pi_i)$], fluid flows continuously from plasma into the interstitium. The oncotic pressure in the interstitium is about 75% of that in the plasma. In addition, σ, the osmotic reflection coefficient, is considerably closer to 1 than to 0. These two observations indicate that the endothelium of the pulmonary microcirculation restricts the passage of plasma proteins relative to water. In other words, the endothelium acts as a *semipermeable membrane*.

Like other semipermeable membranes, the pulmonary microvascular endothelium sieves larger solutes in proportion to the transendothelial pressure gradient. When the hydrostatic driving force ($P_{mv} - P_i$) is increased, the flow of water across the membrane increases more than the flow of protein. Consequently, the concentration of protein in the filtrate decreases (Fig. 14-5). In animal experiments, the protein concentration in the pulmonary interstitium can be reduced to as low as 20% to 30% of the protein concentration in the plasma by increasing the microvascular hydrostatic pressure to high levels. This sieving effect of the microvascular endothelium is an important protective mechanism for the lung, as described later.

THE EDEMA SAFETY FACTORS

At first glance, the Starling equation suggests that pulmonary edema may develop whenever any of the four pressures in the equation (P_{mv}, P_i, Π_{mv}, Π_i) changes in a direction that increases the fluid filtration rate. If that were so, pulmonary edema would occur with alarming frequency. Fortunately, most changes in the Starling forces are rapidly counterbalanced by physiologic compensatory mechanisms that minimize or prevent accumulation of edema fluid.

Consider, for example, what happens when the plasma oncotic pressure is reduced by 50% (Fig. 14-6), such as with rapid intravenous infusion of saline

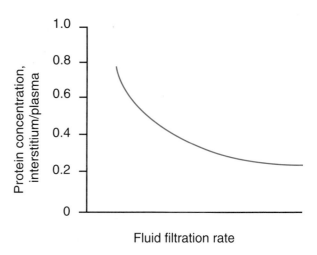

Figure 14-5. Sieving effect of the pulmonary microvascular endothelium. In the healthy lung, the ratio of protein concentration in the interstitium to that in plasma decreases as fluid filtration rate increases. This protective mechanism increases the oncotic pressure gradient and opposes further filtration of fluid.

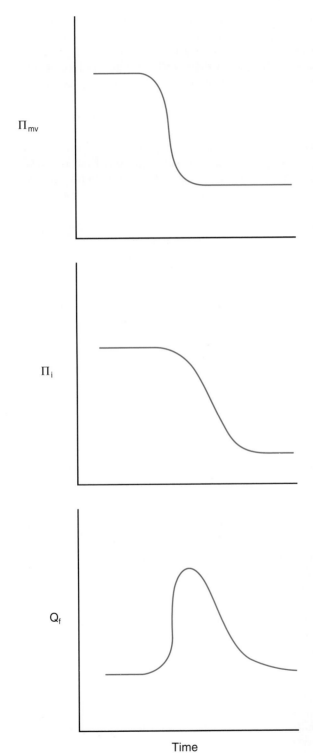

Π_{mv}

Π_i

Q_f

Time

Figure 14-6. Effect of a sudden decrease in plasma oncotic pressure on pulmonary transendothelial filtration rate. The decrease in microvascular oncotic pressure (Π_{mv}) causes a transient increase in fluid filtration rate (Q_f). Q_f returns to baseline as the interstitial oncotic pressure (Π_i) approaches a new equilibrium value and a normal oncotic pressure gradient is restored.

into a patient who has bled massively from a wound. As predicted by the Starling equation, the sudden reduction in pulmonary microvascular oncotic pressure (Π_{mv}) increases fluid filtration (Q_f) into the interstitium. The flow of a protein-poor plasma filtrate into the interstitium, however, reduces the interstitial oncotic pressure (Π_i) and restores the oncotic pressure gradient to normal. Consequently, the fluid filtration rate returns rapidly to baseline. Thus, even a severe reduction in plasma oncotic pressure causes only a transient increase in lung water content that is well tolerated.

The physiologic compensatory mechanisms that protect the lungs from pulmonary edema are known collectively as the *edema safety factors*. Four of these compensatory mechanisms are summarized in Table 14-2. Understanding the edema safety factors is key to understanding changes in lung fluid balance.

THE SIEVING EFFECT

One of the most important edema safety factors is the sieving effect of the pulmonary endothelium. Because the endothelium is semipermeable to protein, an increase in the microvascular hydrostatic pressure (e.g., as occurs in left heart failure) causes a corresponding decrease in interstitial oncotic pressure (see Fig. 14-5). As a result, the increase in the hydrostatic driving force ($P_{mv} - P_i$) is partly counterbalanced by an increase in the oncotic absorption force ($\Pi_{mv} - \Pi_i$), and the net effect on fluid filtration rate (Q_f) is minimized. Only when the interstitial oncotic pressure approaches a minimum value do further increases in microvascular hydrostatic pressure cause a fully proportional increase in fluid filtration.

INCREASE IN INTERSTITIAL HYDROSTATIC PRESSURE

As edema fluid begins to accumulate within the interstitium around the pulmonary microcirculation, transendothelial filtration is also opposed by an

---

TABLE 14-2.   *THE EDEMA SAFETY FACTORS*

Decrease in interstitial oncotic pressure (sieving effect)
An increase in transmicrovascular hydrostatic pressure gradient is partly counterbalanced by a corresponding increase in oncotic pressure gradient.

Increase in interstitial hydrostatic pressure
Hydrostatic pressure in perimicrovascular interstitial space increases as interstitium becomes distended with edema fluid. Transcapillary hydrostatic pressure gradient is reduced, opposing further fluid movement.

Increase in plasma oncotic pressure
In response to sudden, severe increase in pulmonary microvascular hydrostatic pressure, protein concentration in plasma increases as a large quantity of protein-poor fluid is driven into the lungs. Resultant increase in plasma oncotic pressure opposes further fluid movement. Effect declines over time as protein concentration in plasma reequilibrates with systemic extravascular fluid spaces.

Reserve capacity of the lymphatic system
Flow through pulmonary lymphatic system can increase up to 15-fold to compensate for increase in transmicrovascular filtration rate.

increase in the interstitial hydrostatic pressure (P_i). Because the perimicrovascular interstitium is relatively noncompliant, small increases in interstitial fluid volume can cause P_i to increase by 5 mmHg or more. The increase in P_i also increases the rate of flow of fluid from the perimicrovascular interstitium to the bronchovascular interstitium, the site of the terminal lymphatics.

INCREASE IN PLASMA ONCOTIC PRESSURE

A third edema safety factor is clinically important only under extreme circumstances, such as in severe, acute left heart failure, in which 1 to 2 L or more of protein-poor fluid can enter the lungs over a short time. The sudden loss of protein-poor fluid from the circulation increases the plasma oncotic pressure (Π_{mv}), thereby opposing further movement of fluid into the lungs.

LYMPHATIC SYSTEM RESERVE

The fourth edema safety factor is the reserve capacity of the pulmonary lymphatic system. Lung lymph flow is a function of the interstitial hydrostatic pressure, the pumping capacity of the smooth muscle in the collecting lymphatics, and the hydrostatic pressure in the central vein into which the thoracic lymphatics drain. As edema fluid accumulates around the terminal lymphatic vessels, pulmonary lymph flow may increase up to 15-fold to maintain a balance between the rate that fluid enters and leaves the lungs. Edema accumulates in the lungs only when the reserve capacity of the lymphatics is overwhelmed.

Because of the edema safety factors, most perturbations that affect the fluid filtration rate do not cause clinically significant pulmonary edema. In fact, only two mechanisms are known to cause this disorder: (1) an increase in microvascular hydrostatic pressure sufficient to overwhelm the edema safety factors, resulting in hemodynamic pulmonary edema; and (2) an increase in the permeability of the pulmonary microvascular walls, resulting in permeability pulmonary edema.

HEMODYNAMIC PULMONARY EDEMA

The lung is protected from modest increases in pulmonary vascular pressure by the edema safety factors. Hemodynamic edema develops when these physiologic compensatory mechanisms are overwhelmed at microvascular pressure exceeding 25 to 30 mmHg (normal range, 5–12 mmHg). Pulmonary microvascular pressures as high as 40 to 45 mmHg are sometimes observed; these pressures are associated with fulminant alveolar edema.

The most common cause of hemodynamic edema is acute or chronic left heart failure. Other cardiac causes include severe mitral valve disease and certain congenital heart diseases. Isolated right ventricular failure does not cause pulmonary edema. Renal failure can result in hemodynamic pulmonary edema if the ability of the kidneys to excrete urine is reduced (oliguric renal failure). As the intravascular plasma volume increases in a patient with oliguric renal failure, pulmonary microvascular pressure may rise to exceed the threshold for edema formation in the lung.

Hemodynamic pulmonary edema is usually diagnosed by correlation of clinical findings with chest radiographic abnormalities. The patient with moderate or severe pulmonary edema may complain of dyspnea on exertion or at rest. The dyspnea is often increased in the supine position (*orthopnea*) and is partly relieved by sitting upright. Patients with pulmonary edema may also awaken at night with severe shortness of breath (*paroxysmal nocturnal dyspnea*).

On physical examination, end-inspiratory rales are usually heard in both lung bases. Scattered wheezes may be present as well. In fact, pulmonary edema sometimes mimics an acute asthma attack. Increased airway resistance, decreased airflow rate, and turbulent airflow are thought to be potentiated by accumulation of edema fluid within the peribronchial connective tissue and, in some cases, by reactive bronchospasm (see Chaps. 4 and 5).

Chest radiographic findings in hemodynamic pulmonary edema reflect the anatomic and physiologic bases of this disorder. The heart shadow is often enlarged, reflecting dilation of the cardiac chambers. Pulmonary arteries in the upper lung zones appear prominent because high pulmonary vascular pressures increase perfusion to these areas (see Chaps. 12 and 13). Bronchial and vascular markings are widened and blurred, especially near the hila, because of accumulation of edema fluid in the peribronchovascular interstitial spaces. Fluid in the subpleural connective tissue causes visible thickening of the lung fissures. Right-sided or bilateral pleural effusions are often seen in chronic pulmonary edema. In severe alveolar edema, most of these radiographic findings are obscured by dense, fluffy infiltrates that "white-out" both lungs (Fig. 14-7).

PERMEABILITY PULMONARY EDEMA

Pulmonary edema due to increased permeability is caused by acute, widespread injury to the pulmonary microvascular endothelium. The anatomic basis of permeability pulmonary edema has been elucidated by electron micrographic studies of acutely injured lungs. Water and protein leak from the pulmonary

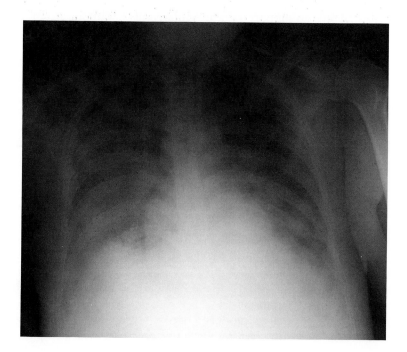

Figure 14-7. Chest radiograph showing bilateral "white-out" caused by severe hemodynamic pulmonary edema.

microcirculation into the adjacent interstitial and alveolar spaces through abnormal gaps between damaged endothelial and epithelial cells. These gaps are probably formed by the fragmentation and sloughing of necrotic cells.

Figure 14-8 illustrates the key physiologic differences between permeability and hemodynamic pulmonary edema. In permeability edema, acute injury to the pulmonary microcirculation increases the filtration coefficient (K_f) and decreases the osmotic reflection coefficient (σ) of the endothelium so that fluid leaks into the lungs at a rate that is disproportionately high relative to the net driving pressure. When the permeability of the alveolar–capillary membrane increases, edema forms even at normal microvascular hydrostatic pressures (8–12 mmHg); severe edema develops at elevated pressures.

In addition to altering the two constants in the Starling equation, acute injury to the microcirculation reduces or eliminates the edema safety factor associated with the sieving effect. Because the damaged microvascular walls are less restrictive to the passage of plasma proteins, the protein content of the filtrate no longer decreases as the filtration rate increases (Fig. 14-9). Consequently, the oncotic absorptive force [$\sigma(\Pi_{mv} - \Pi_i)$] does not increase at higher filtration rates to oppose further filtration of fluid as it does in the normal lung.

Permeability edema also differs from the hemodynamic type with regard to time course. Hemodynamic edema is frequently manifested within minutes of a sudden increase in the pulmonary capillary hydrostatic pressure, as might occur during a myocardial infarction. In contrast, permeability edema may not become clinically apparent for 6 to 48 hours after the onset of acute lung injury. The delay probably reflects the gradually progressive effect of the lung's inflammatory response to the initial injury on capillary permeability.

Permeability and hemodynamic edema also differ in the rate of resolution of lung dysfunction. Hemodynamic edema begins to improve noticeably within hours of restoration of the pulmonary microvascular pressure to normal. Water is actively resorbed from the alveolar air spaces across the intact epithelium by the action of adenosine triphosphate-requiring ion channels. Even severe hemodynamic edema may clear completely within 2 to 4 days. Permeability edema resolves at a more variable, generally slower, rate. The acutely injured alveolar–capillary membrane takes time to heal. Also, the high protein content

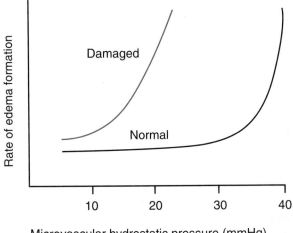

Figure 14-8. Relationship between pulmonary microvascular hydrostatic pressure and rate of edema formation in a patient with normal pulmonary endothelium and a patient with acutely damaged endothelium. See text for discussion.

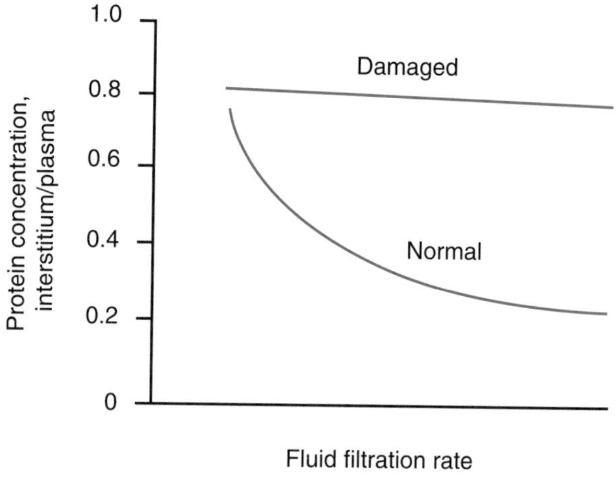

Figure 14-9. Loss of sieving effect in the acutely injured lung. The ratio of protein concentration in the interstitium to that in plasma does not decrease in the injured lung with increasing microvascular hydrostatic pressure because the damaged endothelium is much less restrictive to passage of plasma proteins.

of the edema fluid slows the rate of resolution of the edema, because protein moves back across the epithelium more slowly than salt and water.

ADULT RESPIRATORY DISTRESS SYNDROME

PATHOPHYSIOLOGY

Permeability pulmonary edema is a physiologic derangement of the lung that ranges from asymptomatic to life-threatening in severity. Severe permeability edema is a characteristic early feature of the *adult* (or *acute*) *respiratory distress syndrome* (ARDS). ARDS is not a specific disease; it is a category of acute respiratory failure that is to be distinguished from several others. ARDS is defined clinically as acute lung injury that results in: (1) widespread, bilateral pulmonary infiltrates; (2) severe, refractory hypoxemia; and (3) marked reduction in lung compliance.

ARDS begins with an acute injury to the alveolar–capillary membrane that results in permeability pulmonary edema. The injury may be caused directly by a physical or chemical insult, such as inhalation of toxic fumes or overinflation of the lungs. Alternatively, the injury may be indirect, with the pulmonary endothelium responding to a systemic inflammatory process such as sepsis. In some cases, the lung injury heals quickly and pulmonary function returns to normal over several days. In other instances, the initial injury gives rise to a sustained inflammatory response. Healing then takes place slowly (over weeks or months), if at all.

Lung biopsies obtained more than 2 or 3 weeks after the onset of sustained ARDS no longer show pulmonary edema; instead, they reveal an intense inflammatory reaction accompanied by extensive remodeling of the lungs and widespread fibrosis (see Chap. 7). Fifty percent or more of patients in whom sustained ARDS develops die of respiratory failure or of intercurrent complications, despite the best available intensive care.

CAUSES OF ARDS

An extraordinary variety of disorders cause, or are associated with, ARDS. The most common is sepsis. In severe sepsis, a systemic inflammatory response to a local infection causes acute injury to endothelium throughout the body, including the lungs. This response is called the *systemic inflammatory response syndrome* (SIRS). When SIRS causes severe injury to the pulmonary capillaries, ARDS ensues. Other important causes of ARDS include bacterial and viral pneumonias, aspiration of acidic gastric contents, inhalation of toxic gases, and various adverse drug reactions. Rapid ascent to high altitude sometimes causes ARDS (*high-altitude pulmonary edema*). Fractures of the hip or femur can cause this condition if large quantities of fat from the bone marrow embolize to the lungs (*fat embolism syndrome*). ARDS threatens lung transplant recipients if the transplanted lung is incompletely preserved during the harvesting procedure (*reimplantation syndrome*).

Patients with ARDS complain of sudden dyspnea. Chest radiographs show widespread pulmonary infiltrates that may be indistinguishable from the bilateral "white-out" seen in hemodynamic pulmonary edema. Hypoxemia is invariably present and may be severe. Accumulation of edema fluid and inflammatory cells greatly reduces pulmonary compliance, so that increased effort is required to ventilate the lungs (see Chap. 2). Hypercapnic respiratory failure occurs when the patient is no longer able to maintain an adequate minute ventilation (see Chap. 18).

HEMODYNAMIC VERSUS PERMEABILITY PULMONARY EDEMA

Permeability pulmonary edema resembles hemodynamic edema in many respects. Both are characterized by dyspnea, hypoxemia, and bilateral, dense radiographic infiltrates. How does the clinician distinguish one form of pulmonary edema from the other?

The distinction is often apparent from the clinical circumstances associated with the onset of the pulmonary edema. For example, if a patient known to have heart disease presents to an emergency room with pulmonary edema accompanied by severe chest pain and electrocardiographic evidence of myocardial infarction, the assumption usually is that the edema is hemodynamic in origin. On the other hand, a patient found to have acute pulmonary edema after inhaling chlorine gas in an industrial accident probably has permeability edema.

If the physiologic mechanism of edema formation can not be discerned with confidence from the clinical circumstances, measurement of the pulmonary artery occlusion pressure (PAOP) or pulmonary capillary wedge pressure (PCWP) using a pulmonary artery flotation catheter (Swan-Ganz catheter) is usually performed (see Chap. 12). The PAOP provides a reasonable approximation of pulmonary microvascular hydrostatic pressure. A PAOP less than 15 mmHg suggests permeability pulmonary edema. A PAOP above 20 to 25 mmHg is compatible with hemodynamic edema (see Fig. 14-8).

Even with direct hemodynamic measurements, confusion about the type of pulmonary edema may arise. For example, myocardial ischemia can cause severe, but transient, left ventricular dysfunction. The resulting pulmonary edema lasts for many hours after the PAOP returns to baseline. If the PAOP is first measured when the ischemia has resolved, the clinician might conclude erroneously that the edema was caused by increased permeability.

Confusion may also occur because the finding of an elevated PAOP does not exclude the possibility that permeability injury may also be present. To diagnose permeability edema when the PAOP is elevated, the clinical course of the edema is observed as the PAOP responds to treatment. If pulmonary edema has not improved within 24 to 48 hours after the PAOP has returned to normal, permeability injury has probably occurred, along with hemodynamic edema.

TREATMENT OF PULMONARY EDEMA

The first principle in treating severe pulmonary edema is to ensure satisfactory oxygenation and acid–base balance (see Chap. 10). Arterial blood gases are measured at frequent intervals. A high concentration of O_2 is administered through a tight-fitting face mask. If the face mask does not restore adequate oxygenation, or if respiratory acidosis develops, the patient is intubated and mechanical ventilation is begun.

Hemodynamic pulmonary edema often responds dramatically to administration of diuretics. Patients who are unresponsive to diuretics because of renal failure may require dialysis or ultrafiltration to remove excess fluid. If hemodynamic pulmonary edema is caused by left heart failure, inotropic agents (e.g., dobutamine) and vasodilator drugs (e.g., sodium nitroprusside) may also be used to improve myocardial contractility.

Treatment of permeability pulmonary edema is directed at reversing the underlying cause of the acute lung injury, if possible, and at supporting vital organ function with the hope that the lung will heal. To minimize accumulation of edema fluid in the lungs, every effort is made to keep intravascular volume at a minimum that is consistent with adequate cardiac output (see Fig. 14-8).

SELECTED READING

Demling RH. Current concepts on the adult respiratory distress syndrome. Circ Shock 30:297, 1990.

Fishman, AP. Pulmonary edema. In: Fishman AP, ed. Pulmonary Diseases and Disorders. 2nd ed. New York: McGraw-Hill, 1988:919–952.

Hansen-Flaschen J, Fishman AP. Adult respiratory distress syndrome: Clinical features and pathogenesis. In: Fishman AP, ed. Pulmonary Diseases and Disorders. 2nd ed. New York: McGraw-Hill, 1988:2201–2214.

Rinaldo JE, Christman JW. Mechanisms and mediators of ARDS. Clin Chest Med 11:621–632, 1990.

Taylor AE, Barnard JW, Barman SA, Adkins WK. Fluid balance. In: Crystal RG, West JB, eds. The Lung: Scientific Foundations. New York: Raven Press, 1991: 1147–1161.

Lippincott's Pathophysiology Series: Pulmonary Pathophysiology, edited by Michael A. Grippi. J. B. Lippincott Company, Philadelphia © 1995.

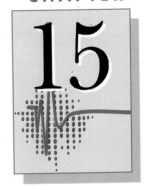

Clinical Presentations: Pulmonary Circulation and Pulmonary Edema

Michael A. Grippi

The following four cases focus on disorders of the pulmonary circulation covered in Chapters 12 through 14. Although not all of the clinical entities discussed are common, each highlights important pathophysiologic concepts related to the pulmonary circulation and its role in gas exchange.

CASE 1

The patient is a 57-year-old man who has smoked two packs of cigarettes daily for the past 30 years. He has an intermittent cough that occasionally is productive of a teaspoon of sputum in the morning. One week before admission to the hospital he noticed a vague feeling of "indigestion." On the day of admission he experienced substernal pressure radiating down his left arm. The pain lasted 30 minutes and was accompanied by shortness of breath. The patient was brought to the emergency room for evaluation.

In the emergency room, the patient appears to be in moderate respiratory distress and is complaining of chest tightness. His blood pressure is 140/90 mmHg, his pulse is 110 beats per minute, and his respirations are 30 breaths per minute. Examination of the chest reveals scattered expiratory wheezes and rales at both bases. The apical cardiac impulse

is palpable in the sixth intercostal space in the midclavicular line. The first and second heart sounds are normal; third and fourth heart sounds are audible. Cyanosis, clubbing, and edema are absent.

The patient has a significant smoking history and, on the basis of the history of chronic sputum production, may have chronic bronchitis. The recent history is very suggestive of acute myocardial infarction. The diagnosis can be substantiated by looking for an injury pattern in the electrocardiogram and an elevation in serum levels of enzyme markers for myocardial necrosis (creatinine phosphokinase and lactate dehydrogenase).

The patient is dyspneic for several reasons, including the development of fluid in the pulmonary interstitium and alveoli—pulmonary edema (see Chap. 14). The cardiomegaly (apical impulse in sixth intercostal space) and third heart sound indicate left ventricular dysfunction as the underlying cause. Rales represent the auscultatory findings of the fluid. Peribronchial edema and heightened airway reactivity result in airway narrowing and audible wheezing (referred to as "cardiac asthma"). These mechanical alterations in the lungs stimulate vagal afferent fibers that, in conjunction with hypoxemia-induced stimulation of carotid body afferents (see Chap. 16), may contribute to the sensation of dyspnea.

The white blood cell count is 15,600 per mm^3. The hemoglobin is 14.3 g/dl. Arterial blood gases obtained while the patient is breathing room air show a pH of 7.47, a Pa_{O_2} of 60 mmHg, and a Pa_{CO_2} of 32 mmHg. The patient's chest radiograph is shown in Figure 15-1; his electrocardiogram is shown in Figure 15-2.

There are several reasons for the patient's hypoxemia. He has a 60 pack-year smoking history and may well have had an increased alveolar—arterial oxygen gradient before the acute myocardial infarction. Left ventricular dysfunction may have led to increased pressure in the pulmonary venous capillaries, producing interstitial edema and alveolar flooding (see Chap. 14). Consequently, ventilation—perfusion mismatch would be accentuated, and areas of physiologic shunting increased (see Chap. 13).

The patient is admitted to the intensive care unit. A pulmonary artery flotation catheter is inserted (see Chap. 12) and the following pressures are measured:

Right atrial (RA)	= 7 mmHg
Right ventricular (RV)	= 40/7 mmHg
Pulmonary arterial (PA)	= 40/22 mmHg
Pulmonary artery occlusion pressure (PAOP) or pulmonary capillary wedge pressure (PCWP)	= 24 mmHg

The patient is treated with supplemental O_2 administered through a mask that delivers an F_{IO_2} of 0.3, intravenous nitroglycerin, and intravenous diuretics. Repeat arterial blood gases show a pH of 7.44, a Pa_{O_2} of 70 mmHg, and a Pa_{CO_2} of 36 mmHg. He improves slowly over the next 24 hours and makes an uneventful recovery.

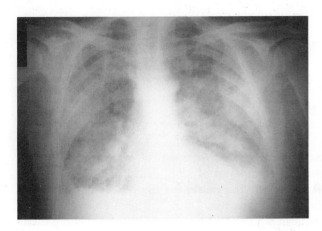

Figure 15-1. Case 1: postero-anterior chest radiograph, showing congestive heart failure.

The hemodynamic measurements demonstrate significant elevation of PAOP, which, in this patient, should provide an accurate reflection of left atrial and left ventricular end-diastolic pressures. The elevation of hydrostatic pressure accounts for the filtration of fluid into the interstitium and alveoli. Right atrial pressure is not elevated significantly, corresponding to the lack of clinical signs of significant right-sided heart failure. Alveolar flooding usually does not occur until PAOP exceeds 25 to 30 mmHg. The measured value of 24 mmHg is probably indicative of the efficacy of treatment in the interval between the patient's arrival in the emergency room and placement of the pulmonary artery flotation (Swan-Ganz) catheter.

The initial alveolar–arterial oxygen gradient is 51 mmHg ([760 − 47]0.21 − 1.2[32] − 60 = 51). If this gradient and the $Paco_2$ remained constant, administration of an Fio_2 of 0.3 should have resulted in an increase in the Pao_2 to 120 mmHg. (Actual gradient is [760 − 47]0.3 − 1.2[36] − 70 = 101 mmHg; if [A–a] Po_2 remained constant at 51 mmHg, Pao_2 should have been [760 − 47]0.3 − 1.2[36] − 51 = 120 mmHg). Therefore, ventilation–perfusion relationships had worsened by the time of the second arterial blood gas.

Measurement of pulmonary function tests in this clinical setting would reveal a restrictive pattern, due to increased lung water. Because of the long smoking history and the presence of wheezing on physical examination, signs of reduced expiratory airflow rates might also be ex-

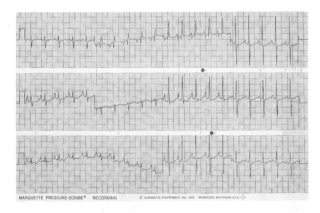

Figure 15-2. Case 1: electrocardiogram, demonstrating acute myocardial infarction.

pected. Alterations in the diffusing capacity are variable in cardiogenic pulmonary edema. Fluid in the airways and interstitium can create a diffusion barrier, reducing DLco. Elevated pressures in the compliant pulmonary vascular bed, however, may increase pulmonary blood volume, thereby increasing DLco (see Chap. 9).

CASE 2

A 28-year-old man first presented for medical evaluation 10 years ago because of an elevated hemoglobin of 19.5 g/dl. Phlebotomies have been performed approximately twice yearly for the last 2 years because of headaches, dizziness, and tachycardia. There has been no mental sluggishness, visual or auditory changes, or bleeding tendencies. The patient reports no exercise intolerance. He has played the trumpet for 20 years.

Physical examination shows no plethora. The blood pressure is 120/80 mmHg. Clubbing of the fingers and toes is noted.

Laboratory data include a hemoglobin of 19 g/dl and normal white blood cell and platelet counts. A bone marrow examination shows no stainable iron; results are otherwise negative. The Pao$_2$ is 55 mmHg (89% saturation). The blood volume is normal. A chest radiograph is interpreted as normal. Because of the hypoxemia, pulmonary function tests are performed. Lung volumes, expiratory airflow rates, maximal voluntary ventilation, and diffusing capacity are within normal limits.

The patient has polycythemia—an abnormal elevation in hemoglobin concentration. His symptoms of headaches, dizziness, and tachycardia are attributable to the elevated hematocrit. Periodic phlebotomies had been performed for relief of symptoms. The findings from the blood counts, bone marrow analysis, and blood volume measurement, coupled with the hypoxemia, indicate secondary polycythemia, rather than polycythemia vera. Furthermore, the negative routine pulmonary function test results exclude generalized lung disease as a cause for the hypoxemia.

Repeat arterial blood gases are measured while the patient is breathing room air, and then while breathing 100% oxygen:

	Room Air	100% O$_2$
Pao$_2$(mmHg)	58	255
Paco$_2$(mmHg)	34	37
pH	7.43	7.40
[HCO$_3^-$](mEq/L)	23	24

Mixed venous Po$_2$, measured while the patient is breathing room air, is 40 mmHg; it increases to 50 mmHg (81% saturation) when the patient breathes 100% O$_2$.

The Pa_{O_2} on room air is low. The relatively low Pa_{O_2} (255 mmHg) while the patient is breathing 100% O_2 indicates a right-to-left shunt. The shunt fraction, Q_S/Q_T, determined on 100% O_2, is calculated as mean pulmonary capillary O_2 content (Cc_{O_2}) minus mean arterial O_2 content (Ca_{O_2}), divided by mean capillary O_2 content minus mixed venous O_2 content ($C\bar{v}_{O_2}$) (see Chaps. 12 and 13):

$$\frac{Q_S}{Q_T} = \frac{(Cc_{O_2} - Ca_{O_2})}{(Cc_{O_2} - C\bar{v}_{O_2})} \qquad [15\text{-}1]$$

In solving equation [15-1], the first step is to calculate the mean alveolar P_{O_2}, because this is assumed to be the same as the mean pulmonary capillary P_{O_2}. Although the mean alveolar P_{O_2} can be calculated using direct measurements of the exhaled N_2, CO_2, and H_2O vapor concentrations, it is more practical to use the alveolar gas equation:

$$P_{AO_2} = (P_B - P_{H_2O}) \cdot F_{IO_2} \qquad [15\text{-}2]$$
$$- P_{ACO_2}\left(F_{IO_2} + \frac{1 - F_{IO_2}}{R}\right)$$

$$P_{AO_2} = (760 - 47)(1.0) - (37)(1.0) = 676 \, mmHg \qquad [15\text{-}3]$$

Next, the O_2 contents of end-capillary (alveolar), arterial, and mixed venous blood are calculated, recalling that the *bound* O_2 content of 1 g of fully saturated hemoglobin is 1.34 ml O_2, and that the *dissolved* O_2 content of blood is 0.003 ml O_2 per dl per mmHg (see Chap. 10):

$$O_2 \, content = [(g \, Hb/dl)(1.34 \, ml \, O_2/g \, Hb)(O_2 \, sat)] \\ + [(Pa_{O_2})(0.003 \, ml \, O_2/dl/mmHg)] \qquad [15\text{-}4]$$

$$Cc_{O_2} = [(19)(1.34)(100\%)] + [(676)(0.003)] \\ = 27.46 \, ml \, O_2/dl \qquad [15\text{-}5]$$

$$Ca_{O_2} = [(19)(1.34)(100\%)] + [(255)(0.003)] \\ = 26.23 \, ml \, O_2/dl \qquad [15\text{-}6]$$

$$C\bar{v}_{O_2} = [(19)(1.34)(81\%)] + [(50)(0.003)] \\ = 20.77 \, ml \, O_2/dl \qquad [15\text{-}7]$$

Thus,

$$\frac{Q_S}{Q_T} = \frac{(27.46 - 26.23)}{(27.46 - 20.77)} = 0.18 \, or \, 18\% \qquad [15\text{-}8]$$

Right heart catheterization shows a pulmonary artery pressure of 25/10 mmHg. Careful reexamination of the chest radiograph reveals an abnormality (Fig. 15-3), prompting performance of a pulmonary angiogram (Fig. 15-4). Subsequently, the abnormality is resected surgically.

Review of the chest radiograph shows an arteriovenous communication. Examination of the surgical specimen establishes the diagnosis of a cavernous pulmonary hemangioma. The hemangioma walls contain abundant elastic tissue and varying amounts of fibrous connective tissue. The vascular channels permit deoxygenated venous blood to bypass alveoli, constituting an anatomic basis for right-to-left shunting.

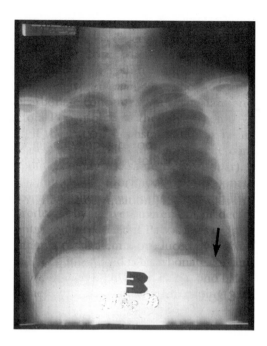

Figure 15-3. Case 2: posteroanterior chest radiograph. A faint, nodular density in the left lower lobe may be seen.

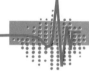

CASE 3

The patient is an 83-year-old man admitted to the hospital with an infected right shoulder joint. Initially, he was treated with antibiotics and surgical drainage and did well. However, after 1 week, wound drainage has stopped and pain has increased. He now has a fever. As the patient is being prepared for repeat surgical drainage, he experiences dizziness and shortness of breath.

The patient's blood pressure is 70/40 mmHg, his pulse is 120 beats per minute, and his temperature is 101°F. The chest is clear; cardiac examination reveals tachycardia and no third heart sound.

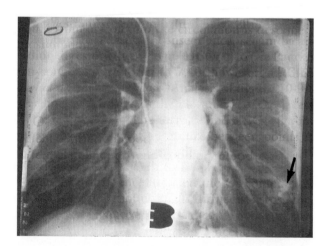

Figure 15-4. Case 2: pulmonary angiogram. An arteriovenous malformation is shown in the left lower lobe.

Intravenous fluids and supplemental O_2 at 2 L/minute are administered. Repeat arterial blood gases show a pH of 7.55, a PaO_2 of 98 mmHg, and a $PaCO_2$ of 26 mmHg. The patient is taken to the operating room for drainage of his infected shoulder.

Fever continues after surgery. The chest radiograph demonstrates new, bilateral, lower lobe infiltrates. On the fifth postoperative day, the patient experiences the sudden onset of severe shortness of breath. The respiratory rate is 44 breaths per minute and the pulse is 130 beats per minute. The blood pressure is 105/80 mmHg. Scattered wheezes are heard throughout the lung fields. An electrocardiogram shows sinus tachycardia but no signs of ischemia. The chest radiograph is unchanged. An arterial blood gas obtained while the patient is breathing 100% O_2 demonstrates a pH of 7.39, a PaO_2 of 77 mmHg, and a $PaCO_2$ of 32 mmHg.

The major considerations in the differential diagnosis include pulmonary embolism, multilobar pneumonia, and pulmonary edema (either cardiogenic or noncardiogenic). The radiographic findings and blood gas abnormalities are consistent with each of these diagnoses. The sudden onset of shortness of breath in a bed-ridden patient several days after surgery raises the strong possibility of pulmonary embolism. Additional studies are necessary to establish the diagnosis.

Because of concerns about pulmonary embolism, a ventilation–perfusion lung scan is performed. The lung scan is "indeterminate," and a pulmonary angiogram is done.

A ventilation–perfusion lung scan may be suggestive of pulmonary embolism, and in the appropriate clinical setting, a "high-probability" scan may be considered diagnostic. Nonetheless, a pulmonary angiogram is the gold standard for establishing the diagnosis.

The pulmonary angiogram demonstrates a large saddle embolus at the bifurcation of the right main pulmonary artery, as well as an embolus in the pulmonary artery to the left lower lobe.

After the pulmonary angiogram, the patient becomes more short of breath. A repeat arterial blood gas shows a further drop in the PaO_2 to 50 mmHg. The patient is intubated and mechanical ventilation is instituted. A repeat arterial blood gas while the patient is breathing 100% O_2 shows a pH of 7.28, a PaO_2 of 78 mmHg, and a $PaCO_2$ of 47 mmHg.

Because of the massive nature of the pulmonary embolus and resultant hemodynamic and respiratory compromise, the patient is treated with a thrombolytic agent. Within 12 hours he is hemodynamically stable, and an arterial blood gas obtained while he is spontaneously breathing 50% O_2 shows a pH of 7.50, a PaO_2 of 93 mmHg, and a $PaCO_2$ of 31 mmHg.

The patient's hemodynamic and respiratory status continues to improve, and a repeat pulmonary angiogram 24 hours later demonstrates considerable dissolution of the emboli. On completing the course of thrombolytic therapy, the patient is given intravenous heparin, and eventually he is discharged on an oral anticoagulant. He makes a slow, complete recovery.

In acute pulmonary embolism, the primary mechanism responsible for hypoxemia is ventilation–perfusion mismatch (see Chaps. 12 and 13). The finding of uncorrected hypoxemia while breathing 100% O_2 (Pao_2 = 78 mmHg), however, denotes an additional component of right-to-left shunt. With major pulmonary embolism, intrapulmonary shunting and intracardiac shunting through a patent foramen ovale may occur as pulmonary artery pressure rises. The underlying mechanisms responsible for the ventilation–perfusion mismatch are not well understood, although neural and humoral agents may be involved in regional redistribution of blood flow and ventilation (see Chap. 12).

The hypocapnia noted in the initial arterial blood gas ($Paco_2$ = 26 mmHg) reflects an increase in alveolar ventilation as part of an increase in overall minute ventilation ($\dot{V}_E$). The increase in $\dot{V}_E$ occurs despite an increase in dead space (V_D) arising from occlusion of the pulmonary capillary bed (increased V_D/V_T). The increased $\dot{V}_E$ may arise from increased respiratory drive, mediated through vagal afferents, or pain associated with the embolism (e.g., from pulmonary infarction).

With occluded vessels supplying some alveoli, alveolar Po_2 (Pao_2) is similar in perfused and nonperfused alveoli, because the source of O_2 (inspired air) is the same for all alveoli. The alveolar Pco_2 ($Paco_2$) is different in perfused and non-perfused alveoli, however, because the source of alveolar CO_2 is the blood. The $Paco_2$ of perfused alveoli is normal, fluctuating between the Pco_2 of mixed venous blood (45 mmHg) arriving at the alveoli, and the Pco_2 of pulmonary arterial blood (40 mmHg) departing from perfused alveoli. The $Paco_2$ in nonperfused alveoli rapidly equilibrates with the only other source of CO_2—inspired air, in which the Pco_2 is essentially zero. Thus, ventilation of these nonperfused alveoli may represent a tremendous increase in physiologic dead space.

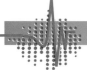

CASE 4

The patient is a 37-year-old woman referred for evaluation of progressive exertional dyspnea and right ventricular failure. Her past medical history is significant for a pulmonary embolism 10 years ago, treated with 1 week of intravenous heparin, followed by 6 months of an oral anticoagulant. She had no further symptoms until 1 year ago, when exertional dyspnea developed. Her walking is now limited to two blocks.

Physical examination shows a young woman in no distress. Chest examination is remarkable for scattered expiratory wheezes throughout both lung fields. Cardiac examination reveals that the second heart sound is widely split; the pulmonic component is increased.

The patient's past history is notable for a pulmonary embolism 10 years ago. She received standard treatment—heparin, followed by an oral anticoagulant, warfarin. The physical examination shows expiratory wheezing, suggesting airway narrowing. Accentuation of the pulmonic component of the second heart sound raises the possibility of pulmonary hypertension as the basis for the right ventricular failure.

Chest radiography demonstrates hyperinflation, clear lung fields, and prominent pulmonary arteries. A diagnosis of chronic obstructive

pulmonary disease (COPD) is made and the patient is advised to stop smoking. Bronchodilators are prescribed. Over the next several months, the patient continues to have gradually worsening exertional dyspnea. She cannot walk 50 yards without stopping. Lower extremity edema and tenderness in the right upper abdominal quadrant develop.

Repeat physical examination shows a dyspneic patient with a blood pressure of 96/78 mmHg, a pulse of 108 beats per minute, and a respiratory rate of 22 breaths per minute. The chest is clear to auscultation. The jugular venous pressure is estimated at 11 cm H_2O. The right ventricular impulse is palpable. The pulmonic component of the second heart sound is markedly increased, and a loud murmur of tricuspid regurgitation is heard. The liver is enlarged and tender to palpation. Moderate pitting edema of the lower extremities is noted.

Because of "hyperinflation" and prominent pulmonary arteries seen on chest radiography, a diagnosis of COPD is made. The patient is only 37 years old, and a diagnosis of COPD with secondary pulmonary hypertension would be very unusual, even in patients with underlying α_1-antitrypsin deficiency (see Chap. 6). The patient now has peripheral edema, hepatic enlargement (right upper quadrant abdominal tenderness), and right ventricular hypertrophy with tricuspid regurgitation (i.e., cor pulmonale).

An electrocardiogram shows evidence of right ventricular hypertrophy. The chest radiograph reveals dilated pulmonary arteries and enlargement of the right heart. The right upper and left lower lung fields appear hypovascular. Pulmonary function tests demonstrate mild airway obstruction, hyperinflation, and a mild gas transfer abnormality, with a DLCO of 66% of predicted. Arterial blood gases obtained while the patient is breathing room air show a pH of 7.52, a Pao_2 of 55 mmHg, and a $Paco_2$ of 33 mmHg.

The electrocardiographic findings are consistent with cor pulmonale. Pulmonary function tests show obstruction and hyperinflation, consistent with obstructive airway disease. The reduced DLCO, however, is *not* indicative of a *specific* pulmonary disorder. Many factors affect the DLCO: alveolar surface area, hemoglobin concentration, hemoglobin affinity for O_2, and pulmonary capillary blood volume (see Chap. 9).

A lung scan (Fig. 15-5) demonstrates multiple segmental perfusion defects and is read as "high probability" for pulmonary emboli. A pulmonary angiogram is performed. At the time of the angiogram, the pulmonary artery pressure is 104/45 mmHg (mean, 66 mmHg). The pulmonary artery occlusion pressure is 10 mmHg, and the cardiac output is 3 L/minute. Evidence of chronic pulmonary emboli is demonstrated during contrast injection (Fig. 15-6).

Although the reduced DLCO was initially attributed to loss of lung parenchyma from COPD (emphysema), the angiogram and scan findings suggest that the DLCO is better explained by loss of pulmonary capillaries and reduced gas exchange across the alveolar–capillary membrane.

The hemodynamic data demonstrate severe pulmonary hypertension

Figure 15-5. Case 4: Lung scan, posterior view. Perfusion and ventilation studies are shown. Multiple segmental and subsegmental perfusion defects are seen on the left; perfusion is absent on the right and in the left upper lung field. The perfusion defects are not matched by defects in the ventilation scan.

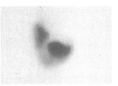

Perfusion

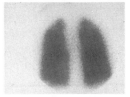

Ventilation

(PAP = 104/45 mmHg), normal left atrial filling pressure (PAOP = 10 mmHg), and reduced cardiac output (3 L/minute). Pulmonary vascular resistance (PVR) is also markedly increased (see Chap. 12):

$$PVR = \frac{\overline{PAP} - LAP}{C.O.} \cdot 79.9 \qquad [15\text{-}9]$$

$$PVR = \frac{66 - 10}{3} \cdot 79.9 = 1492 \, dyne \cdot sec \cdot cm^{-5} \qquad [15\text{-}10]$$

Clinical diagnoses of severe pulmonary hypertension and right ventricular failure secondary to chronic, unresolved pulmonary emboli are established. Pulmonary thromboendarterectomy is performed, a surgical procedure in which clots and underlying fibrous plaques in the pulmonary artery are removed (Fig. 15-7). Subsequently, the patient is discharged on an oral anticoagulant.

One year after surgery, an arterial blood gas obtained while the patient is breathing room air shows a pH of 7.42, a Pao$_2$ of 95 mmHg,

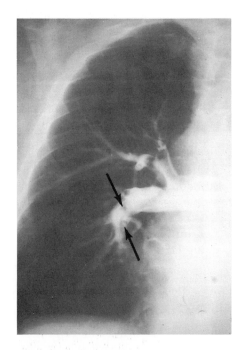

Figure 15-6. Case 4: Pulmonary angiogram. Filling defects, indicating pulmonary emboli to the right lung, are seen (*arrows*).

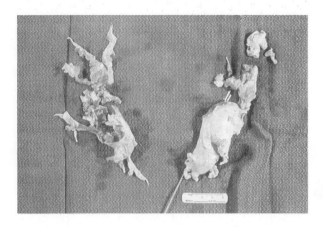

Figure 15-7. Case 4: surgical specimens from pulmonary thromboendarterectomy.

and a Pa_{CO_2} of 36 mmHg. Right heart catheterization reveals a pulmonary artery pressure of 44/20 mmHg (mean, 30 mmHg), pulmonary artery occlusion pressure of 7 mmHg, and cardiac output of 5 L/minute. A lung scan (Fig. 15-8) and pulmonary angiogram (Fig. 15-9) demonstrate improved lung perfusion.

Unlike the previous case of *acute* pulmonary embolism (case 3), this case demonstrates *chronic* pulmonary emboli. Although the patient is only 37 years old, she carried a diagnosis of chronic obstructive pulmonary disease because of the clinical and radiographic findings of cor pulmonale. The rapid progression of her symptoms, the presence of findings consistent with marked pulmonary hypertension, and a clinical suspicion of pulmonary embolic disease prompted a lung scan and, subsequently, a pulmonary angiogram. The diagnosis established eventually was chronic pulmonary

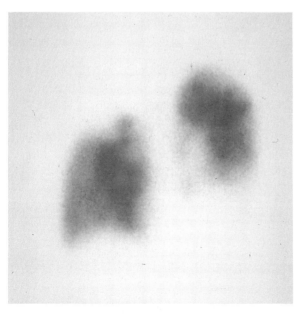

Figure 15-8. Case 4: postoperative perfusion lung scan. The blood flow pattern is markedly improved.

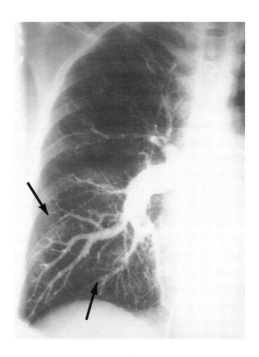

Figure 15-9. Case 4: postoperative pulmonary angiogram. Perfusion is reestablished in previously abnormal areas (*arrows*).

embolism. The patient experienced dramatic improvement after pulmonary thromboendarterectomy.

The postthromboendarterectomy hemodynamic data show mild pulmonary hypertension, normal left atrial filling pressure, and normal cardiac output. The pulmonary vascular resistance is markedly reduced:

$$PVR = \frac{30 - 7}{5} \cdot 79.9 = 368 \, dyne \cdot sec \cdot cm^{-5} \qquad [15\text{-}11]$$

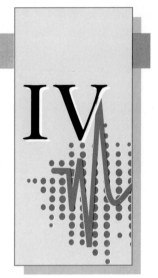

INTEGRATED RESPIRATORY FUNCTIONS: CONTROL OF BREATHING, RESPIRATORY FAILURE, AND EXERCISE

Lippincott's Pathophysiology Series: Pulmonary Pathophysiology, edited by Michael A. Grippi. J. B. Lippincott Company, Philadelphia © 1995.

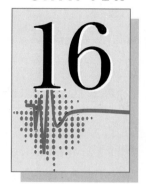

Chemical and Neural Control of Respiration

Scott Manaker

In previous chapters, the functional anatomy, mechanics, and biophysics that govern the exchange of O_2 and CO_2 between inspired air and circulating blood are discussed. To accommodate wide fluctuations in O_2 consumption and CO_2 production engendered by activities of daily life, and to maintain Pao_2 and $Paco_2$ within a narrow range, minute ventilation ($\dot{V}E$) must be finely adjustable. A complex respiratory control system has evolved to achieve this homeostatic regulation.

This chapter focuses on the chemosensors and mechanoreceptors of the respiratory control system. In addition, the integrated responses of the respiratory control system to several major pathophysiologic derangements are considered.

OVERVIEW OF THE RESPIRATORY CONTROL SYSTEM

As with many physiologic control systems, that governing respiration is organized as a negative feedback loop (Fig. 16-1). Inspired gas flows through airways to the alveoli, where it participates in gas exchange at the alveolar–capillary membrane (see Chap. 9). Sensors detect information about mechanical events (e.g., lung inflation) and chemical parameters (e.g., prevailing Pao_2 and $Paco_2$). This information is integrated in a *central controller* in the medulla that modulates neural output to motoneurons innervating the respiratory muscles. Coordinated firing of respiratory motoneurons results in synchronous contraction of the respiratory muscles, generating airflow.

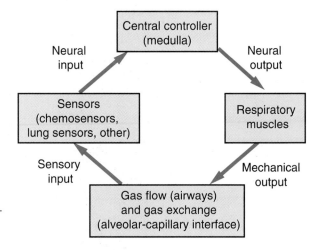

Figure 16-1. The respiratory control system as a negative feedback loop. See text for description.

When chemical perturbations like hypoxia or hypercapnia are sensed, signals to the controller eventuate in increased neural output to the respiratory motoneurons and a rise in minute ventilation. Arterial hypocapnia produces a decrease in ventilation.

CHEMICAL CONTROL OF RESPIRATION

The respiratory system maintains adequate levels of O_2 in arterial blood in support of the metabolic activity of peripheral tissues and prevents the accumulation of CO_2 arising from that activity. Highly specialized tissues monitor the O_2 level in arterial blood and the CO_2 level in a richly perfused organ, the brain. These two separate sensing mechanisms allow for rapid ventilatory responses to alterations in gas exchange.

CENTRAL CHEMORECEPTORS

Of the several chemosensors that monitor gas exchange, the responsibility for detecting alterations in CO_2 homeostasis rests primarily with the *central chemoreceptors*. Although neurons whose firing rates and excitability are modulated by alterations in P_{CO_2} are found in many regions of the central nervous system, cells with these properties, which relay information to the respiratory controller, have been localized to the medulla.

The central chemoreceptors may reside near the ventral medullary surface, where the hypoglossal nerve rootlets exit the brain stem. Although their exact location, neural connectivity, and neurochemistry are unknown, the chemosensitive cells appear to be distinct from nearby neurons that contribute to respiratory rhythmogenesis and constitute the central controller.

The chemosensitive cells respond to alterations in $[H^+]$ and P_{CO_2} in the extracellular fluid of the intracerebral interstitial space. In the past, measurements on cerebrospinal fluid were used as an approximation of the chemistry of the intracerebral interstitial space. More recently, application of sensitive pH electrodes has shown that increases in minute ventilation are closely coupled to corresponding elevations in $[H^+]$ of extracellular fluid, not cerebrospinal fluid.

As local [H$^+$] increases (equivalent to a fall in pH), central chemoreceptors signal the central controller to increase ventilation. Alterations in extracellular [H$^+$], however, are not a unique stimulus to the central chemoreceptors. In fact, an increase in minute ventilation in response to an isolated elevation in extracellular fluid [H$^+$], in the absence of changes in Pco_2 (isocapnic metabolic acidosis), evolves more slowly. In addition, the response is smaller in magnitude (Fig. 16-2) than that elicited solely by an elevation in Pco_2 (respiratory acidosis).

One explanation for the rapidity of the ventilatory response to hypercapnia is the ease with which CO$_2$ diffuses across the blood–brain barrier. In contrast, the blood–brain barrier is relatively impermeable to the ionic species, H$^+$ and HCO$_3$$^-$. Furthermore, an elevated Pco_2 produces vasodilation, particularly in the cerebral circulation, thereby promoting diffusion of CO$_2$ across the blood–brain barrier. Hence, diffusion of CO$_2$ represents another primary transduction mechanism for relaying alterations in acid–base status to the central chemoreceptors.

In respiratory acidosis, the elevated Paco_2 produces an increase in CO$_2$ diffusion across the blood–brain barrier. The elevated CO$_2$ results in an increase in [H$^+$] around the central chemoreceptors, which detect the change and signal the central controller to increase ventilation, compensating for the respiratory acidosis. Because the ventilatory response to a CO$_2$-induced increase in [H$^+$] in the extracellular fluid is greater than the response to an identical alteration in [H$^+$] produced in the absence of an increase in Pco_2 (see Fig. 16-2), Pco_2 and [H$^+$] must represent *independent* stimuli to the central chemoreceptors. At a molecular level, whether [H$^+$] and Pco_2 constitute different stimuli to a single sensor mechanism, or individual stimuli to different sensor mechanisms, remains unknown.

Finally, because acidification of the cerebral interstitial fluid is an important step in central chemoreception, important factors affecting this process should be noted.

Unlike blood, cerebral interstitial fluid contains very little protein. Without the buffering capacity of protein, pH shifts in the intracerebral, extracellular

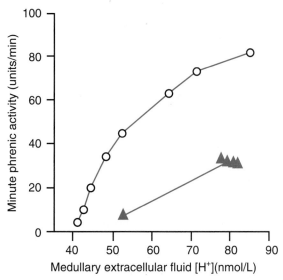

Figure 16-2. Relationship between medullary extracellular fluid [H$^+$] and respiration, measured as firing frequency or "minute activity" of the phrenic nerve. Medullary extracellular fluid [H$^+$] was elevated by creation of a respiratory acidosis (open circles) or metabolic acidosis from HCl infusion (closed triangles). The ventilatory response is greater to hypercapnia than to metabolic acidosis, despite a similar alteration in medullary extracellular fluid [H$^+$]. (From Eldridge FL, Kiley JP, Millhorn DE. Respiratory responses to medullary hydrogen ion changes in cats: Different effects of respiratory and metabolic acidoses. J Physiol 358:285–297, 1985.)

fluid occur more rapidly than in blood. In addition, the compensatory ventilatory response to chronic acidification of the cerebral extracellular fluid (as is seen in chronic hypercapnia) is more rapid than that of the blood. Movement of HCO_3^- from the blood, across the blood–brain barrier, into the cerebral interstitial fluid occurs within 24 to 48 hours. In contrast, renal retention of HCO_3^- in response to plasma acidification requires 48 to 72 hours.

THE CAROTID BODIES

Whereas monitoring of P_{CO_2} occurs in the brain stem, sensing of P_{O_2} occurs exclusively in the *carotid bodies* (Fig. 16-3). The carotid bodies are located at the bifurcation of each of the common carotid arteries into the internal and external carotids (see Fig. 16-3A). Despite their tiny size, the carotid bodies have an enormous blood flow, estimated at 1.4 to 2.0 L/minute/100 g of tissue; this large flow is consistent with the organs' critical role as the primary oxygen sensor.

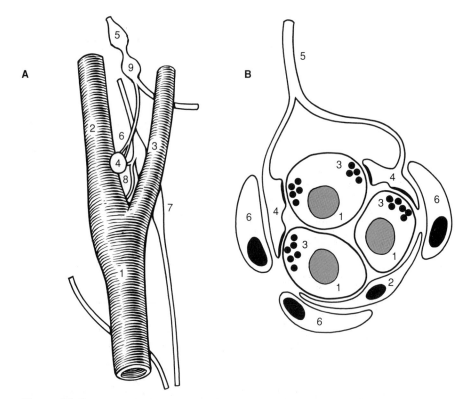

Figure 16-3. Carotid body. **(A)** Frontal view of right carotid artery bifurcation. Common carotid artery (1) divides into the internal (2) and external (3) carotid arteries. The carotid body (4) is innervated by sensory fibers originating in the petrosal ganglion (5) and travelling through the carotid sinus nerve (6). The superior cervical ganglion (7) also innervates the carotid body, by way of the ganglioglomerular nerves (8). The nodose ganglion (9) is external to the internal carotid artery. **(B)** Carotid body cell cluster, consisting of chemoreceptor (1) and sustentacular (2) cells. Chemoreceptor cells have, in their cytoplasm, synaptic vesicles (3), which are usually located near contacts with sensory nerve endings (4) originating from branching fibers of the carotid sinus nerve (5). Capillaries (6) surround the clusters. (From González C, Almaraz L, Obeso A, Rigual R. Oxygen and acid chemoreception in the carotid body chemoreceptors. Trends in Neuroscience 154:146–153, 1992.)

Cell Types in the Carotid Body

The carotid bodies are composed of several cell types (see Fig. 16-3B). The primary cell is the *glomus cell* (type I cell), which contains several neurotransmitters, including large quantities of dopamine and other catecholamines, serotonin, acetylcholine, and several neuropeptides. Glomus cells are considered the actual chemosensing cells.

Groups of glomus cells are enveloped by *sustentacular cells* (type II cells); usually, there are three to six glomus cells per sustentacular cell. The physiologic role of the sustentacular cells is unknown, but the cells are thought to be related ultrastructurally and functionally to the glia of the central nervous system. Groups of glomus cells, surrounded by sustentacular cells, are enmeshed in a rich network of capillaries, providing an optimal arrangement for oxygen chemosensation.

Carotid Body Function

Glomus cells form synapses with afferent fibers of the *carotid sinus nerve.* A sensory branch of the glossopharyngeal nerve, the carotid sinus nerve innervates the carotid body and carotid sinus baroreceptors. Glossopharyngeal afferents originate mainly in sensory neurons of the petrosal ganglion. In response to arterial hypoxia, glomus cells release dopamine in proportion to the decrement in Pao_2. Dopamine release is modulated by alterations in pH produced by metabolic or respiratory acidosis and produces a large increase in the tonic activity of carotid body sensory afferents. These afferent fibers demonstrate some degree of tonic activity under normoxic, or even hyperoxic, conditions; they are silenced only in the presence of marked arterial hyperoxia and hypocapnia (Fig. 16-4).

When Pao_2 falls below 60 mmHg, activity of the carotid body afferents increases exponentially (see Fig. 16-4A). Because the firing rate of a single carotid body afferent fiber is 5 to 25 impulses per second, the carotid body responds quickly to changes in Pao_2 occurring within or between individual breaths.

The critical role of the carotid body in regulation of oxygenation is highlighted by total abolition of the hypoxic ventilatory response in humans after bilateral resection or denervation of the carotid body. In some nonhuman species, similar oxygen-sensing organs are also present in the aortic arch. These *aortic bodies* have a response that is functionally similar to that of the carotid bodies.

In contrast to its critical role in oxygen sensing, the carotid body contributes relatively little to the ventilatory response to changes in $Paco_2$. Although the firing rate of carotid body afferents clearly varies with $Paco_2$ (see Fig. 16-4B), additional afferent activity in response to metabolic or respiratory stimuli does not augment elevations in minute ventilation produced by the central chemoreceptors. Furthermore, carotid body denervation reduces the ventilatory response to elevation in $Paco_2$ by less than 20%, providing additional evidence that the carotid body plays a minor role in mediating the ventilatory response to acidosis.

NEURAL CONTROL OF RESPIRATION

The central respiratory controller also receives proprioceptive and nociceptive stimuli from the lungs. This information is relayed by pulmonary vagal

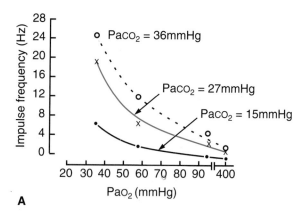

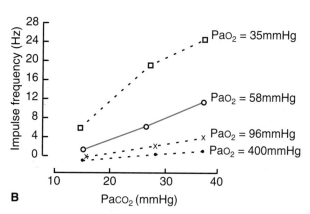

Figure 16-4. Carotid body activity, as a function of PaO_2 or $PaCO_2$. (A) Activity of a single carotid body afferent fiber versus PaO_2 at three different levels of $PaCO_2$. (B) Activity of a single carotid body afferent fiber versus $PaCO_2$ at four different levels of PaO_2. (From Cherniack NS, Pack AI. Control of ventilation. In: Fishman AP, ed. Pulmonary Diseases and Disorders. New York: McGraw-Hill, 1988:133. [Figure is replotted data from Lahiri S, DeLaney R. Respir Physiol 24:249–266, 1975].)

afferents whose cell bodies lie in the *nodose ganglion*. The sensory terminals of these vagal afferents terminate at various loci within the lung, whereas the central endings synapse in the *nucleus of the solitary tract* within the medulla. Major categories of pulmonary vagal afferents include: (1) slowly adapting stretch receptors, (2) rapidly adapting receptors, and (3) C-fibers.

SLOWLY ADAPTING STRETCH RECEPTORS

Slowly adapting stretch receptors are an important group of pulmonary *mechanoreceptors*. These vagal afferents consist of large, myelinated fibers, whose sensory terminals lie within airway smooth muscle. The discharge rate of slowly adapting stretch receptors increases with lung inflation (Fig. 16-5). During maintained inflation, receptor activity persists, albeit at a minimally reduced rate (see Fig. 16-5A), providing continued input to the central controller regarding the lung's inflation status. The slowly adapting stretch receptors have an important physiologic role in the *Hering-Breuer reflexes,* which terminate inspiration and prolong expiration.

Rapid inflation of the lung during *inspiration* increases the firing rates of slowly adapting stretch receptors, which ultimately leads to termination of the inspiration. Under experimental conditions, rapid lung inflation during (neural) *expiration* increases stretch receptor firing rates, thereby prolonging the expiratory phase and inhibiting the onset of the next inspiration. Therefore, progres-

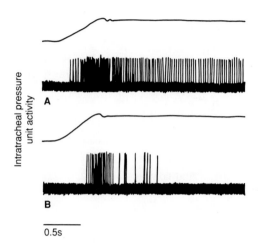

Figure 16-5. Responses of two different types of pulmonary vagal afferents to maintained lung inflation. In each panel, the upper tracing represents lung inflation measured by intratracheal pressure; the lower tracing represents unit activity over time. **(A)** Slowly adapting stretch receptor. **(B)** Rapidly adapting receptor. (From Knowlton GC, Larrabee MG. A unitary analysis of pulmonary volume receptors. Am J Physiol 147: 100–114, 1946.)

sive lung inflation *shortens* inspiration and *lengthens* expiration, depending on when the inflation occurs in the neural respiratory cycle.

The Hering-Breuer reflexes may be operative when tidal volumes are greater than 1 L (e.g., in exercising adults), but not during resting tidal ventilation. Furthermore, these reflexes may be more important for respiratory timing in newborns than in adults.

Lung denervation, such as that produced with bilateral lung transplantation, has relatively little effect on respiratory control, although increases in tidal volume may be demonstrated (Fig. 16-6). This finding is consistent with loss of volume-related feedback to the central controller.

RAPIDLY ADAPTING RECEPTORS

Rapidly adapting receptors, also known as *irritant receptors,* constitute a second major category of lung mechanoreceptors. The sensory terminals of these large, myelinated vagal afferent fibers lie between airway epithelial cells. Rapidly adapting receptors are stimulated by inhaled noxious compounds, such as dust, certain gases, and cold air. They also respond to lung inflation, but their firing rates quickly decrease during maintained inflation (see Fig. 16-5B)—hence, the designation, "rapidly adapting." In addition, stimulation of rapidly adapting receptors produces bronchoconstriction and tachypnea, resulting in rapid, shallow breathing. Stimulation of these receptors is an important mechanism for cough and tachycardia and may be clinically significant in the pathogenesis of asthma and reactive airway disease (see Chap. 5).

C-FIBERS

Classification and Activity

The third major group of lung mechanoreceptors are the *C-fibers*—small, nonmyelinated fibers that are slowly conducting vagal afferents. C-fibers terminate in the lung parenchyma, airways, and blood vessels. Therefore, they are accessible to mediators present in capillary or bronchial arterial blood.

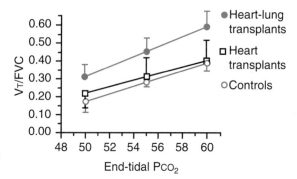

Figure 16-6. Relationship between tidal volume (adjusted for forced vital capacity) and end-tidal CO_2 during hypercapnic gas inhalation in healthy subjects (open circles), heart transplant recipients (open squares), and heart–lung transplant recipients (filled circles). Lung denervation in heart–lung transplantation is associated with an increase in tidal volume at rest and during periods of increased minute ventilation, consistent with loss of inhibitory volume-related feedback to the central controller. (From Duncan SR, Kagawa FT, Vaughn AS, Theodore J. Hypercarbic ventilatory responses of human heart–lung transplant recipients. Am Rev Respir Dis 144:126–130, 1991.)

There are two types of C-fibers: *pulmonary C-fibers* and *bronchial C-fibers.* The pulmonary C-fibers terminate in the lung parenchyma and are stimulated experimentally by substances injected into the pulmonary artery. Bronchial C-fibers terminate in the large airways and blood vessels and are stimulated experimentally by substances injected into the bronchial artery circulation. C-fibers may be activated by exogenous chemicals (e.g., capsaicin or phenyldiguanide) or endogenous substances (e.g., bradykinin).

The activity of C-fibers is independent of the respiratory phase, and C-fibers have little role in normal tidal breathing. The fibers are stimulated by the inhalation of irritants, such as noxious gases or particulates, and by mechanical irritation of the airways. In general, C-fiber activation produces a rapid, shallow breathing pattern, a pattern that appears to limit the dissemination of potentially toxic agents within the tracheobronchial tree. C-fibers may also be important in mediating the sensation of dyspnea in a variety of clinical settings, such as pulmonary edema, pneumonia, or toxic inhalations. Their stimulation produces bradycardia and mucus secretion; the latter may be important in the pathogenesis of obstructive airway disease.

J-receptors

Pulmonary C-fibers include the *J-receptors,* which terminate in the lung parenchyma adjacent to the capillaries (*juxta*capillary) and are stimulated by the development of interstitial edema (see Chap. 14). Activation of J-receptors elicits laryngeal closure and apnea, followed by rapid, shallow breathing. J-receptors may also be important in mediating the sensation of dyspnea, not only in pulmonary edema, but also in pneumonia and pulmonary embolism.

ADDITIONAL RESPIRATORY SENSORS

In addition to central and peripheral chemoreceptors and lung mechanoreceptors, a wide variety of other sensors provide input to the central respiratory controller.

Upper Airway Receptors

Receptors in the nose and upper airway respond to both mechanical and chemical stimuli. These receptors are very similar to the rapidly adapting receptors in the lung parenchyma, and their stimulation produces coughing, sneezing, bronchoconstriction, and laryngeal spasm.

Proprioceptive Afferents

Proprioceptive afferents in peripheral joints and muscles may play an important role in the increased ventilation that occurs with exercise. Similarly, muscle spindle organs and gamma motoneurons may play a role in the control of respiratory muscles.

Muscle Spindles

Muscle spindle organs are critical in regulating the strength of muscle contraction through spinal reflexes; these organs likely play an identical role in regulating the force of respiratory muscle contraction. The one exception to this rule is the diaphragm, the major inspiratory muscle, which has few, if any, muscle spindles. Although dyssynchrony of muscle spindle afferents during respiratory muscle contraction has been suggested as a possible cause of dyspnea, muscle spindles may be more important in the generation of maximal expiratory force for clearing airway obstructions.

Visceral and Cutaneous Sensory Afferents

Finally, visceral and cutaneous sensory afferents also provide information to the central respiratory controller, because both pain and elevation in skin temperature produce hyperventilation.

RESPIRATORY NEURONS AND RESPIRATORY RHYTHMOGENESIS

During wakefulness, respiration may be consciously controlled, as during exercise or speaking. When a subject is asleep or unconscious, however, breathing persists "automatically," in the same way as cardiac and intestinal contractions. The neural circuitry of respiratory control is distinct from that modulating autonomic functions and controlling motor activities.

RESPIRATORY NEUROANATOMY

The broad range of respiratory sensory afferents provides much information to the medullary central controller. In the early 20th century, studies showed that transection of the nervous system at the pontomedullary border did not eliminate spontaneous respiration; however, transection at the medullospinal border did.

Although "automatic" respiration resides in the medulla, voluntary or behaviorally controlled respiration requires medullary integration of signals descending from the cerebral cortex, diencephalon, and other rostral brain structures. Complicated acts like speaking, exercise, and "anticipatory" breathing (e.g., that preceding exercise) are examples of such behaviorally controlled respiration.

The exact neurons responsible for respiratory rhythmogenesis remain controversial. At least three groups of cells have been identified; each is composed of neurons whose timing patterns are closely linked with the respiratory cycle (Fig. 16-7).

One group is located in the *Kölliker-Fuse nucleus* in the rostrolateral pons. These neurons are not essential for automatic respiration, but they probably

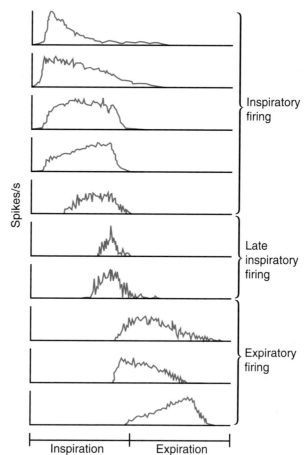

Figure 16-7. Respiratory neuron firing patterns during a respiratory cycle. Each plot represents a typical discharge pattern for an individual brain stem respiratory neuron. Each type of neuron fires in one of three respiratory phases: inspiration, late inspiration, or expiration. The pattern may be one of either incremental or decremental activity during the respiratory phase. (From Feldman JL. Neurophysiology of breathing in mammals. In: Bloom FE, ed. Handbook of Physiology: The Nervous System IV: Intrinsic Regulatory Systems of the Brain. Washington, DC: American Physiological Society, 1986:463–524.)

play a role in adaptation of the respiratory rhythm to physiologic and behavioral activities.

A second group is located in the lateral subdivision of the *nucleus of the solitary tract* in the dorsal medulla. This *dorsal respiratory group* is composed mainly of neurons that fire predominantly during inspiration.

A third group of respiratory neurons lies in the *ventrolateral medulla* near the nucleus ambiguus. This group is composed principally of expiratory neurons. Although the major firing patterns and connectivity among these three groups are known, the exact mechanism of respiratory rhythmogenesis remains controversial.

MECHANISMS OF RESPIRATORY RHYTHMOGENESIS

Two principal theories have been proposed for respiratory rhythmogenesis.

According to one theory, firing of so-called *conditional pacemaker cells* residing in the medulla is synchronized with the phases of the respiratory cycle. Rhythmic activity persists within these cells in the absence of any synaptic inputs, much like the activity of cells constituting components of the cardiac conduction system.

According to the major alternative theory, no single pacemaker nucleus or pacemaker cells exist. Rather, within major clusters of respiratory neurons is a collection of cells whose *pooled* firing patterns produce inspiration and expiration—an *oscillating respiratory network*.

CENTRAL INTEGRATION OF AFFERENT INPUTS

As described, a complex array of sensors provides information about the upper and lower respiratory tracts, gas exchange, and muscle activity. In addition, the respiratory system responds to three clinically important ventilatory stimuli: alterations in Pa_{CO_2} and Pa_{O_2}, and acid–base disturbances.

RESPONSE TO CHANGES IN Pa_{CO_2}

Perhaps the most important factor regulating resting minute ventilation is the level of Pa_{CO_2}, detected by the central chemoreceptors. When a healthy subject breathes in a closed chamber in which expired CO_2 is allowed to accumulate, rebreathing of CO_2 results in a rise in Pa_{CO_2} at a rate of approximately 4 mmHg per minute. If arterial O_2 content is kept constant, minute ventilation increases approximately 2 to 3 L per minute for each 1 mmHg increase in Pa_{CO_2} (Fig. 16-8). Reducing the concentration of O_2 in the inhaled gas mixture (thereby lowering Pa_{O_2}) increases not only the minute ventilation for a given level of Pa_{CO_2}, but also the *slope or rate of increase* in minute ventilation with rising Pa_{CO_2} (synergistic relationship). The respiratory controller detects changes in both Pa_{O_2} and P_{CO_2}, and the combination of hypoxia and hypercapnia produces a greater increase in minute ventilation than either stimulus alone.

Although increases in Pa_{CO_2} produce an increase in minute ventilation, reductions in Pa_{CO_2} are also detected by the central chemoreceptors, resulting in a reduction in the central drive to breathe. Therefore, lowering Pa_{CO_2} (e.g., during mechanical ventilation) may produce a reduction in minute ventilation. Although hyperventilation does not result in apnea in an awake subject, a reduction in Pa_{CO_2} by hyperventilation may produce apnea in a sleeping subject (see Chap. 17). Decreased central chemosensitivity, rather than a decline in the actual level of Pa_{CO_2}, can also produce a decrease in minute ventilation. It is through this mechanism that drugs (e.g., narcotics), increasing age, and athletic training result in a lower minute ventilation, both at rest and in response to inhalation of CO_2-enriched gas mixtures.

When considering the ventilatory responses to hypocapnia and hypercapnia, it is important to distinguish between the "drive to breathe" and the effectiveness of ventilation. For example, breathing through a straw increases the work of breathing. Measurements of the minute ventilatory response to hypercapnic gas mixtures inspired through the straw, however, demonstrate a *reduced* ventilatory response to CO_2, despite the increase in drive to breathe produced by the hypercapnia. Similarly, the minute ventilatory response to a hypercapnic gas mixture is reduced in a wide range of obstructive and restrictive pulmonary diseases, not because of reduced central chemosensitivity, but because of a limitation in the mechanics of ventilation (see Chaps. 2–7).

RESPONSE TO CHANGES IN Pa_{O_2}

In the presence of a normal Pa_{CO_2}, minute ventilation does not increase until Pa_{O_2} is less than 60 mmHg (Fig. 16-9). This observation might be expected

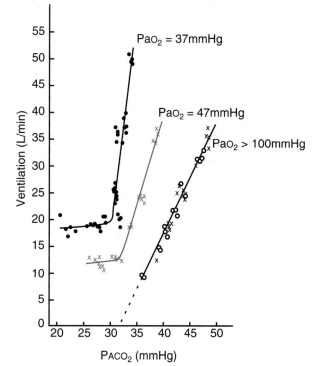

Figure 16-8. Ventilatory response to rebreathing of CO_2 at three different levels of Pa_{O_2}. The slope of the relationship increases with progressive hypoxemia. (From Neilson M, Smith H. Studies on the regulation of respiration in acute hypoxia. With an appendix on respiratory control during prolonged hypoxia. Acta Physiol Scand 24:293–313, 1951.)

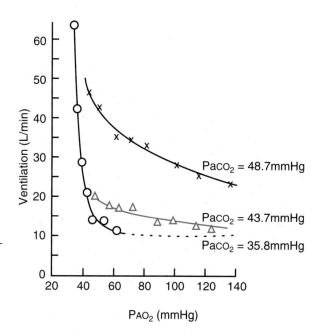

Figure 16-9. Ventilatory response to hypoxia. In the presence of hypocapnia (Pa_{CO_2} = 35.8 mmHg), no ventilatory response occurs until the Pa_{O_2} is less than 60 mmHg. (From Loeschcke HH, Gertz KH. Intracranielle Chemorezeptoren mit Wirkung auf die Atmung. Pflügers Archiv 267:460–477, 1958.)

on the basis of the minimal change in carotid body activity that is seen when Pa_{O_2} is greater than 60 mmHg. As is evident from the previously described studies of the integrated respiratory response to hypercapnia, elevations in Pa_{CO_2} increase minute ventilation at any given Pa_{O_2}. During activities of daily life, hypoxia does not play an important role in stimulating minute ventilation in healthy adults. The ventilatory response to hypoxia, however, becomes critically important in certain environments, such as high altitude, or in the hypoxia resulting from respiratory diseases. The ventilatory response to hypoxia may play an important role in maintaining gas exchange and homeostasis in a wide variety of diseases of the lung parenchyma, airways, pulmonary vasculature, and chest bellows.

RESPONSE TO METABOLIC ACIDOSIS AND METABOLIC ALKALOSIS

As discussed in Chapter 10, H^+ and HCO_3^- are in equilibrium with H_2O and CO_2 in the blood. An increase in $[H^+]$ (e.g., lactic acidosis) shifts the equilibrium and increases Pa_{CO_2}. Hence, there are two independent drives to increase minute ventilation: increased $[H^+]$ and increased Pa_{CO_2}.

During pure metabolic acidosis, however, an elevated Pa_{CO_2} is observed only if V_D/V_T and minute ventilation remain constant. The increase in $[H^+]$ in metabolic acidosis causes hyperventilation as compensation for the pH changes; consequently, Pa_{CO_2} is reduced.

In contrast to metabolic acidosis, the respiratory compensation for metabolic alkalosis—hypoventilation—is relatively weak and highly variable among subjects.

SELECTED READING

Eldridge FL, Kiley JP, Millhorn DE. Respiratory responses to medullary hydrogen ion changes in cats: Different effects of respiratory and metabolic acidoses. J Physiol 358:285–297, 1985.

Feldman JL. Neurophysiology of breathing in animals. In Bloom FE, ed. Handbook of Physiology: The Nervous System IV: Intrinsic Regulatory Systems of the Brain. Washington, DC: American Physiological Society, 1986:463–524.

González C, Almaraz L, Obeso A, Rigual R. Oxygen and acid chemoreception in the carotid body chemoreceptors. Trends in Neurosciences 15:146–153, 1992.

Richter DW, Ballantyne D, Remmers J. How is the respiratory rhythm generated? A model. News in Physiologic Sciences 1:109–112, 1986.

Lippincott's Pathophysiology Series: Pulmonary Pathophysiology, edited by Michael A. Grippi. J. B. Lippincott Company, Philadelphia © 1995.

Control of Respiration During Sleep

Richard J. Schwab

The principles of chemical and neural control of respiration discussed in Chapter 16 do not take into account variations in the "state" of the subject. So-called "state dependence" of physiologic control mechanisms is an important consideration in respiration, and sleep constitutes the most notable special state.

Although we spend up to one third of our lives sleeping, relatively little is known about the function of sleep or its role in health and disease. A number of physiologic alterations in the control and mechanics of breathing characterize sleep. These sleep-induced changes may disrupt normal sleep and contribute to the pathogenesis of cardiopulmonary disease, including the development of hypoxemia, alveolar hypoventilation, pulmonary hypertension, and cor pulmonale. In addition, many disorders, including asthma (see Chap. 5), chronic obstructive pulmonary disease (see Chap. 6), restrictive lung diseases (see Chap. 7), and cardiovascular diseases may become worse during the night secondary to changes in the control of ventilation during sleep.

This chapter presents an overview of sleep and accompanying physiologic changes in the control of respiration. In addition, two clinically important disorders of respiratory control are highlighted—central and obstructive sleep apnea.

PHYSIOLOGY OF SLEEP

Although sleep appears to be a passive condition, it is actually an amalgam of complex processes and profound physiologic changes. Two distinct states characterize normal sleep: (1) *nonrapid eye movement (NREM) sleep,* also known as quiet or slow-wave sleep; and (2) *rapid eye movement (REM) sleep,* also known as paradoxical or active sleep. Each is characterized by unique physiologic and electroencephalographic (EEG) hallmarks.

Sleep onset is characterized by NREM sleep, which, according to EEG criteria, is divided into four stages (Fig. 17-1). Each successive stage represents a deeper stage of sleep; the arousal threshold is lowest in stage 1 and highest in stage 4 (delta sleep). Normally, on falling asleep a human adult passes successively through stages 1 through 4, entering stage 4 approximately 35 minutes after sleep onset (Fig. 17-2). Periods of REM sleep punctuate repetitive cycling through stages 1 through 4 of NREM sleep. NREM sleep comprises 75% to 80% of total sleep time.

REM sleep is characterized by increased metabolic activity of the central

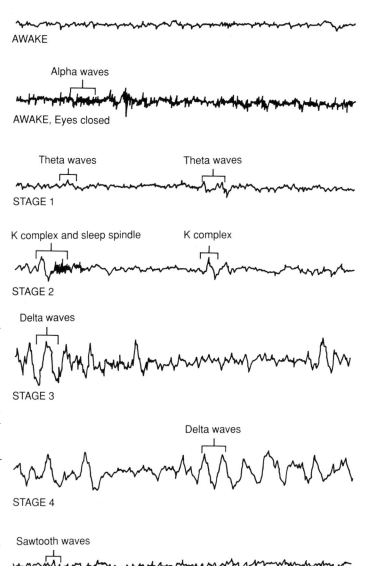

Figure 17-1. Polysomnographic tracings showing EEG patterns in wakefulness, NREM sleep (stages 1–4), and REM sleep. Characteristic wave patterns for each stage are noted. K complexes are large waves, lasting a minimum of 0.5 second; they consist of an upward deflection followed by a downward deflection. K complexes are characteristic of stage 2 sleep and are usually triggered by a defined stimulus, such as noise. Sleep spindles, also characteristic of stage 2 sleep, are intermittent bursts of activity in the range of 12 to 14 cycles per second that last for a minimum of 0.5 second. (From Schwab RJ, Getsy JE, Pack AI. Central nervous system failure including sleep disorders. In: Carlson RW, Geheb MA, eds. The Principles and Practice of Medical Intensive Care. Philadelphia: WB Saunders, 1993:775.)

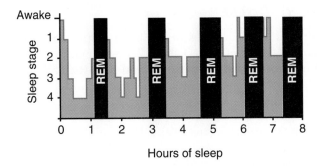

Figure 17-2. Cycling of sleep stages in a healthy young subject. NREM sleep predominates in the first one third of the night; REM sleep becomes more prominent in the last one third of the night. Time intervals between REM periods shorten as the night progresses. NREM sleep comprises 75% to 80% of sleep, whereas REM sleep comprises 20% to 25%.

nervous system and is the stage when dreaming principally occurs. REM sleep is characterized by episodic rapid eye movements and EEG activity that is similar to that in wakefulness (see Fig. 17-1). The rapid eye movements are associated with increased central neuron activity. This activity does not usually result in peripheral movements, however, because there is active suppression of motoneuron activity in REM sleep (muscle atonia). Periodic, "phasic" twitching of the extremities in REM sleep may be seen.

As noted, REM alternates with NREM sleep throughout the night in a cyclical fashion. Cycles of REM sleep occur approximately every 90 to 110 minutes and typically last 10 to 30 minutes. As the night progresses, REM cycles lengthen (see Fig. 17-2). REM sleep comprises approximately 20% to 25% of total sleep time, occurring in four to six discrete episodes during the night.

OVERALL CONTROL OF RESPIRATION DURING SLEEP

The control of respiration during sleep in healthy subjects and in patients with sleep-related respiratory disorders is a complicated process. Respiration is believed to be controlled by a *central respiratory pattern generator,* situated in the medulla. The primary function of this respiratory center is maintenance of respiratory homeostasis, that is, preservation of normal arterial blood gases. The respiratory center receives information from three areas: (1) higher cortical centers, (2) mechanical receptors in the chest wall and lung, and (3) central and peripheral chemoreceptors (see Chap. 16).

The higher cortical centers may override the central respiratory pattern generator, and cortical inputs may affect ventilation during wakefulness (e.g., anxiety can cause hyperventilation). Similarly, during dreaming, the cortical centers may have a significant impact on medullary respiratory neurons.

As noted in Chapter 16, receptors in the chest wall and lung provide information to the respiratory center. Pulmonary receptors, including stretch, rapidly adapting, and C-fiber receptors, are affected by a variety of stimuli, including lung inflation, lung deflation, and inhalation of noxious agents. Stimulation of rapidly adapting and C-fiber receptors results in rapid, shallow breathing secondary to decreases in tidal volume and inspiratory time.

Finally, the central pattern generator also receives input from the carotid body, the major peripheral chemoreceptor that senses primarily changes in Pa_{O_2}. The carotid body responds quickly to changes in Pa_{O_2} and is responsible for the increase in ventilation during hypoxia. Changes in P_{CO_2} and pH are sensed principally by the medullary chemoreceptors (see Chap. 16).

BREATHING PATTERN DURING SLEEP

Several important physiologic consequences of sleep on respiration are sleep stage-dependent (Table 17-1). As noted in Table 17-1 and Figure 17-3, the normal breathing pattern may be periodic in stages 1 and 2, particularly in elderly subjects; however, the pattern becomes regular in stages 3 and 4. The mechanisms underlying these ventilatory oscillations during the lighter stages of NREM sleep are unknown.

In REM sleep, the pattern of respiration is distinctly irregular. A small number of apneas may be observed, even in healthy subjects. The irregularity is most pronounced during flurries of rapid eye movements, with hypoventilation well documented during periods of dense rapid eye movements. The variability not only affects the timing of inspiration and expiration, but also the amplitude of the ventilatory movements (Fig. 17-4). The irregular breathing pattern appears to be centrally mediated, because the irregularities persist despite manipulations of afferent stimuli, such as induction of hypoxia or hypercapnia, carotid body resection, or vagotomy.

VENTILATORY PARAMETERS DURING SLEEP

A number of ventilatory parameters are predictably altered during sleep. Several have significant physiologic consequences, particularly in patients with underlying lung disease. Most notable are changes in alveolar ventilation and accompanying changes in arterial blood gases, oxygen consumption, upper airway resistance, and lung volume.

Alveolar Ventilation

Alveolar ventilation decreases during sleep primarily because of a decrease in tidal volume. As a result, $PaCO_2$ increases and PaO_2 decreases (see Table 17-1; Fig. 17-5). The hypercapnia and hypoxemia are more significant in REM than NREM sleep (Figs. 17-5 and 17-6).

The ventilatory response to hypoxia and to hypercapnia is reduced during

TABLE 17-1. *EFFECTS OF SLEEP ON NORMAL RESPIRATION**

RESPIRATORY VARIABLE	NREM SLEEP	REM SLEEP
Breathing pattern	Periodic in stages 1 & 2; regular in stages 3 & 4	Irregular, with or without apneas
Arterial oxygen tension	↓ (3–10 mmHg)	↓ ↓
Arterial carbon dioxide tension	↑ (2–8 mmHg)	↑ ↑
Alveolar ventilation	↓	↓ ↓
Tidal volume	↓	↓ ↓
Hypoxic ventilatory response	↓	↓ ↓
Hypercapnic ventilatory response	↓	↓ ↓
Oxygen consumption	↓ ↓ (15%–25%)	↓
Upper airway resistance	↑	↑ ↑

NREM, nonrapid eye movement; REM, rapid eye movement.
*Changes compared to wakefulness.

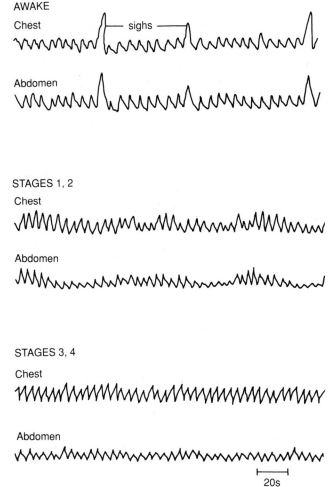

Figure 17-3. Breathing pattern in a healthy elderly subject during wakefulness and NREM sleep, assessed using respiratory inductance plethysmography (RIP). RIP is a noninvasive technique used to measure chest wall and abdominal wall excursion; changes in the electrical inductance of elastic bands encircling the rib cage and abdomen are converted into volume measurements. Except for intermittent sighs, during wakefulness the ventilatory pattern is regular. Periodic breathing is noted in stages 1 and 2, but regular breathing occurs in stages 3 and 4. (From Pack AI, Kline LR, Hendricks JC, Morrison AR. Control of respiration during sleep. In: Fishman AP, ed. Pulmonary Diseases and Disorders. New York: McGraw-Hill, 1988:146.)

sleep compared with the awake state. Reductions are greater in REM than NREM sleep (Figs. 17-7 and 17-8). Although diaphragm activity is also reduced in REM sleep, the activity is adequate to maintain ventilation.

Upper Airway Resistance

Upper airway resistance is also increased in sleep—a major contributing factor to the reduction in minute ventilation. The upper airway dilator muscles become hypotonic or atonic during REM sleep. As a consequence, upper airway resistance increases significantly.

Oxygen Consumption

In healthy subjects, O_2 consumption decreases by 15% to 25% during sleep. O_2 consumption appears to be greater in REM than NREM sleep, but this finding may be more dependent on circadian rhythm than on sleep stage.

Lung Volume

During REM sleep, chest wall muscle atonia causes a decrease in functional residual capacity (FRC), which, in turn, results in ventilation–perfusion mismatching (see Chap. 13).

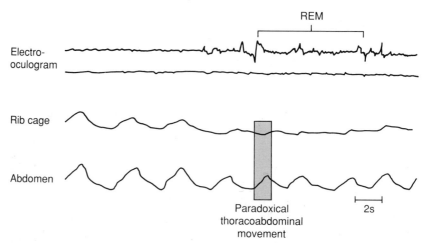

Figure 17-4. Breathing pattern in a healthy young subject during REM sleep, assessed using respiratory inductance plethysmography. The electrooculogram demonstrates phasic rapid eye movements characteristic of REM sleep. During REM sleep, irregularities in timing and amplitude of ventilatory movements are noted. In this example, respiration becomes paradoxical (i.e., the rib cage moves *inward* when the abdomen moves outward). (From Pack AI, Kline LR, Hendricks JC, Morrison AR. Control of respiration during sleep. In: Fishman AP, ed. Pulmonary Diseases and Disorders. New York: McGraw-Hill, 1988:150.)

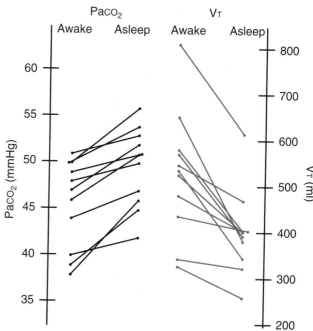

Figure 17-5. Comparison of changes in $Paco_2$ and tidal volume (V_T) in wakefulness and sleep. Tidal volume decreases and $Paco_2$ increases during sleep. (From Birchfield RI, Sieker HO, Heyman A. Alterations in respiratory function during natural sleep. *J Lab Clin Med* 54:216–222, 1959.)

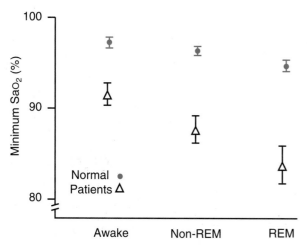

Figure 17-6. Changes in arterial O_2 saturation during wakefulness, NREM sleep, and REM sleep in healthy subjects and patients with cystic fibrosis. The mean arterial O_2 saturation is lower in REM than NREM sleep in both groups. The mean arterial O_2 saturation is highest during wakefulness. (From Muller NL, Francis PW, Gurwitz D, Levison H, Bryan AC. Mechanism of hemoglobin desaturation during rapid-eye-movement sleep in normal subjects and in patients with cystic fibrosis. Am Rev Respir Dis 121:463–469, 1980.)

Effects in Disease States

In general, these sleep-related physiologic changes in ventilatory parameters do not have major clinical significance in healthy subjects. In patients with underlying pulmonary diseases, however, they may have important implications. Studies have demonstrated significant hypoxemia and hypercapnia associated with REM and NREM sleep in patients with cystic fibrosis, chronic obstructive pulmonary disease (see Chap. 6), and idiopathic pulmonary fibrosis (see Chap. 7).

Patients with these disorders also have blunted responses to hypoxia and

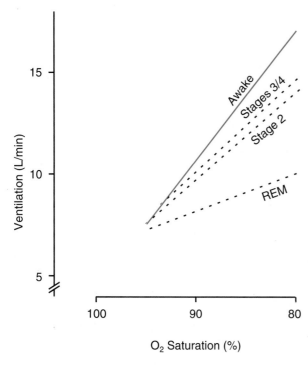

Figure 17-7. Ventilatory response to hypoxia during wakefulness and sleep in healthy subjects. The hypoxic ventilatory response is lowest in REM sleep and highest during wakefulness. (Figure modified from Douglas NJ. Control of ventilation during sleep. Clin Chest Med 6:563–572, 1985.)

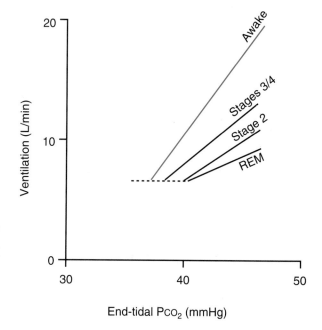

Figure 17-8. Ventilatory response to hypercapnia during wakefulness and sleep in healthy subjects. The hypercapnic ventilatory response is lowest in REM sleep and highest during wakefulness. (Figure modified from Douglas NJ. Control of ventilation during sleep. Clin Chest Med 6:563–572, 1985.)

hypercapnia during sleep, which contribute to the development of nocturnal respiratory acidosis (see Chap. 10). A decline of 10% to 35% in arterial hemoglobin saturation during sleep may occur in patients with chronic obstructive pulmonary disease (COPD). Many patients may not be hypoxemic during wakefulness; however, they readily desaturate during sleep because hemoglobin saturation lies near the inflection point on the oxyhemoglobin dissociation curve (Fig. 17-9). Hypoxemic episodes are especially significant during REM sleep. Therefore, patients with COPD or, for that matter, any type of chronic respiratory disease, are at risk for significant gas exchange abnormalities during sleep.

HEMODYNAMIC CHANGES DURING SLEEP

Physiologic changes in the circulation during sleep may be significant; selected examples are listed in Table 17-2. In general, blood pressure is reduced during NREM sleep and fluctuates considerably during REM sleep. At times, blood pressure during REM sleep may be elevated over that in wakefulness.

Pulmonary artery pressure increases during sleep, but systemic vascular resistance decreases. Heart rate also decreases by 5% to 10% during NREM sleep, with considerable variability during REM sleep. Similarly, cardiac output decreases in NREM sleep and is variable in REM sleep.

These hemodynamic changes are unlikely to be significant in healthy subjects; however, they may be important in hypotensive patients and in patients with disorders characterized by low cardiac output.

SLEEP APNEA SYNDROMES

Sleep apnea is a disorder originally identified in the 1960s when investigators noted repetitive pauses in breathing during sleep in patients complaining of

Normal

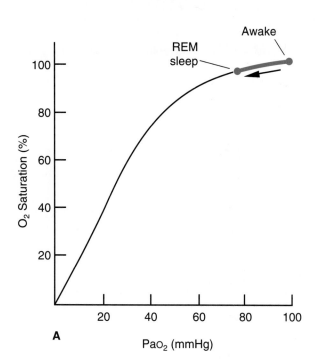

A

Lung disease
(COPD or interstitial)

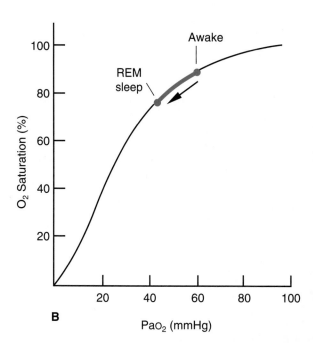

B

Figure 17-9. Oxyhemoglobin dissociation curve during wakefulness and sleep in healthy subjects **(A)** and in patients with lung disease **(B)**. Hypoventilation during REM sleep in patients with lung disease results in hypoxemia. These patients may not be hypoxemic during wakefulness; however, they may readily desaturate during sleep because hemoglobin saturation lies near the inflection point of the curve. (From Pack AI, Kline LR, Hendricks JC, Morrison AR. Control of respiration during sleep. In: Fishman AP, ed. Pulmonary Diseases and Disorders. New York: McGraw-Hill, 1988:153.)

TABLE 17-2.   *NORMAL HEMODYNAMIC CHANGES DURING SLEEP**

HEMODYNAMIC VARIABLE	NREM SLEEP	REM SLEEP
Blood pressure	↓ (10%–15%)	Variable; blood pressure higher than in NREM
Heart rate	↓ (5%–10%)	Variable or resting level
Cardiac output	↓ (10%)	Variable or decreased
Systemic vascular resistance	↓	↓
Pulmonary artery pressure	↑	↑

NREM, nonrapid eye movement; REM, rapid eye movement.
*Changes compared to wakefulness.

excessive daytime sleepiness. *Apnea* is defined as the cessation of breathing for more than 10 seconds. *Hypopnea* is defined as a decrement in airflow (of the order of 50%) associated with a 4% drop in hemoglobin saturation or an EEG "arousal." Both apneas and hypopneas contribute to the *respiratory disturbance index* (RDI), defined as the number of apneas plus hypopneas per hour of sleep. An RDI greater than 15 is diagnostic of sleep apnea. Apneas during sleep may be obstructive, central, or mixed. Mixed apneas have features of both central and obstructive apneas.

CENTRAL SLEEP APNEA

Central sleep apnea is defined as repeated episodes of apnea during sleep *in the absence of respiratory muscle effort.* The pathogenesis is based on abolition of central drive to the respiratory pump muscles. Recurrent episodes of hypoxia, hypercapnia, and acidemia occur during the apneas.

Central sleep apnea may be idiopathic; however, it is associated with a number of neurologic disorders that affect the central respiratory control centers (e.g., autonomic dysfunction, neuromuscular disease, bulbar poliomyelitis, myasthenia gravis, encephalitis, and brain stem infarction). The clinical features range from sleep fragmentation and daytime sleepiness to end-stage pulmonary hypertension and right heart failure (see Chap. 12). The diagnosis of central sleep apnea is based on polysomnography, which demonstrates recurrent episodes of apnea without chest wall or abdominal wall movement (Fig. 17-10).

Treatment strategies for patients with central sleep apnea include administration of supplemental O_2 and nasal continuous positive airway pressure (CPAP; see later). Although CPAP is reasonable first-line therapy, the mechanism by which CPAP corrects central apneas remains unclear. In patients with severe central sleep apnea, treatment is directed toward correcting nocturnal alveolar hypoventilation by using positive-pressure, noninvasive ventilation delivered through a nasal mask during sleep.

OBSTRUCTIVE SLEEP APNEA

Obstructive sleep apnea syndrome (OSAS) is a common clinical disorder, with a prevalence of at least 2% to 4% in the middle-aged population. It is defined as recurrent episodes of apnea during sleep *caused by upper airway occlusion.*

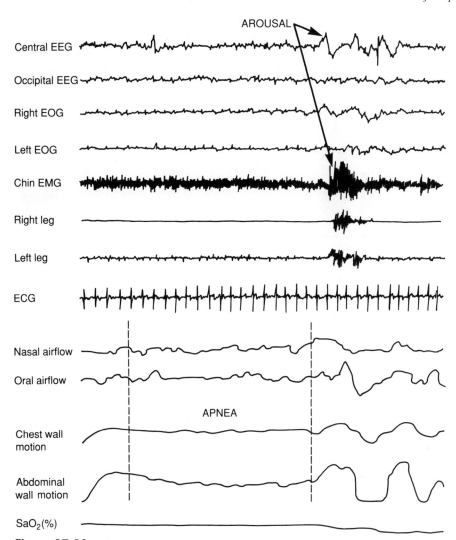

Figure 17-10. Polysomnogram from a patient with central sleep apnea syndrome. Nasal and oral airflows are absent when the chest wall and abdomen are motionless during the apnea. The absence of chest wall and abdominal motion indicates lack of respiratory effort. At the end of the central apnea, an arousal occurs, as noted by an increase in EMG activity. (From Schwab RJ, Getsy JE, Pack AI. Central nervous system failure including sleep disorders. In: Carlson RW, Geheb MA, eds. The Principles and Practice of Medical Intensive Care. Philadelphia: WB Saunders, 1993:777.)

Patients with OSAS show respiratory effort (i.e., chest wall and abdominal wall movement), unlike patients with central sleep apnea in whom there is no respiratory drive. Airflow is absent, however, because of occlusion of the upper airway. The diagnosis of OSAS is based on polysomnography, which demonstrates repeated apneic events, arousals, and hemoglobin desaturations (Fig. 17-11).

The primary determinants of upper airway caliber are the level of activity of the upper airway dilator muscles and the intraluminal pressure. The extrathoracic location of the upper airway exposes it to negative intraluminal pressure during inspiration and positive intraluminal pressure during expiration. During wakefulness, inspiratory activity of the upper airway dilator muscles counterbal-

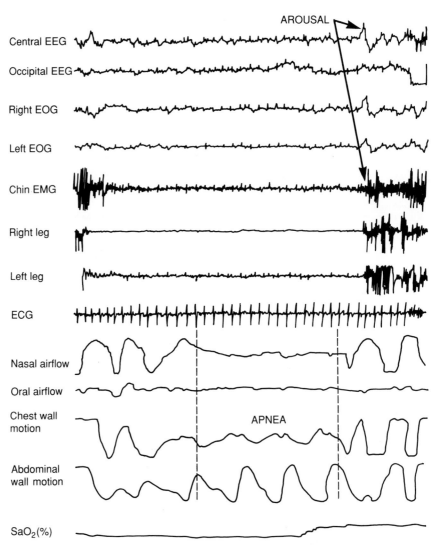

Figure 17-11. Polysomnogram from a patient with obstructive sleep apnea syndrome. Nasal and oral airflow are absent, despite persistent chest wall and abdominal motion during the apnea. Hemoglobin saturation (Sao_2) declines during the apnea. In addition, abdominal and chest wall paradoxical movements are evident. At the end of the apnea, arousal occurs, as noted by an increase in EMG activity. (From Schwab RJ, Getsy JE, Pack AI. Central nervous system failure including sleep disorders. In: Carlson RW, Geheb MA, eds. The Principles and Practice of Medical Intensive Care. Philadelphia: WB Saunders, 1993:778.)

ances the negative intraluminal pressure generated by chest wall muscle contraction (see Chap. 2). Activity of the upper airway dilator muscles decreases during sleep, particularly during REM sleep, a period when obstructive events are often most severe. With the reduction in upper airway dilator muscle activity, negative intraluminal pressure during inspiration may promote upper airway closure.

An obstructive apnea is usually resolved by moving from a deeper stage of sleep (e.g., REM) to a lighter stage (or wakefulness) with an arousal. Upper airway dilator activity is increased by moving to a lighter stage of sleep. The cycle repeats itself as the patient falls back to sleep. This sleep–apnea cycle may occur hundreds of times each night, resulting in repetitive episodes of hemoglobin desaturation and severe sleep fragmentation.

The most common symptoms of OSAS are excessive daytime sleepiness and loud snoring. Witnessed apneic episodes are commonly reported. Patients may fall asleep at inappropriate times, such as in the middle of a conversation or while operating a motor vehicle. Pulmonary hypertension and right heart failure develop in 10% to 15% of patients with severe OSAS.

The treatment of choice for OSAS is nasal CPAP. Nasal CPAP provides a "pneumatic splint" for the airway, preventing collapse during sleep when upper airway dilator muscle activity and airway caliber are reduced.

CLINICAL DISORDERS EXACERBATED DURING SLEEP

In patients with underlying pulmonary or cardiovascular abnormalities, sleep has profound physiologic effects on ventilatory function. Respiratory disturbances during sleep may induce or aggravate a number of pulmonary or cardiovascular disorders. Asthma, chronic obstructive pulmonary disease, restrictive lung disease, coronary artery disease, arrhythmias, and congestive heart failure may be exacerbated during sleep.

ASTHMA

Nocturnal bronchoconstriction is common in asthma, although its cause is unclear. Patients with asthma may manifest nocturnal falls in expiratory airflow rates of 50%. Nocturnal asthma attacks are not related to any specific sleep stage. Patients hospitalized for asthma should be expected to experience drops in expiratory flow rates during sleep. Long-acting bronchodilators may be helpful in minimizing nocturnal bronchoconstriction (see Chap. 5).

CHRONIC OBSTRUCTIVE PULMONARY DISEASE

In patients with COPD, hemoglobin saturation during sleep may fall by 10% to 35% compared with wakefulness (see Fig. 17-9B). Hypoxemia is especially significant during REM sleep. Hypercapnia may also be exacerbated during sleep in patients with COPD; the Pa_{CO_2} is higher in REM than NREM sleep.

Cardiac arrhythmias and ischemia have been reported during periods of nocturnal hypoxemia in patients with COPD. Oxygen administration usually reverses most of these cardiac abnormalities.

Patients with other lung diseases (e.g., cystic fibrosis, interstitial fibrosis, and other restrictive lung disorders) also have been noted to become hypoxemic during sleep. As a general rule, any patient with significant lung disease is at risk for development of nocturnal hypoxemia.

CARDIOVASCULAR DISEASES

Little is known about the interaction of cardiovascular disease and sleep, although cardiac ischemia and arrhythmias often occur during sleep. Nocturnal angina occurs in both REM and NREM sleep, although there is no predominance in any specific sleep stage. Epidemiologic studies have demonstrated an increased risk for myocardial infarction between 6:00 AM and 12:00 noon, but

Figure 17-12. Cheyne-Stokes respiration. Periods of hyperpnea alternate with periods of apnea. Respiration waxes and wanes smoothly in a crescendo–decrescendo pattern. Normally, the hyperpneic phase of Cheyne-Stokes respiration is longer than the apneic phase. (Figure modified from Plum F, Posner JB. The pathologic physiology of signs and symptoms of coma. In: The Diagnosis of Stupor and Coma. 3rd ed. Philadelphia: FA Davis, 1982:34.)

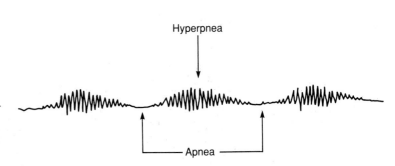

the relationship to sleep physiology remains unclear. The incidence of ventricular arrhythmias has not been correlated with specific sleep stages.

Patients with severe, but stable, congestive heart failure may demonstrate nocturnal hypoxemia, despite normal hemoglobin saturation during wakefulness. Hemoglobin desaturation during sleep has been associated with *Cheyne-Stokes respiration,* a pattern of periodic breathing characterized by episodes of apnea and hypopnea that alternate with hyperpnea (Fig. 17-12). Cheyne-Stokes respiration in patients with congestive heart failure occurs primarily in stages 1 and 2 of NREM sleep; it is rarely found in the deeper stages (delta sleep) or during REM sleep. Hypoxemic episodes in patients with congestive heart failure may exacerbate cardiac dysfunction and disrupt sleep, resulting in frequent nocturnal arousals, fatigue, and daytime hypersomnolence. A reduction in the frequency and severity of nocturnal hypoxemia is achieved with successful treatment. Nasal CPAP and administration of supplemental O_2 may be helpful additions to the standard pharmacologic treatment of congestive heart failure.

SELECTED READING

Bradley TD, Phillipson EA. Central sleep apnea. *Clin Chest Med* 13:481–492, 1992.

Carskadon MA, Dement WA. Normal human sleep: An overview. In: Kryger MH, Roth T, Dement C, eds. Principles and Practice of Sleep Medicine. Philadelphia: WB Saunders, 1989:3–13.

Hudgel DW, Cherniak NS. Sleep and breathing. In: Fishman AP, ed. Update: Pulmonary Diseases and Disorders. New York: McGraw-Hill, 1992:249–261.

Kaplan J, Staats BA. Obstructive sleep apnea. Mayo Clin Proc 65:1087–1094, 1990.

Schwab RJ, Getsy JE, Pack AI. Central nervous system failure including sleep disorders. In: Carlson RW, Geheb MA, eds. The Principles and Practice of Medical Intensive Care. Philadelphia: WB Saunders, 1993:773–786.

Shepard JW Jr. Cardiopulmonary consequences of obstructive sleep apnea. Mayo Clin Proc 65:1250–1259, 1990.

Lippincott's Pathophysiology Series: Pulmonary Pathophysiology, edited by Michael A. Grippi. J. B. Lippincott Company, Philadelphia © 1995.

CHAPTER

18

Pathophysiology of Respiratory Failure

Paul N. Lanken

The preceding chapters focus on selected functional components of the respiratory system. Abnormalities in *any* of these components, including the lung parenchyma, chest wall, pulmonary circulation, alveolar–capillary membrane, or neural or chemical control systems, may result in clinically apparent disease. Through a variety of mechanisms, severe respiratory dysfunction may disrupt homeostasis, with life-threatening consequences.

Respiratory failure, defined broadly as severe impairment of respiratory gas exchange, is categorized as one of two types: *hypercapnic* or *hypoxemic* (Table 18-1). Either may arise acutely or chronically, and each is defined by characteristic changes in arterial blood gases.

HYPERCAPNIC AND HYPOXEMIC RESPIRATORY FAILURE

Hypercapnic respiratory failure is defined as a Pa_{CO_2} greater than 45 mmHg (the upper limit of normal for Pa_{CO_2}). The term "pump failure" has also been used to describe hypercapnic failure; it comprises disorders in which alveolar ventilation is limited relative to the rate of CO_2 production (see section on Balance Between Ventilatory Supply and Demand, later).

Hypoxemic respiratory failure is defined as clinically significant hypoxemia despite therapy with high (and potentially toxic) concentrations of supplemental O_2. In general, hypoxemic failure is characterized by a Pa_{O_2} less than 55 mmHg while the patient is inspiring gas with an F_{IO_2} of 0.6 or greater. Hypoxemic

TABLE 18-1.	CLASSIFICATION OF RESPIRATORY FAILURE
CATEGORY OF RESPIRATORY FAILURE	**DEFINITION**
Hypercapnic	Pa_{CO_2} >45 mmHg
Acute	Develops in minutes to hours
Chronic	Develops over several days or more
Hypoxemic	Pa_{O_2} <55 mmHg while inspiring O_2 at 60% or greater concentration
Acute	Develops in minutes or hours
Chronic	Develops over several days or more

respiratory failure constitutes "lung failure" or failure of the O_2 exchange mechanism.

As noted, life-threatening respiratory failure may arise from a variety of causes. Because treatment varies widely, an understanding of the underlying mechanisms is important. Consideration of the functional components of the respiratory system and of prototypic diseases constitutes a practical approach to the topic.

FUNCTIONAL COMPONENTS OF THE RESPIRATORY SYSTEM

Normal gas exchange depends on the integration of several functional components of the respiratory system—an "interlocking" system that must adapt to exercise (see Chap. 19) and a variety of pathologic conditions. The four major functional components (Fig. 18-1) include (1) the central nervous system (CNS); (2) the chest bellows, which includes the peripheral nervous system, muscles of respiration, and chest wall; (3) the airways; and (4) the alveolar gas-exchanging units.

Operation of the respiratory system as a feedback loop is illustrated schematically in Figure 18-2. By means of peripheral and central chemoreceptors (see Chap. 16), the CNS component monitors the levels of P_{O_2} and P_{CO_2} in blood and cerebrospinal fluid. These gas tensions represent the "output" (or controlled variables) of the respiratory system. Information on gas tensions is integrated with other sensory input and modulates neural output controlling the level and pattern of ventilation. This neural output results in inspiratory muscle contraction, which, in turn, produces cyclic changes in pleural pressure and lung inflation (see Chap. 2).

Lung inflation and deflation necessitate gas flow into and out of the gas-exchanging regions, where passive diffusion of O_2 and CO_2 across the alveolar–capillary membrane occurs (see Chap. 9). In effect, "pump failure" refers to dysfunction of the CNS, chest bellows, or airways, whereas "lung failure" refers to dysfunction of the alveoli, pulmonary capillaries, and alveolar–capillary membrane (see Fig. 18-1).

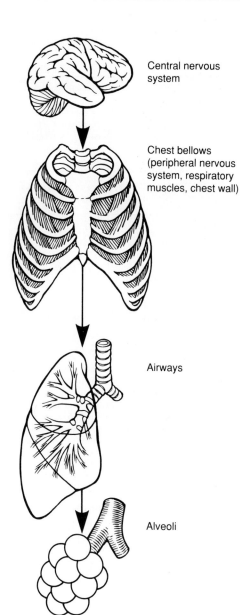

Central nervous
system

Chest bellows
(peripheral nervous
system, respiratory
muscles, chest wall)

Airways

Alveoli

Figure 18-1. Functional components of the respiratory system. The neural drive for respiration originates in the central nervous system at the level of the medulla. Efferent neural activity is carried by way of the phrenics and other motoneurons of the peripheral nervous system to the respiratory muscles. Changes in intrathoracic pressure effected by inspiratory muscle contraction result in airflow and delivery of gas to the alveoli. (From Lanken PN. Weaning from mechanical ventilation. In: Fishman AP, ed. Update: Pulmonary Diseases and Disorders. New York: McGraw-Hill, 1982:367.)

BALANCE BETWEEN VENTILATORY SUPPLY AND DEMAND

Hypercapnic respiratory failure results, ultimately, from a continuing imbalance between a subject's ventilatory *supply*—defined as the maximal amount of ventilation that can be sustained—and the ventilatory *demand*—defined as the overall level of ventilation specified by the CNS controller. This concept of a dynamic balance between supply and demand is illustrated in Figure 18-3.

Normally, the respiratory system has considerable physiologic reserve for ventilatory supply. For example, a healthy 30-year-old man of average height,

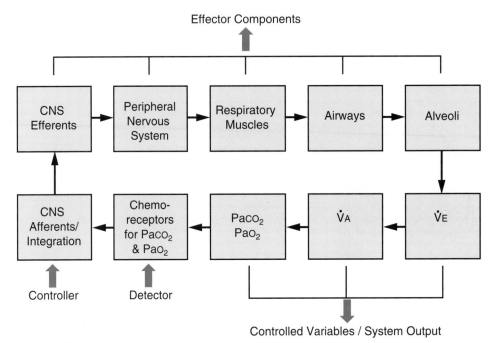

Figure 18-2. The respiratory control system as a feedback loop. The central nervous system controller receives afferent information, including input from chemoreceptors, which monitor levels of P_{O_2} and P_{CO_2} in arterial blood and cerebrospinal fluid. The controller integrates the afferent input and generates the central neural drive to breathe. The neural drive is transduced into motor activity, which eventuates in gas exchange in alveoli. The major controlled variables are total minute ventilation ($\dot{V}E$), alveolar ventilation ($\dot{V}A$), and arterial levels of P_{O_2} and P_{CO_2}. (From Lanken PN. Respiratory failure: An overview. In: Carlson RW, Geheb MA, eds. The Principles and Practice of Medical Intensive Care. Philadelphia: WB Saunders, 1993:755.)

weighing 70 kg, has a resting minute ventilation ($\dot{V}E$) of approximately 6 to 7 L/minute. However, the maximal level of ventilation that he can sustain, that is, the *maximal sustainable ventilation* (MSV), is about 90 L/minute—15 times his resting ventilation.

VENTILATORY SUPPLY

As noted, a subject's ventilatory supply is the MSV, defined as the minute ventilation that can be sustained indefinitely without development of respiratory muscle fatigue. In healthy subjects, the MSV is approximately 50% of the maximal voluntary ventilation (MVV) (see Chap. 4). In patients with lung disease, the MSV may equal or exceed 50% of their MVV. Factors that decrease the MVV also decrease the MSV (Table 18-2).

VENTILATORY DEMAND

Ventilatory demand (i.e., $\dot{V}E$) may be expressed in the following two equations:

$$\dot{V}E = \frac{\dot{V}A}{(1 - V_D/V_T)} \qquad [18\text{-}1]$$

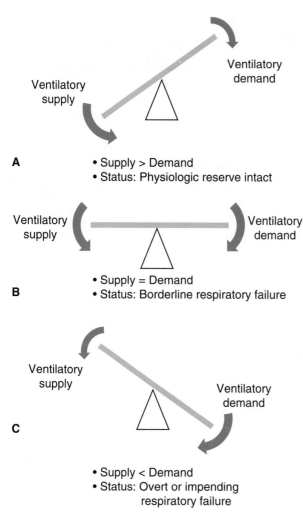

A
- Supply > Demand
- Status: Physiologic reserve intact

B
- Supply = Demand
- Status: Borderline respiratory failure

C
- Supply < Demand
- Status: Overt or impending respiratory failure

Figure 18-3. Dynamic balance between ventilatory supply (maximal sustainable ventilation) and ventilatory demand (overall level of ventilation specified by the central nervous system controller). Relative size of the arrows indicates levels of supply and demand in each of the three circumstances illustrated. **(A)** Normal. Ventilatory supply greatly exceeds demand. **(B)** Disorder characterized by decreased supply and increased demand (e.g., acute asthma attack). **(C)** Disorder in which ventilatory demand exceeds ventilatory supply (e.g., sepsis in a patient with COPD), leading to respiratory muscle fatigue and hypercapnic respiratory failure.

and

$$\dot{V}_A = K \cdot \frac{\dot{V}_{CO_2}}{Pa_{CO_2}} = K \cdot \dot{V}_{O_2} \cdot \frac{RQ}{Pa_{CO_2}} \qquad [18\text{-}2]$$

where:

$\dot{V}_E$ = expired minute ventilation (ventilatory demand)
$\dot{V}_A$ = alveolar minute ventilation
V_D/V_T = ratio of dead space to tidal volume
K = a constant
$\dot{V}_{CO_2}$ = minute CO_2 production
$\dot{V}_{O_2}$ = minute O_2 consumption
RQ = respiratory quotient ($\dot{V}_{CO_2}/\dot{V}_{O_2}$)

Analysis of equations [18-1] and [18-2] indicates that only a limited number of variables determine the level of ventilatory demand. In common disorders of

TABLE 18-2.   *FACTORS THAT ADVERSELY AFFECT VENTILATORY SUPPLY*

FACTOR	CLINICAL EXAMPLES
Abnormal respiratory mechanics	
Airflow obstruction	Asthma, chronic obstructive pulmonary disease
Chest wall deformities	Kyphoscoliosis, flail chest
Loss of lung volume	Pneumonia, interstitial lung disease, large pleural effusion
Decreased respiratory muscle strength and endurance	
Disorders of the phrenic nerves	Guillain-Barré syndrome, poliomyelitis
Disorders of neuromuscular transmission	Myasthenia gravis
Respiratory muscle atrophy	Ventilator dependency, malnutrition
Respiratory muscle weakness	Electrolyte abnormalities, hypoxemia, acidosis
Altered diaphragmatic force–length relationship	Hyperinflation and diaphragm flattening

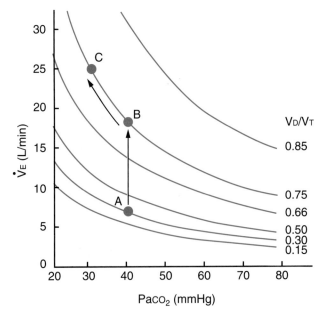

Figure 18-4. The effect of increased V_D/V_T and hypocapnia on ventilatory demand. The relationship between $\dot{V}_E$ and Pa_{CO_2} is shown for a series of V_D/V_T isopleths (i.e., constant level of V_D/V_T). Point A represents normal values for V_D/V_T, Pa_{CO_2}, and $\dot{V}_E$. Point B denotes the effect on $\dot{V}_E$ of increasing V_D/V_T from 0.3 to 0.75; $\dot{V}_E$ would need to increase from 7 L/minute to 18 L/minute to maintain Pa_{CO_2} constant at 40 mmHg. Point C denotes the additional effect on $\dot{V}_E$ of hypocapnia; a $\dot{V}_E$ of 25 L/minute would be necessary to maintain Pa_{CO_2} at 30 mmHg. (Modified from Selecky PA, Wasserman K, Klein M, Ziment I. A graphic approach to assessing interrelationships among minute ventilation, arterial carbon dioxide tension and ratio of physiologic dead space to tidal volume in patients on respirators. Am Rev Respir Dis 117:181–184, 1978.)

respiratory failure, one of the most important factors is an increase in V_D/V_T (see Chap. 3). The normal ratio of 0.3 may increase to 0.6 or higher. Figure 18-4 illustrates the effects of an increase in V_D/V_T on $\dot{V}_E$. Factors adversely affecting ventilatory demand are listed in Table 18-3.

FAILURE OF THE CENTRAL NERVOUS SYSTEM

When the central neural drive for respiration decreases, $\dot{V}_E$ declines because of reductions in respiratory rate (f) and tidal volume (V_T). As a consequence, according to equation [18-1], if V_D/V_T remains constant (or increases, as is more likely, because V_T decreases without a substantial change in anatomic dead space), alveolar ventilation ($\dot{V}_A$) must also decrease. According to equation [18-2], the decrease in $\dot{V}_A$ results in a rise in Pa_{CO_2} if $\dot{V}_{CO_2}$ remains constant. When Pa_{CO_2} exceeds 45 mmHg, the criterion for hypercapnic ventilatory failure is met. Under these circumstances, the imbalance between ventilatory supply and demand is the result almost exclusively of a decrease in supply.

CHANGES IN ARTERIAL BLOOD GASES

In respiratory failure due to disorders of the CNS, characteristic changes are observed in arterial blood gases. A rise in Pa_{CO_2} and secondary fall in pH occur, as described by the Henderson-Hasselbalch equation. As a consequence, respiratory acidosis develops (see Chap. 10). In addition, a secondary fall in Pa_{O_2} arises, as determined by the alveolar gas equation (Fig. 18-5).

In cases where neural respiratory drive is depressed *acutely,* serum bicarbonate concentration rises slightly, due to a mass action effect from the increase in Pa_{CO_2} and dissociation of H_2CO_3 into HCO_3^- and H^+ (see Chap. 10). When the hypercapnia develops gradually (over days or weeks), the fall in pH is tempered by an elevation in serum bicarbonate concentration, mediated by the kidneys. In the absence of lung disease (e.g., atelectasis or pneumonia), the normal alveolar–arterial oxygen difference is maintained. Table 18-4 summarizes these changes.

PULMONARY FUNCTION TESTS

Pulmonary function testing is not easily performed in cases of acute respiratory failure due to CNS dysfunction; the patient is frequently unable to follow instructions. Pulmonary mechanics, per se, may be normal.

TABLE 18-3. *FACTORS THAT ADVERSELY AFFECT VENTILATORY DEMAND*

FACTOR	CLINICAL EXAMPLES
Increased V_D/V_T	Asthma, chronic obstructive pulmonary disease, pulmonary emboli
Increased O_2 consumption	Increased work of breathing, fever
Increased respiratory quotient	Excessive carbohydrate feeding
Decreased Pa_{CO_2}	Hypoxemia, metabolic acidosis

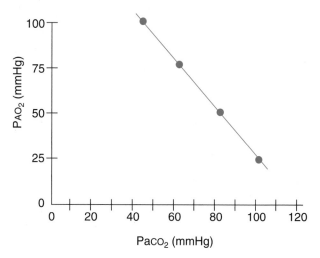

Figure 18-5. Graphic representation of the alveolar gas equation, illustrating effect of increasing Pa_{CO_2} on PA_{O_2}. Assuming a normal difference between PA_{O_2} and Pa_{O_2} of 10 to 20 mmHg, one can estimate the effect of hypoventilation on Pa_{O_2}. If the alveolar–arterial oxygen difference exceeds 20 mmHg, the adverse effect of hypoventilation on arterial oxygenation is even more pronounced.

TABLE 18-4. ACUTE RESPIRATORY FAILURE: CHANGES IN ARTERIAL BLOOD GASES, ALVEOLAR–ARTERIAL O₂ GRADIENT, AND VENTILATION

FAILED RESPIRATORY SYSTEM COMPONENT	PHYSIOLOGIC PARAMETER					
	pH	Pa_{CO_2}	Pa_{O_2}	$(A - a)P_{O_2}$	$\dot{V}_E$	$\dot{V}_A$
Central nervous system	↓	↑	↓	NL	↓	↓
Peripheral nervous system or chest bellows	↓	↑	↓	NL or ↑ *	↓	↓
Airways						
Asthma						
Early phase (before respiratory failure)	↑	↓	NL	↑	↑	↑
Crossover point	NL	NL	NL to ↓	↑	↑	NL
Respiratory muscle fatigue	↓	↑	↓	↑	↑	↓
Chronic obstructive pulmonary disease						
Non-CO₂ retainer	↓	↑ **	↓	↑	↑	↓
CO₂ retainer						
Baseline	NL to ↓	↑	↓	↑	NL	↓
Flare	↓ ↓	↑ ↑	↓ ↓	↑	NL or ↑	↓
Alveoli						
Before respiratory muscle fatigue	↑	↓	↓ ↓	↑ ↑	↑	↑
After respiratory muscle fatigue	↓	↑	↓ ↓	↑ ↑	↓	↓

↑, increased; ↑ ↑, markedly increased; ↓, decreased; ↓ ↓, markedly decreased; NL, in normal range; ↑ *, commonly seen when atelectasis or pneumonia occur; ↑ **, Pa_{CO_2} normal at baseline, but increases during exacerbation.

CLINICAL CORRELATIONS

The differential diagnosis of *acute* respiratory failure due to CNS depression includes sedative or opiate overdose and diseases of the medullary respiratory control centers, such as encephalitis and brain stem stroke. The differential diagnosis of *chronic* respiratory failure due to CNS disease includes depression of central respiratory drive (e.g., sleep apnea syndrome; see Chap. 17) and chronic opiate use.

Treatment is directed at the underlying etiology (e.g., use of an opiate antagonist in the case of narcotic overdose). In addition, supportive care is provided, including intubation and mechanical ventilation, until the cause of the respiratory failure is reversed.

FAILURE OF THE CHEST BELLOWS

Disorders of motoneurons innervating the respiratory muscles, or weakness of the respiratory muscles, may result in a diminished $\dot{V}_E$, despite preservation of central ventilatory drive. As respiratory muscle weakness progresses, a decline in transpulmonary pressure generated with each breath eventually leads to a diminished tidal volume. Lack of sufficient muscle strength to achieve periodic, spontaneous, large tidal volumes (sighs) further exacerbates the situation.

Sighs are critical in maintaining normal surfactant activity (see Chap. 2). Lack of sighs results in "microatelectasis" (i.e., atelectasis at the alveolar level), followed by "macroatelectasis" (i.e., atelectasis at the segmental or lobar level). Both types of atelectasis, if extensive, decrease the static compliance of the lungs and the respiratory system. The end result is a smaller tidal volume relative to transpulmonary pressure (Fig. 18-6).

As in the case of respiratory failure due to CNS disease, decreased respiratory muscle strength produces decreased ventilatory supply and an imbalance between ventilatory supply and demand. Ventilatory demand changes little, except under two circumstances: (1) $\dot{V}_{O_2}$ may increase modestly if the patient is febrile (e.g., due to pneumonia); and (2) $\dot{V}_{O_2}$ may increase due to an increase in the elastic work of breathing (see Fig. 18-6) if the patient's lung or respiratory system compliance is substantially reduced.

Clinical disorders associated with a reduction in respiratory system compliance include kyphoscoliosis and other significant anatomic distortions of the chest wall, and restriction to downward excursion of the diaphragm, such as from tense ascites. Normally, the O_2 expenditure ascribable to the work of breathing is modest, representing only 2% to 3% of the total $\dot{V}_{O_2}$. In pathologic states, however, it may increase up to 10-fold.

CHANGES IN ARTERIAL BLOOD GASES

The underlying pathophysiologic mechanisms in failure of the chest bellows are similar to those in failure of the CNS. Consequently, changes in arterial blood gases are similar. A rise in Pa_{CO_2}, fall in arterial pH, and respiratory acidosis are seen. Pa_{O_2} is also reduced (see Table 18-4). The alveolar–arterial oxygen gradient is commonly increased, however, due to concomitant atelectasis or pneumonia. The serum bicarbonate level is usually normal or only slightly elevated in cases of acute respiratory failure, depending on the degree of hyper-

Figure 18-6. Static and dynamic pressure–volume curves and work of breathing. **(A)** Static and dynamic pressure–volume curves for a healthy lung (solid lines) and for a lung with decreased compliance (broken lines). In the healthy lung, an inspired tidal volume of 1000 ml requires a transpulmonary pressure of 12 cm H_2O (blue arrow). When compliance is decreased by 50%, the same transpulmonary pressure (black arrow) effects a tidal volume of only 500 ml. **(B)** Work of breathing and lung compliance. In the healthy lung, the elastic work of breathing necessary to effect a tidal volume of 1000 ml is indicated by the darkly stippled area. In contrast, the elastic work of breathing necessary to effect the same tidal volume when compliance is reduced by 50% is indicated by the hatched area. In **(A)** and **(B)**, the blue circles represent the end-inspiratory (alveolar) pressure of the lung with normal compliance; the open circles represent the end-inspiratory pressure of the lung with decreased compliance.

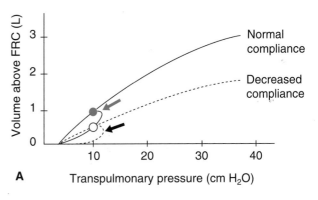

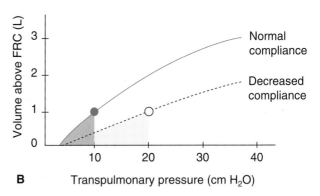

capnia. Patients with chronic hypercapnia demonstrate renal compensation and an elevated serum bicarbonate concentration.

PULMONARY FUNCTION TESTS

With respiratory muscle weakness, maximal inspiratory and expiratory pressures are diminished. The FVC is reduced, whereas the $FEV_1/FVC\%$ remains normal. The MVV is decreased in proportion to the decrease in FEV_1. The pattern is characteristic of restrictive disorders (see Chap. 4).

CLINICAL CORRELATIONS

The differential diagnosis of weakness of the respiratory muscles includes (1) disorders of respiratory motoneurons (e.g., Guillain-Barré syndrome); (2) disorders of the neuromuscular junction (e.g., myasthenia gravis or use of neuromuscular blocking agents); and (3) primary disorders of the muscles (e.g., polymyositis).

Fatigue of the respiratory muscles may also produce weakness acutely. Muscle fatigue is defined as the inability of a muscle to sustain a set level of motor output over a specified period of time. Fatigue is characterized by loss of power output and, eventually, muscle weakness. If the muscle is allowed to rest, gradual recovery of motor function is expected. The MSV, described previously, may also be defined as the maximal level of ventilation achievable without development of respiratory muscle fatigue. Clinical variables affecting respiratory muscle strength and endurance are summarized in Table 18-2.

Treatment of respiratory failure due to neuromuscular weakness varies according to the disorder. If specific interventions (e.g., use of pharmacologic agents to treat myasthenia gravis) are unavailable or are unsuccessful, supportive care, including mechanical ventilation, is used.

RESPIRATORY FAILURE DUE TO AIRWAY DISEASE

The mechanisms underlying respiratory failure due to airway disease include a severe limitation in ventilatory supply and substantial increase in ventilatory demand.

The limitation of ventilatory supply arises from narrowing of the airways. Expiratory and inspiratory airflow rates and exhaled lung volume (e.g., FEV_1) are diminished. These changes directly limit the MSV. FRC is increased, and the diaphragm is flattened due to hyperinflation. As a result, the force–length relationship of the diaphragm is altered (see Chap. 2); the diaphragm is less efficient and is predisposed to fatigue.

Ventilatory demand is increased, primarily because of three pathophysiologic developments: (1) increased V_D/V_T, (2) increased $\dot{V}_{O_2}$, and, occasionally, (3) hypocapnia.

In acute airway obstruction, such as an asthma attack or exacerbation of chronic obstructive pulmonary disease, V_D/V_T may exceed 0.6 (Fig. 18-4) because of profound mismatching of ventilation and perfusion (see Chap. 13).

The resistive work of breathing is increased (see Chap. 2), resulting in a marked increase in minute O_2 consumption of the respiratory muscles. Respiratory muscle O_2 consumption may represent up to 25% of total $\dot{V}_{O_2}$ under these conditions.

Finally, in the early phase of an acute asthma attack, Pa_{CO_2} is usually reduced because the CNS controller has lowered the normal "set-point" for Pa_{CO_2}, largely in response to vagal afferent signals from the lung (see Chap. 16). Lowering the set-point to 30 to 35 mmHg necessitates a higher $\dot{V}_E$, as evident from equation [18-2], and as illustrated in Figure 18-4.

CHANGES IN ARTERIAL BLOOD GASES

In airway disorders, changes in arterial blood gas measurements may be complex. Distinctions between the two major clinical entities—asthma and chronic obstructive pulmonary disease (COPD)—provide insight into the pathophysiology.

Asthma

In an acute flare of asthma leading to respiratory failure, three "phases" can be defined on the basis of the Pa_{CO_2} (see Chap. 5). The first phase of mild hyperventilation (acute respiratory alkalosis) is followed by a middle phase in which the Pa_{CO_2} may be normal. Subsequently, a third phase of overt respiratory failure, with an elevated Pa_{CO_2}, is seen (see Table 18-4).

An asthmatic attack may not progress beyond the first phase if the flare is treated successfully. Similarly, although the second phase may not progress to the third, a normal Pa_{CO_2} (referred to as the "crossover point") in an asthmatic patient in respiratory distress should prompt concern, because it may be a harbinger of incipient respiratory failure. The patient should be observed closely.

Chronic Obstructive Pulmonary Disease

In a patient experiencing an acute flare of COPD, the baseline Pa_{CO_2} may be normal or elevated. When elevated, the patient is said to be a "chronic CO_2 retainer."

Changes in arterial blood gases during an acute flare differ in asthma and COPD (see Table 18-4). In COPD, determination of the degree of *acute* deterioration may be difficult to assess solely on the basis of the Pa_{CO_2}, without knowledge of the patient's baseline value. Consequently, judgment about the severity of the attack is based on the degree of respiratory acidosis. Patients who have a blood pH below 7.25 are usually regarded as critically ill; they have a strong indication for institution of mechanical ventilation.

PULMONARY FUNCTION TESTS

Patients with respiratory failure due to airflow obstruction have characteristic obstructive changes in pulmonary function tests (see Chap. 4). The FEV_1, FVC, and $FEV_1/FVC\%$ are decreased. Maximal static pressures may be normal, unless respiratory muscle fatigue has developed.

CLINICAL CORRELATIONS

The differential diagnosis is limited to asthma, COPD, and other much less common forms of upper airway obstruction (e.g., tracheal or laryngeal cancer). Therapy is directed at the underlying cause of the obstruction. In asthma, treatment is aimed at relief of bronchospasm and mucosal inflammation (see Chap. 5). In COPD, bronchodilators are also used, and treatment is focused on lower respiratory tract infection, if present, and reduction of increased respiratory secretions (see Chap. 6).

FAILURE OF ALVEOLAR GAS EXCHANGE

Failure of alveolar gas exchange, which leads to hypoxemic respiratory failure, is usually caused by disorders in which there is diffuse alveolar disease. Perfusion of poorly ventilated or unventilated alveoli persists, creating areas of low $\dot{V}/\dot{Q}$ (<1 or 0), as discussed in Chapter 13. Alveoli with $\dot{V}/\dot{Q} = 0$ constitute a right-to-left shunt; that is, blood from the right side of the circulation (right-sided heart chambers or pulmonary artery) enters the left side of the circulation without prior oxygenation. The effect of a pure right-to-left shunt on Pa_{O_2} is illustrated in Figure 18-7. The magnitude of the right-to-left shunt is calculated using the shunt equation (see Chap. 12, Table 12-5).

Ventilation is increased because of the direct effect of hypoxemia in stimulating carotid arterial chemoreceptors, and the effect of vagal afferents stimulated by inflammatory exudate and edema in the lung parenchyma (see Chap. 16). Ventilatory demand is also markedly increased due to an elevation in V_D/V_T. Finally, $\dot{V}_{O_2}$ is increased because of an elevated resistive work of breathing due to low lung compliance (see Chap. 2).

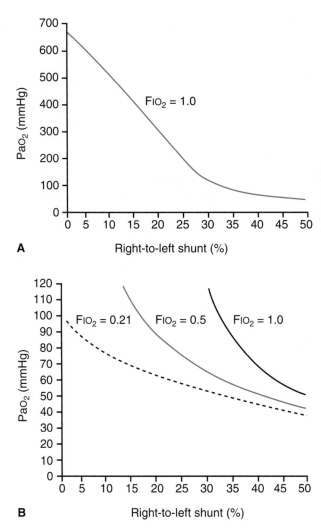

Figure 18-7. Effects of right-to-left shunt on arterial oxygenation. **(A)** Relationship between increasing right-to-left shunt and Pao_2 while breathing 100% O_2. This is a graphic representation of the shunt equation. The following assumptions are made: (1) cardiac output, hemoglobin concentration, and Pao_2 are normal; and (2) hypoventilation, diffusion block, and ventilation–perfusion mismatching are absent. **(B)** Effect of administration of supplemental O_2 on Pao_2 in the presence of right-to-left shunt. At the highest shunt level, Pao_2 increases by only about 12 mmHg, despite an increase in partial pressure of inspired O_2 from 150 mmHg to 760 mmHg. (From Lanken PN. Adult respiratory distress syndrome: Clinical management. In: Carlson RW, Geheb MA, eds. The Principles and Practice of Medical Intensive Care. Philadelphia: WB Saunders, 1993:830.)

Ventilatory supply decreases with widespread alveolar flooding in cardiogenic and noncardiogenic pulmonary edema (see Chap. 14), with resultant limitations in tidal volume and vital capacity.

CHANGES IN ARTERIAL BLOOD GASES

The pathophysiologic hallmark in failure of alveolar gas exchange is a decreased Pao_2. Secondary changes in $Paco_2$ and pH arise from acute respiratory alkalosis in the early phase of these disorders (see Table 18-4). If ventilatory demand exceeds ventilatory supply for a sufficiently long period, respiratory muscle fatigue develops and acute respiratory acidosis ensues.

PULMONARY FUNCTION TESTS

Pulmonary function tests are difficult to obtain in patients in acute respiratory distress. If performed, however, they show a decreased tidal volume and vital capacity, without evidence of reduced airflow. Respiratory muscle strength is preserved unless respiratory muscle fatigue has developed.

CLINICAL CORRELATIONS

The most common clinical disorders that produce hypoxemic respiratory failure are cardiogenic and noncardiogenic pulmonary edema (adult respiratory distress syndrome), severe pneumonia, and massive pulmonary embolism.

Therapy is directed at the underlying etiology. Although supplemental O_2 is part of routine treatment, the hypoxemia is characteristically refractory to O_2 therapy because of a high right-to-left shunt fraction (see Fig. 18-7). Patients with severe, diffuse disease usually require mechanical ventilation.

SELECTED READING

Cournand A, Richards DW Jr, Bader RA, et al. The oxygen cost of breathing. Trans Assoc Am Physicians 67:162–173, 1954.

Donahoe M, Rogers RM, Wilson DO, et al. Oxygen consumption of the respiratory muscles in normal and in malnourished patients with chronic obstructive pulmonary disease. Am Rev Respir Dis 140:385–391, 1989.

Kelly B, Luce J. The diagnosis and management of neuromuscular diseases causing respiratory failure. Chest 99:1485–1494, 1991.

Lanken PN. Weaning from mechanical ventilation. In: Fishman AP, ed. Update: Pulmonary Diseases and Disorders. New York: McGraw-Hill, 1982:366–386.

Otis AB. The work of breathing. In: Fenn WO, Rahn H, eds. Handbook of Physiology: Respiration, vol I, section 3. Washington, DC: American Physiological Society, 1964:463–476.

Roussos C, Macklem PT. The respiratory muscles. N Engl J Med 307:786–797, 1982.

Selecky PA, Wasserman K, Klein M, Ziment I. A graphic approach to assessing interrelationships among minute ventilation, arterial carbon dioxide tension and ratio of physiologic dead space to tidal volume in patients on respirators. Am Rev Respir Dis 117:181–184, 1978.

Lippincott's Pathophysiology Series: Pulmonary Pathophysiology, edited by Michael A. Grippi. J. B. Lippincott Company, Philadelphia © 1995.

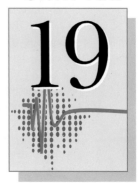

CHAPTER

19

Exercise Physiology

Basil J. Petrof and Michael A. Grippi

The physiology of exercise is based on coordinated functioning of the respiratory, cardiovascular, and musculoskeletal systems. Limitations in any of these systems may result in impaired exercise tolerance. Conversely, because exercise constitutes a performance stress, exercise testing may uncover subtle cardiopulmonary disease that is "masked" by the body's reserve capacity.

This chapter focuses on the basics of normal and abnormal exercise physiology and the application of exercise testing in evaluation of known or suspected cardiopulmonary disease.

OVERVIEW OF EXERCISE PHYSIOLOGY AND CLINICAL EXERCISE TESTING

During normal exercise, profound physiologic changes are observed in multiple organ systems, including the respiratory system. Increases in airflow rate and tidal volume result in greater resistive and elastic loads on the lung. Respiratory muscle O_2 consumption increases, and increases in venous return, heart rate, and catecholamine release raise cardiac output and pulmonary blood flow. Dilation and recruitment of pulmonary blood vessels and reduction in pulmonary vascular resistance (see Chap. 12) facilitate the increase in blood flow.

In the periphery, blood vessels in skeletal muscles are recruited, and peripheral blood flow is preferentially redistributed to active muscle groups. O_2 extraction by working muscles increases. If maximal energy use by the muscles exceeds that which can be supported by the available O_2 supply, anaerobic metabolism ensues. The resulting increase in blood lactate and hydrogen ion concentrations stimulates the carotid bodies (see Chap. 16), resulting in a disproportionate increase in $\dot{V}E$ as compensation for the fall in pH.

Obviously, then, exercise is an extremely complex phenomenon that requires the coordination of many physiologic processes (Fig. 19-1). Since the early 1980s, the popularity of exercise testing for the diagnosis of underlying cardiopulmonary disease and assessment of exercise capacity has grown. The most frequent indications for cardiopulmonary exercise testing are to (1) establish a specific diagnosis and elucidate the factors causing exercise limitation; (2) objectively assess a subject's functional work capacity; (3) follow disease progression or the effects of therapy; and (4) assess the need for specific treatment (e.g., administration of supplemental O_2 during exercise).

OXYGEN UPTAKE AS AN INDEX OF WORKLOAD

In determining whether the cardiopulmonary response to exercise is normal, the *workload* presented to the exercising subject must be quantified. Workload may be expressed in customary units of work and power; however, a more commonly used measure of workload in a clinical context is the level of O_2 consumption. The basis for this "oxygen equivalence of power" is described in the following sections.

WORK AND POWER

Work is performed when force moves through a distance. One unit of work, the *joule* (J), denotes a force of 1 Newton acting through a distance of 1 meter.

Power is the rate of work, or work performed per unit time. A commonly used unit of power is the *watt,* which is 1 joule per second. Clinically, another frequently used unit of power is the *met,* defined as a multiple of the resting metabolic O_2 requirement: one met equals 3.5 ml O_2/minute/kg body weight. In clinical exercise testing, the rate of O_2 consumption or O_2 uptake is determined from expired gas measurements and is used as an index of power output by the exercising subject.

OXYGEN EQUIVALENCE OF POWER

Measurements of O_2 uptake ($\dot{V}O_2$) during exercise are useful for a number of reasons. During whole-body exercise (e.g., exercise on a treadmill or bicycle ergometer), $\dot{V}O_2$ is linearly related to power output up to the point at which maximal O_2 uptake ($\dot{V}O_{2\,max}$) is reached (Fig. 19-2). Beyond this point, anaerobic metabolism sustains further increases in work briefly, but only at the expense of development of a lactic acidosis. Changes in the level of $\dot{V}O_2$ can, therefore, be used as an index of changes in power output during exercise.

In addition, $\dot{V}O_2$ is a better indicator of the "challenge" to the system than is the actual physical workload performed, because the latter may be affected by factors like anxiety and lack of familiarity with the exercise technique. To the extent that $\dot{V}O_{2\,max}$ represents the maximal amount of O_2 delivered to tissues during physical work, it provides a measure of the ability of the entire O_2 delivery system to cope with maximal stress.

Although the slope of the relationship between $\dot{V}O_2$ and power output is linear and independent of age, sex, and height, these variables do affect $\dot{V}O_{2\,max}$;

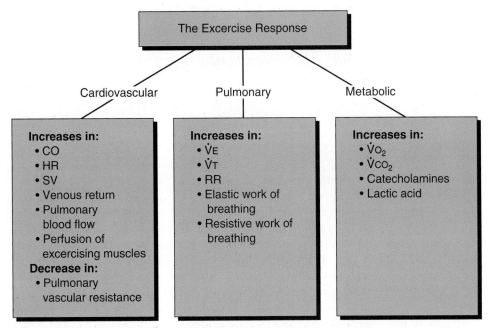

Figure 19-1. Physiologic and biochemical changes in exercise. Coordinated changes in cardiovascular, pulmonary, and metabolic functions facilitate increases in O_2 uptake and CO_2 production over a wide range of exercise loads.

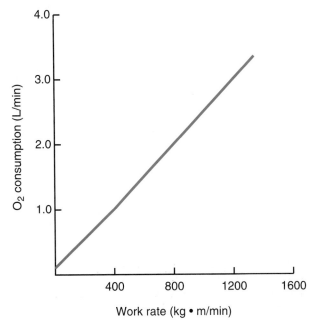

Figure 19-2. Oxygen equivalence of power. The relationship between work rate (power) and O_2 consumption is linear. See text for details.

increasing age, female sex, and smaller stature are associated with decreases in $\dot{V}_{O_2 \max}$. Therefore, appropriate corrections must be made when deriving predicted values. To what degree these variables are independent of other factors known to decrease $\dot{V}_{O_2 \max}$, such as lack of training and reduced muscle mass, is unclear.

COMPONENTS OF THE OXYGEN DELIVERY SYSTEM

Conceptually, the O_2 delivery system comprises several elements: (1) *respiratory function,* including pulmonary mechanics and respiratory muscle performance (see Chap. 2), ventilatory control mechanisms (see Chap. 16), ventilation–perfusion relationships (see Chap. 13), oxygen diffusion (see Chap. 9), and oxygen–hemoglobin affinity (see Chap. 10); (2) *cardiac function,* including the heart rate response to exercise and factors that determine stroke volume (preload, afterload, and cardiac contractility); (3) *control of the peripheral circulation,* that is, the ability to apportion blood flow to exercising muscles at the expense of metabolically less active tissues; and (4) *muscle metabolism,* including oxidative and glycolytic enzyme functions. A significant abnormality in any one of these elements, although often subtle or undetectable at rest due to the large reserve capacity of the system, is more likely to be evident as a reduction in $\dot{V}_{O_2 \max}$. Of course, even a normal $\dot{V}_{O_2 \max}$ does not completely exclude an abnormality in any of the elements.

METHODOLOGY USED IN CLINICAL EXERCISE TESTING

The apparatus used in clinical exercise testing varies from relatively simple to complex. In addition, the extent of data collection can be limited or extensive. Most clinical exercise testing laboratories, however, use similar technology and provide useful information based on a few basic measurements.

MEASUREMENTS AND INSTRUMENTATION

In standard clinical exercise testing, four primary measurements are made: O_2 and CO_2 concentrations in expired gas, minute ventilation, and heart rate.

O_2 concentration is measured using a fuel cell or mass spectrometer, whereas CO_2 concentration is determined using a mass spectrometer or infrared analyzer. Determination of O_2 and CO_2 concentrations in expired gas and knowledge of their concentrations in inspired air permit calculation of O_2 consumption (oxygen uptake) and carbon dioxide production.

Airflow rate is assessed using a pneumotachograph, mass flow sensor, or other device. Tidal volume can be derived electronically from the airflow signal. $\dot{V}_E$ is calculated from measurements of tidal volume and respiratory rate.

Continuous electrocardiographic monitoring of blood pressure measurements and noninvasive determination of arterial oxyhemoglobin saturation using pulse or ear oximetry are also part of the standard exercise test. In certain clinical circumstances, measurements of arterial blood gases and hemodynamics using a Swan-Ganz catheter (see Chap. 12) may be warranted.

TYPES OF EXERCISE TESTS

Although many of the measurements and calculations derived from exercise studies are based on an assumption of steady-state conditions (i.e., a constant workload), true *steady-state exercise protocols* are not needed to obtain reliable data. Accordingly, *progressive, incremental exercise protocols* are most often used in clinical practice. In progressive exercise testing, the workload is gradually increased in a stepwise fashion. Progressive tests have the advantage of providing information about a patient's response to several different workloads. A number of protocols have been devised for both the treadmill and bicycle ergometer.

Progressive incremental exercise studies usually are terminated when the patient is no longer able to continue exercising because of symptoms. The reason for a subject stopping exercise is important. For example, stopping exercise because of shortness of breath has very different implications than stopping because of knee pain. Alternatively, an exercise test may be terminated because of development of chest pain, electrocardiographic abnormalities, arterial oxyhemoglobin desaturation, or an abnormal fall or elevation in blood pressure.

THE NORMAL CARDIOVASCULAR RESPONSE TO PROGRESSIVE EXERCISE

The normal cardiovascular response to dynamic exercise is fairly stereotypical. Three general areas should be considered: (1) changes in O_2 consumption, cardiac output and its determinants, and arteriovenous O_2 difference; (2) changes with aging; and (3) changes in hemodynamics.

OXYGEN CONSUMPTION, CARDIAC OUTPUT, AND ARTERIOVENOUS OXYGEN DIFFERENCE

Cardiac output (the product of heart rate and stroke volume) may increase fivefold during exercise (Fig. 19-3). In healthy subjects, exercise capacity is constrained by cardiovascular, rather than respiratory, limitations to further delivery of O_2 to tissues.

According to the *Fick principle* (see Chaps. 10 and 12):

$$\dot{V}O_2 = \text{C.O.} \cdot (CaO_2 - C\bar{v}O_2) \qquad [19\text{-}1]$$

where C.O. is cardiac output and CaO_2 and $C\bar{v}O_2$ are the oxygen contents of arterial and mixed venous blood, respectively. The *arteriovenous oxygen content difference* ($CaO_2 - C\bar{v}O_2$) reflects tissue oxygen extraction. Redistribution of arterial blood to working muscles, normally amounting to about 80% of the cardiac output during exercise, largely determines the magnitude of this difference.

The arteriovenous oxygen content difference increases approximately threefold at maximal workloads and is relatively constant among healthy subjects. Hence, cardiac output normally rises linearly with $\dot{V}O_2$, as does heart rate. Because cardiac output is the product of heart rate and stroke volume, the ratio of $\dot{V}O_2$ and heart rate, $\dot{V}O_2/HR$—the *oxygen pulse*—is an index of stroke volume at peak exercise:

$$\dot{V}O_2/\text{Heart Rate} = \text{Stroke Volume} \cdot (CaO_2 - C\bar{v}O_2) \qquad [19\text{-}2]$$

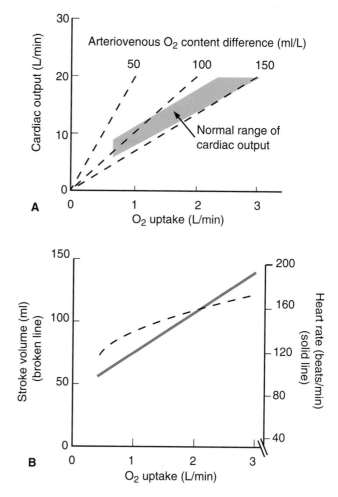

Figure 19-3. Cardiovascular response to progressive exercise. **(A)** Cardiac output increases linearly with O_2 uptake (shaded band). **(B)** Increases in cardiac output are accomplished through increases in stroke volume and heart rate at lower levels of exercise. With progressive increases in O_2 uptake, further increases in cardiac output are achieved through increases in heart rate alone. (From Jones NL. Clinical Exercise Testing. 3rd ed. Philadelphia: WB Saunders, 1988:43–44.)

CHANGES WITH AGING

Maximal heart rate decreases with increasing age (Fig. 19-4) and is the same among age-matched subjects. It can be estimated using the following formula:

$$\text{Maximal Heart Rate} = 210 - [0.65 \cdot \text{Age (yrs)}] \qquad [19\text{-}3]$$

The age-related decline in maximal heart rate is largely responsible for the decrease in cardiac output and $\dot{V}_{O_2 max}$ seen in older subjects. Differences in cardiac output among healthy people of a similar age are caused by differences in stroke volume. Stroke volume tends to be greater in men, larger subjects, and trained subjects. During progressive exercise, stroke volume increases by as much as 50%, a development that occurs at relatively low workloads. Further increments in cardiac output are achieved almost exclusively through increases in heart rate.

CHANGES IN HEMODYNAMICS

The augmentation in cardiac output and associated increase in pulmonary blood flow during exercise cause a mild increase in pulmonary artery pressure.

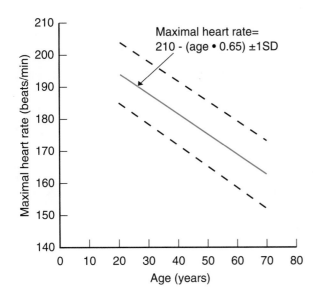

Figure 19-4. Maximal heart rate as a function of age. Maximal heart rate declines linearly with age. The age-related limitation in maximal O_2 consumption is a function of this relationship. Shown is mean heart rate ± SD. (From Jones NL. Clinical Exercise Testing. 3rd ed. Philadelphia: WB Saunders, 1988:45.)

Increased recruitment and dilation of the pulmonary vasculature, however, lead to a considerable fall in pulmonary vascular resistance (see Chap. 12). As a result, a rise in pulmonary artery pressure usually is not observed until cardiac output has increased two- or threefold.

Systolic blood pressure may rise as high as 220 mmHg at peak exercise, whereas diastolic pressure normally does not exceed 90 mmHg. Accordingly, mean arterial pressure increases by approximately 50 mmHg at maximal exercise. A fall in systemic blood pressure during exercise is abnormal.

THE NORMAL VENTILATORY RESPONSE TO PROGRESSIVE EXERCISE

Just as the normal cardiovascular response to exercise is stereotypical, so, too, is the ventilatory response. Changes in minute ventilation, tidal volume, and respiratory rate are quite predictable, as is the alveolar–arterial oxygen gradient. In addition, important changes in the distribution of ventilation, as reflected in the ratio of dead space to tidal volume (V_D/V_T), facilitate marked increases in O_2 and CO_2 fluxes during exercise.

CHANGES IN MINUTE VENTILATION, TIDAL VOLUME, AND RESPIRATORY RATE

The respiratory system has a huge reserve capacity; minute ventilation can be increased 20 times above resting values in healthy subjects. During exercise, minute ventilation increases to meet the need for higher levels of O_2 uptake and CO_2 elimination (Fig. 19-5).

At low and moderate levels of exercise, increased minute ventilation is achieved primarily through increases in tidal volume; tidal volume reaches a maximal value of approximately two thirds of the vital capacity. At higher levels of exercise, further increments in minute ventilation are achieved primarily through increases in respiratory rate; tidal volume remains relatively stable. Te-

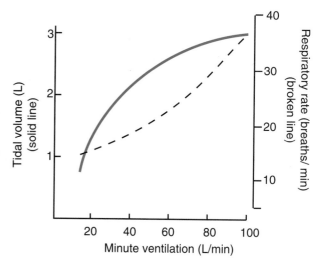

Figure 19-5. The ventilatory response to progressive exercise. The increase in ventilation with progressive exercise is accomplished initially through increases in tidal volume and respiratory rate. At higher levels of exercise, further increases in ventilation are achieved through increases in respiratory rate alone. (From Jones NL. Clinical Exercise Testing. 3rd ed. Philadelphia: WB Saunders, 1988:39.)

leologically, this response makes sense, because generation of tidal volumes larger than 75% of vital capacity requires increased respiratory muscle work due to decreased respiratory system compliance at larger lung volumes (see Chap. 2). An increase in respiratory rate becomes a more "cost-effective" strategy for achieving increased ventilation at higher levels of exercise.

Determination of whether a patient's exercise limitation is the result of a ventilatory impairment requires measurement of the maximal voluntary ventilation (MVV; see Chaps. 4 and 18). Although the MVV may be measured directly, it is usually estimated, based on the empiric relationship:

$$MVV = FEV_1 \cdot 35 \qquad [19\text{-}4]$$

In healthy subjects, the minute ventilation at $\dot{V}_{O_2 max}$ is usually 60% to 70% of the MVV. The additional 30% to 40% of the MVV that is "unused" is the *breathing reserve*. The mere existence of the breathing reserve is consistent with the fact that, in healthy subjects, maximal exercise is limited due to cardiovascular, rather than ventilatory, factors.

CHANGES IN THE DISTRIBUTION OF VENTILATION

Exercise is accompanied by changes in the distribution of ventilation between lung regions that participate in gas exchange and those that do not. As described in Chapter 3, this distribution is expressed as the ratio of dead space (V_D) to tidal volume (V_T), or V_D/V_T (Fig. 19-6).

Normally, V_D/V_T decreases from approximately 0.30 at rest to 0.20 at peak exercise. The decline is caused partly by increased perfusion of apical lung units that typically have high ventilation–perfusion ratios, resulting in better ventilation–perfusion matching within the lung (see Chap. 13). Moreover, the larger tidal volumes accompanying exercise result in a relatively small increase in anatomic dead space compared with the increase in alveolar ventilation.

As discussed in Chapter 3, V_D/V_T can be calculated using the *Bohr equation:*

$$V_D/V_T = \frac{Pa_{CO_2} - P\bar{E}_{CO_2}}{Pa_{CO_2}} \qquad [19\text{-}5]$$

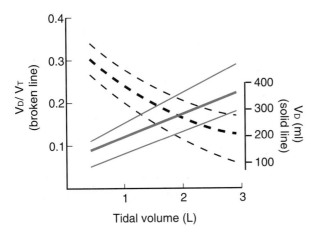

Figure 19-6. Changes in V_D/V_T during exercise. Normal resting V_D/V_T is approximately 0.30. With progressive exercise, V_D rises. V_T rises to a greater extent, however, resulting in a progressive decline in V_D/V_T. The efficiency of CO_2 elimination is enhanced—an important development in the setting of increased CO_2 production during exercise. Shown are the means and ranges for V_D/V_T and V_D. (From Jones NL. Clinical Exercise Testing. 3rd ed. Philadelphia: WB Saunders, 1988:41.)

where Pa_{CO_2} and $P\bar{E}_{CO_2}$ are the partial pressures of CO_2 in arterial blood and mixed expired gas, respectively. Failure of V_D/V_T to fall during exercise is evidence of underlying lung disease.

CHANGES IN THE ALVEOLAR–ARTERIAL OXYGEN GRADIENT

The alveolar–arterial oxygen gradient remains normal at low levels of exercise, but increases to approximately 30 mmHg at maximal workloads (Fig. 19-7). Widening of the gradient occurs despite improvement in ventilation–perfusion matching during exercise. This phenomenon is probably the result of augmented O_2 extraction by exercising muscles, resulting in a lower mixed venous O_2 content and corresponding decrease in Pa_{O_2}.

THE ANAEROBIC THRESHOLD

Normal resting metabolism is an aerobic process. Significant levels of dynamic exercise are also aerobic. With a large workload, or in the presence of cardiopulmonary disease, however, metabolism may become significantly anaerobic. The transition phase from aerobic to anaerobic metabolism constitutes a physiologically interesting and clinically useful point for study in exercise testing.

DEFINITION OF THE ANAEROBIC THRESHOLD

The *anaerobic threshold* is defined as the level of exercise above which aerobic metabolism is no longer able to fully meet energy requirements; anaerobic metabolism ensues. At values of $\dot{V}_{O_2}$ below the anaerobic threshold, exercise can be sustained for prolonged periods; above the anaerobic threshold, exercise becomes symptom-limited.

When the O_2 requirements of working muscles exceed the O_2 supply, intermediary metabolism results in the conversion of pyruvate to lactate. The lactic acid is buffered by bicarbonate ions, leading to increased carbon dioxide production (see Chap. 10). These changes, coupled with the ventilatory response to increasing lactic acidosis, lead to characteristic alterations in gas exchange that permit identification of the anaerobic threshold by noninvasive means (see later).

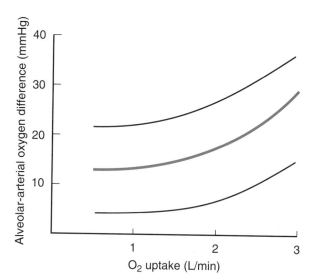

Figure 19-7. The alveolar–arterial oxygen gradient during exercise. The gradient is normal at low levels of exercise and increases modestly at high levels of oxygen uptake. Shown are mean (thick line) and range. (From Jones NL. Clinical Exercise Testing. 3rd ed. Philadelphia: WB Saunders, 1988:42.)

At workloads below the anaerobic threshold, O_2 consumption, CO_2 production, and minute ventilation increase linearly and in parallel (Fig. 19-8). More complex changes occur at the anaerobic threshold, as discussed in the following sections.

METABOLIC PHASES OF THE ANAEROBIC THRESHOLD

During progressive exercise, two metabolic phases follow attainment of the anaerobic threshold (see Fig. 19-8).

In the first, the *isocapnic phase,* the increase in $\dot{V}_{CO_2}$ becomes nonlinear and elicits a proportionate rise in $\dot{V}_E$. Pa_{CO_2}, and its indirect measure, end-tidal P_{CO_2}, remain normal. Although the increase is matched to the increase in $\dot{V}_{CO_2}$, it is disproportionately high relative to $\dot{V}_{CO_2}$, which continues to rise linearly with the workload. Accordingly, at this stage, the ratio of $\dot{V}_E$ to $\dot{V}_{CO_2}$, $\dot{V}_E/\dot{V}_{CO_2}$—also known as the *ventilatory equivalent for CO_2*—and end-tidal P_{CO_2} remain constant. On the other hand, the ratio of $\dot{V}_E$ to $\dot{V}_{O_2}$, $\dot{V}_E/\dot{V}_{O_2}$—also known as the *ventilatory equivalent for O_2*—and end-tidal P_{O_2} begin to increase. These findings constitute the most widely accepted criteria for identification of the anaerobic threshold.

The second phase, the *hypocapnic phase,* represents the response to increasing metabolic acidosis as a result of further increases in workload. The progressive decline in pH promotes even greater increases in $\dot{V}_E$ through stimulation of the carotid bodies (see Chap. 16). Consequently, $\dot{V}_E/\dot{V}_{CO_2}$ increases, and arterial and end-tidal P_{CO_2} fall; both $\dot{V}_E/\dot{V}_{O_2}$ and end-tidal P_{O_2} continue to rise.

THE ANAEROBIC THRESHOLD IN HEALTH AND DISEASE

Healthy subjects usually reach the anaerobic threshold at 50% to 60% of their predicted $\dot{V}_{O_2 max}$. An anaerobic threshold of less than 40% predicted $\dot{V}_{O_2 max}$ usually is considered abnormal.

Determination of the anaerobic threshold is used clinically to help differentiate conditions associated with exercise intolerance.

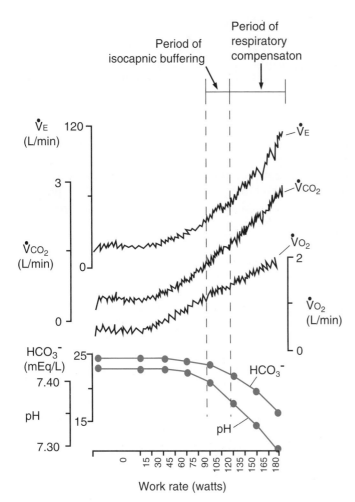

Figure 19-8. Changes in minute ventilation, minute CO_2 production, and minute O_2 consumption during exercise. See text for details. (From Wasserman K, Whipp BJ, Koyal SN, et al. Anaerobic threshold and respiratory gas exchange during exercise. *J Appl Physiol* 35:236–243, 1973.)

If both $\dot{V}_{O_2 max}$ and the anaerobic threshold are normal, the patient is normal or has limited exercise capacity due to decreased exercise efficiency (i.e., increased $\dot{V}_{O_2}$ for a given level of work), such as in obesity. Alternatively, a patient with these findings may have subclinical pulmonary or cardiovascular disease that causes symptoms, despite the fact that physiologic measurements fall within normal limits.

When the $\dot{V}_{O_2 max}$ is low, but the anaerobic threshold is normal, several possibilities should be considered: (1) poor patient effort, (2) lung disease causing ventilatory limitation, or (3) cardiac disease causing pulmonary edema. The development of pulmonary edema may occur without a significant fall in cardiac output; this condition also results in an abnormal ventilatory response.

When both $\dot{V}_{O_2 max}$ and the anaerobic threshold are reduced, a cardiovascular limitation to exercise is suggested. Most often, the limitation is secondary to one of the following: (1) decreased cardiac output, (2) pulmonary vascular disease, (3) peripheral vascular disease, (4) anemia, or (5) sedentary status and poor general fitness.

Finally, training is associated with an increase in the anaerobic threshold, making measurement of the anaerobic threshold a useful tool for following the progress of subjects in training programs.

THE EXERCISE RESPONSE IN PULMONARY DISEASE

Occasionally, the clinical distinction between cardiovascular and pulmonary disease is difficult, because some degree of overlap often exists. For instance, in patients with congestive heart failure, increased left-sided filling pressures and pulmonary edema may develop during exercise. Conversely, patients with chronic obstructive pulmonary disease may have cor pulmonale and pronounced exercise-induced pulmonary hypertension. Despite these caveats, exercise testing can be useful in ascertaining whether the major limitation to exercise is of pulmonary origin. It may also provide clues on the nature of any underlying lung disease. Obviously, this information must be evaluated in the broader context of the patient's clinical history and other diagnostic studies, such as pulmonary function tests (see Chap. 4). Normal exercise-related changes in important physiologic variables in a healthy subject are shown in Fig. 19-9.

THE BREATHING RESERVE IN PULMONARY DISEASE

The most characteristic feature of a ventilatory limitation to exercise is loss of breathing reserve (Fig. 19-10). As noted, healthy subjects usually reach their $\dot{V}o_{2\,max}$ when $\dot{V}E$ reaches 60% to 70% of the MVV. In contrast, patients with a ventilatory limitation are not able to achieve their predicted $\dot{V}o_{2\,max}$ because a ventilatory "ceiling" prevents further exercise. Hence, minute ventilation approaches MVV, and breathing reserve is 15% or less at the conclusion of exercise. The limitation is usually related to abnormal pulmonary mechanics, evident as reductions in FEV_1 and MVV. In addition, increases in VD/VT necessitate a higher level of minute ventilation for any given workload, altering the slope of the relationship between $\dot{V}E$ and $\dot{V}o_2$. To the extent that patients with significant pulmonary disease are frequently sedentary and deconditioned, they may also demonstrate an early anaerobic threshold, which then drives ventilation to nonsustainable levels.

Although patients with pulmonary disease do not usually attain their predicted maximal heart rate, their heart rate may, in fact, be higher than predicted for a given $\dot{V}o_2$. This reflects a reduced stroke volume, evident as a decreased O_2 pulse. Contributing factors include general deconditioning, pulmonary hypertension, and impaired right ventricular function. Although these abnormalities tend to favor the premature onset of anaerobic metabolism, in severe pulmonary disease the ventilatory ceiling is frequently reached before the anaerobic threshold is attained.

EXERCISE LIMITATION IN CHRONIC OBSTRUCTIVE PULMONARY DISEASE

In chronic obstructive pulmonary disease, increased airway resistance and loss of lung elastic recoil cause a reduction in expiratory airflow rate (see Chap. 6), severely limiting the capacity to meet the ventilatory demands of exercise. At higher levels of ventilation, insufficient time for full expiration to FRC results in progressive air trapping. Consequently, the respiratory muscles operate at a mechanical disadvantage (see Chap. 2). Furthermore, the increased work of breathing may promote respiratory muscle fatigue. Ventilation–perfusion mismatching usually results in values of VD/VT of 0.40 or greater at rest, which fail

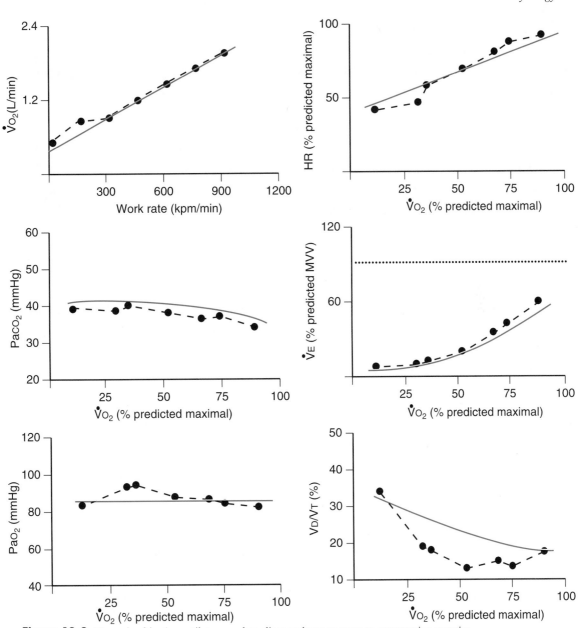

Figure 19-9. Normal subject's ventilatory and cardiovascular responses to progressive exercise. Predicted responses are shown as solid lines. The horizontal dotted line in the graph of $\dot{V}E$ vs. $\dot{V}O_2$ represents the maximal sustainable ventilation (MSV). (Modified from Younes M. Interpretation of clinical exercise testing in respiratory disease. *Clin Chest Med* 5:189–206, 1984.)

to decrease with progressive exercise. This may lead to a rise in $PaCO_2$. A fall in arterial oxyhemoglobin saturation may also be observed.

EXERCISE LIMITATION IN INTERSTITIAL LUNG DISEASE

In patients with interstitial lung disease, lung elastic recoil is increased (see Chap. 7). To minimize the high elastic work of breathing associated with large

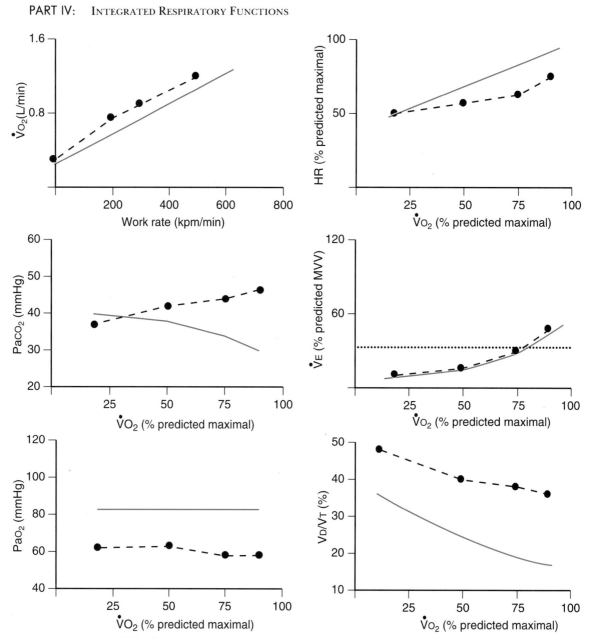

Figure 19-10. Abnormal ventilatory response to exercise in a patient with obstructive airway disease. $\dot{V}_{O_2}$ is excessive at all work rates. Pa_{CO_2} rises with progressive exercise, and Pa_{O_2} remains abnormally low throughout exercise. The patient's minute ventilation at approximately 75% of predicted maximal $\dot{V}_{O_2}$ exceeds the maximal sustainable ventilation. V_D/V_T declines with progressive exercise, but it is elevated throughout the test. (Modified from Younes M. Interpretation of clinical exercise testing in respiratory disease. *Clin Chest Med* 5:189–206, 1984.)

tidal volumes under these circumstances, patients increase $\dot{V}E$ by increasing respiratory frequency, rather than tidal volume. A rapid, shallow breathing pattern is more characteristic of interstitial than obstructive lung disease. Whereas Pa_{CO_2} is more often elevated in obstructive disease, a significant fall in Pa_{O_2} during exercise is more frequent in interstitial disease.

THE EXERCISE RESPONSE IN CARDIOVASCULAR DISEASE

In the absence of a fixed-rate pacemaker, cardiac conduction defects, or drugs that limit heart rate, the pulse rate usually is normal or elevated during exercise in patients with primary cardiac disease. Limitations in cardiac output are caused by a reduction in stroke volume. The limited cardiac output is partially offset by greater tissue O_2 extraction, resulting in an increase in the arteriovenous oxygen difference. The effectiveness of this compensation is limited, however, and, ultimately, anaerobic metabolism occurs at a lower percentage of predicted $\dot{V}O_{2\,max}$. In addition, the low O_2 content of mixed venous blood under these conditions results in magnification of the reduction in Pa_{O_2} due to physiologic shunting (see Chap. 13).

In cardiovascular disease accompanied by low cardiac output during exercise, the following are observed: (1) reduced $\dot{V}O_{2\,max}$, (2) normal breathing reserve, (3) increased heart rate for a given level of $\dot{V}O_2$, (4) decreased O_2 pulse (reflecting diminished stroke volume), and (5) early anaerobic threshold (Fig. 19-11). Furthermore, in patients with substantial impairment of left ventricular function, systemic blood pressure may fail to rise or may even fall during exercise.

CORONARY ARTERY DISEASE

Patients with significant coronary artery disease may demonstrate impaired cardiac contractility with a fall in stroke volume or development of pulmonary venous congestion. In addition, rhythm disturbances, electrocardiographic changes, or angina may lead to termination of the study before maximal heart rate has been achieved.

PERIPHERAL VASCULAR DISEASE

Subjects with peripheral vascular disease, or those who are generally deconditioned, will also demonstrate a decreased $\dot{V}O_{2\,max}$, reduced O_2 pulse, and early anaerobic threshold. In the presence of peripheral vascular disease, maximal heart rate is often not reached due to the development of muscle pain that limits further exercise.

PULMONARY VASCULAR DISEASE

Primary pulmonary vascular disease is characterized by cardiovascular and pulmonary abnormalities that, together, result in diminished $\dot{V}O_{2\,max}$ and work capacity. Cardiac output and O_2 pulse are usually reduced, whereas heart rate tends to remain normal or elevated for a given level of $\dot{V}O_2$. These alterations are accompanied by an early anaerobic threshold. Loss of the pulmonary capillary bed (e.g., due to an obliterative pulmonary vascular disease like primary

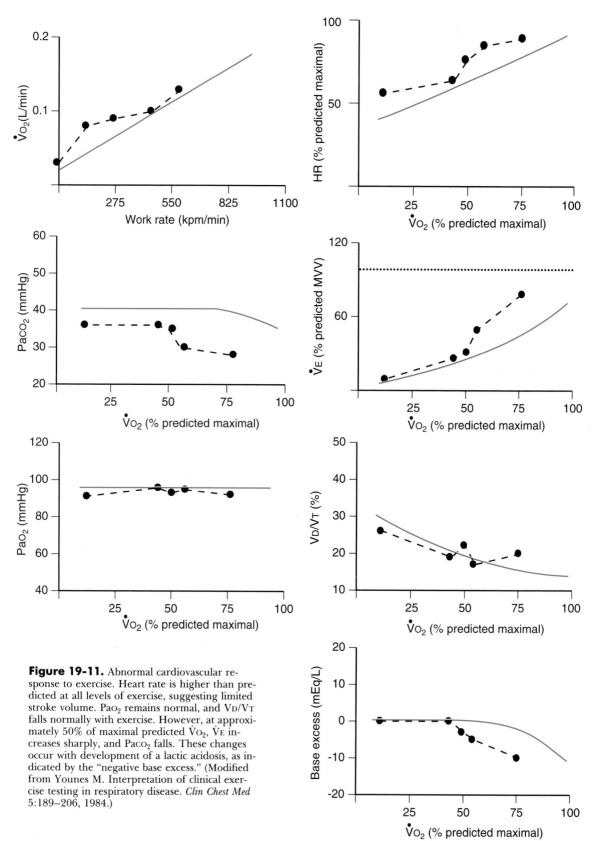

Figure 19-11. Abnormal cardiovascular response to exercise. Heart rate is higher than predicted at all levels of exercise, suggesting limited stroke volume. Pa_{O_2} remains normal, and V_D/V_T falls normally with exercise. However, at approximately 50% of maximal predicted $\dot{V}_{O_2}$, $\dot{V}_E$ increases sharply, and Pa_{CO_2} falls. These changes occur with development of a lactic acidosis, as indicated by the "negative base excess." (Modified from Younes M. Interpretation of clinical exercise testing in respiratory disease. *Clin Chest Med* 5:189–206, 1984.)

pulmonary hypertension; see Chap. 12) causes an increase in V_D/V_T at rest that fails to decline normally with progressive exercise. The increase in dead space ventilation is reflected in a Pa_{CO_2} that is higher than end-tidal P_{CO_2}, indicating significant impairment of gas exchange.

LIMITATIONS IN THE INTERPRETATION OF EXERCISE STUDIES

In clinical practice, submaximal exercise studies in which no clear pulmonary or cardiovascular limitation can be identified are not uncommon. This does not necessarily imply a lack of motivation or malingering on the part of the patient, although these possibilities must be considered.

When performing an exercise test, it is important to note the nature of the limiting symptom and whether the patient appears to be in genuine distress. The onset of angina or joint pain can obviously account for premature termination of a study. If the symptom is referable to the cardiovascular or respiratory systems and abnormalities are noted that cannot be ascribed readily to voluntary control (e.g., heart rate response to progressive exercise, onset of the anaerobic threshold, or development of abnormal gas exchange), the study can be assumed to be "maximal." Test results should be interpreted according to the pattern of abnormalities.

Abnormalities in parameters that can be voluntarily manipulated (e.g., minute ventilation, tidal volume, or respiratory rate) should be considered suspect if there is no evidence of true distress at the conclusion of exercise. Otherwise, psychogenic hyperventilation, exercise-induced pulmonary venous congestion, occult interstitial lung disease, or pulmonary vascular disease should be considered. Any of these conditions may be associated with hyperventilation or rapid, shallow breathing as the earliest detectable abnormality.

Finally, as noted, the information gained from exercise testing must be interpreted in light of the overall clinical picture. Repeated studies over the course of a patient's disease frequently are more useful than measurements made at a single point in time.

SELECTED READING

Bye PTP, Anderson SD, Woolcock AJ, et al. Bicycle endurance performance of patients with interstitial lung disease breathing air and oxygen. *Am Rev Respir Dis* 126:1005–1012, 1982.

Jones NL. Clinical Exercise Testing. 3rd ed. Philadelphia: WB Saunders, 1988.

Killian KJ, Campbell EJM. Dyspnea and exercise. *Annu Rev Physiol* 45:465–479, 1983.

Minh VD, Lee HM, Dolan GF, et al. Hypoxemia during exercise in patients with chronic obstructive pulmonary disease. *Am Rev Respir Dis* 120:787–794, 1979.

Wasserman K, Whipp BJ, Davis JA. Respiratory physiology of exercise: Metabolism, gas exchange, and ventilatory control. *Int Rev Physiol* 23:149–211, 1981.

Wasserman K, Whipp BJ, Koyal SN, et al. Anaerobic threshold and respiratory gas exchange during exercise. *J Appl Physiol* 35:236–243, 1973.

Weber KT, Kinasewitz GT, Janicki JS, et al. Oxygen utilization and ventilation during exercise in patients with chronic cardiac failure. *Circulation* 65:1213–1223, 1982.

Lippincott's Pathophysiology Series: Pulmonary Pathophysiology, edited by Michael A. Grippi. J. B. Lippincott Company, Philadelphia © 1995.

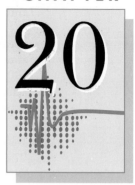

Clinical Presentations: Disorders of Respiratory Control and Respiratory Failure

Michael A. Grippi

The following three cases are based on pathophysiologic concepts developed in Chapters 16 through 19. The scenarios are somewhat more complicated than those presented in the three previous chapters on clinical presentations (Chaps. 8, 11, and 15). Each, however, highlights common clinical problems and direct application of the principles discussed.

CASE 1

The patient is a 33-year-old man with a long-standing history of asthma. Previous asthma attacks have been precipitated by exposure to pollens, upper respiratory tract infections, and anxiety. The patient frequently comes to the emergency room whenever he experiences shortness of breath or wheezing. Four days before admission to the hospital, a sore throat, sneezing, and a temperature of 101.2°F developed. The next day, he began coughing and wheezing. Despite taking his asthma medications, the patient has become progressively more short of breath and comes to the emergency room.

On arrival in the emergency room the patient appears to be in moderate respiratory distress. He has inspiratory and expiratory wheezing and is using accessory muscles of respiration. His blood pressure is 130/85 mmHg, his pulse is 110 beats per minute, and his respiratory rate is 30 breaths per minute. Chest examination shows inspiratory and expiratory wheezing. Cardiac examination is normal.

Frequently, an upper respiratory tract infection or exposure to allergens triggers an asthma attack. In this case, the inciting event appears to have been an infection (sore throat, fever). The patient is in status asthmaticus, which can be defined as an asthmatic episode that fails to respond to aggressive bronchodilator administration in the outpatient setting. Status asthmaticus is potentially life threatening. The mainstay of treatment is high-dose, intravenous corticosteroids. Once given, intravenous corticosteroids often take 6 to 8 hours to produce a beneficial effect (see Chap. 5).

The patient is treated with an inhaled β-agonist. Over the next 4 hours, the following arterial blood gases are obtained:

Time	F_{IO_2}	pH	Pa_{O_2} (mmHg)	Pa_{CO_2} (mmHg)
7:00 PM	0.21	7.47	57	34
8:00 PM	0.30	7.45	81	35
9:00 PM	0.30	7.40	69	40
11:00 PM	0.30	7.28	45	55

The initial arterial blood gas shows hypoxemia and a respiratory alkalosis (see Chap. 10). The hypoxemia is most likely caused by ventilation–perfusion mismatching (see Chap. 13) from bronchoconstriction and mucus plugging of the airways. The respiratory alkalosis occurs because of increased ventilation due to increased drive to breathe. Although hypoxemia may directly stimulate ventilation, asthmatics hyperventilate even when the hypoxemia is corrected, probably as a result of stimulation of vagal afferents (see Chap. 16).

At the time the second arterial blood gas was obtained, the patient was still hyperventilating, as indicated by the continued respiratory alkalosis and hypocapnia. His clinical condition is probably worse, because the alveolar–arterial oxygen gradient has widened further:

Time	F_{IO_2}	Pa_{O_2} (mmHg)	Pa_{CO_2} (mmHg)	P_{AO_2} (mmHg)	Alveolar–Arterial Oxygen Gradient (mmHg)
7:00 PM	0.21	57	34	108	51
8:00 PM	0.30	81	35	172	91

If the alveolar–arterial oxygen gradient had remained the same, the patient should have had a PaO_2 of 121 mmHg while breathing 30% oxygen.

At 11:00 PM, the patient is obtunded and breathing at a rate of 8 breaths per minute. Shortly thereafter, arterial blood gases are obtained while the patient is breathing 50% O_2; they show a pH of 7.01, a PaO_2 of 51 mmHg, and a $PaCO_2$ of 84 mmHg. The patient is intubated, but he cannot be ventilated effectively. A cardiopulmonary arrest ensues and the patient cannot be resuscitated. An autopsy is performed (Fig. 20-1).

From the time of the third arterial blood gas (9:00 PM) to the time of the patient's death shortly after the last arterial blood gas, he tired progressively. Eventually, the patient was unable to oxygenate his blood effectively or eliminate CO_2. With the rise of $PaCO_2$, he became more acidemic, and CO_2 narcosis ensued.

It could have been anticipated that the patient was going to do poorly from the time of the third arterial blood gas. The pH and $PaCO_2$ normalized as the alveolar–arterial oxygen gradient increased. Physical examination likely would have revealed that the patient was tachypneic and moving very little air. In fact, his chest may have been wheeze-free.

As discussed in Chapter 5, the severity of an asthma attack can be graded according to changes in arterial blood gas values (N = normal):

Stage of Asthma	Alveolar–Arterial Oxygen Gradient	PaO₂	PaCO₂	pH
Normal (0)	N	N	N	N
Very mild (I)	↑	N	N or ↓	N or ↑
Moderate (II)	↑ ↑	↓	↓ ↓	↑
Moderately severe (III)	↑ ↑ ↑	↓ ↓	↓	N or ↑
Severe (IV)	↑ ↑ ↑	↓ ↓ ↓	N	N or ↑
Life threatening (V)	↑ ↑ ↑ ↑	↓ ↓ ↓ ↓	↑	↓

At the time of the third arterial blood gas, more intensive bronchodilator and corticosteroid therapy should have been initiated. In addition, early, elective intubation should have been considered, because the patient did not improve rapidly. This patient's airways were totally occluded by mucus plugs, as evident in the autopsy specimen.

CASE 2

A 71-year-old man complains of a 2-year history of marked daytime sleepiness. The hypersomnolence occurs while the patient is watching television, reading, or driving. The patient is a loud snorer and complains of frequent early morning headaches. His weight has gradually increased over the last 3 years from 210 to 233 pounds. There is a history of hypertension and asthma.

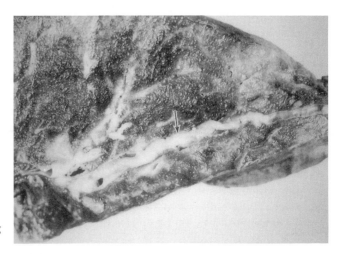

Figure 20-1. Case 1: extensive mucus plug seen in lung specimen obtained at autopsy.

Physical examination reveals a mildly obese man, 5 feet 7 inches in height, weighing 233 pounds. His blood pressure is 150/95 mmHg; his pulse is 72 beats per minute, and his respiratory rate is 18 breaths per minute. Examination of the throat shows a large tongue and excessive pharyngeal soft tissue folds. He has a short, thick neck (collar size, 16.5 inches). His neck veins are distended to 7 cm above the sternal angle. Cardiac examination shows a prominent second heart sound and a systolic murmur at the lower left sternal border. The chest is clear. The abdomen is obese. There is marked pitting edema of the lower extremities.

The patient has a classic history for Pickwickian syndrome, with manifestations of both obstructive sleep apnea and alveolar hypoventilation (see Chap. 17). The physical examination and laboratory findings reveal significant pulmonary hypertension and cor pulmonale, suggesting that the patient has had sleep-disordered breathing and nocturnal oxyhemoglobin desaturations for some time.

There are both anatomic and neural components to this patient's airway obstruction. Anatomic abnormalities, such as macroglossia and enlarged uvula and soft palate, contribute to the disease process. In addition, a neural component of reduced muscle tone during sleep, particularly rapid eye movement (REM) sleep, is a contributing factor. This reduction in muscle activity during REM sleep may be total, as in the atonia of axial skeletal musculature, or partial, as in the case of the diaphragm and upper airway. On the other hand, the mechanisms underlying the alveolar hypoventilation syndrome are not understood.

The white blood cell count is 7700 per mm^3; the hemoglobin is 16.7 g/dl. Arterial blood gases obtained while the patient is breathing room air show a pH of 7.37, a PaO_2 of 52 mmHg, a PaCO_2 of 49 mmHg, and a [HCO$_3^-$] of 30 mEq/L. An electrocardiogram shows right ventricular hypertrophy. The chest radiograph is unremarkable. An all-night sleep study shows repetitive episodes of obstructive apneas (Fig. 20-2) and

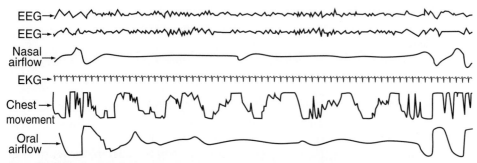

Figure 20-2. Case 2: polysomnogram. Cessation of airflow, despite repetitive chest wall movements, characterizes obstructive apneas.

mixed apneas lasting an average of 30 to 40 seconds in non-REM sleep. Oxygen saturation falls from a baseline of 90% to 72%.

The arterial blood gas reveals hypoxemia and a compensated, chronic respiratory acidosis (see Chap. 10). The hypoxemia is caused partially by hypoventilation, but the alveolar–arterial oxygen gradient is slightly increased (38 mmHg), implying other mechanisms, such as shunt, diffusion barrier, or ventilation–perfusion mismatch. Obese patients have basilar atelectasis, contributing to both ventilation–perfusion imbalance and shunting; atelectasis is likely to play a role in this patient. With a chronically elevated Pa_{CO_2}, acid–base balance is achieved by increased bicarbonate anion reabsorption in the renal proximal tubules.

If pulmonary artery catheterization were performed in this patient, hemodynamic findings would probably include a normal pulmonary artery occlusion pressure (PAOP) and elevated central venous, right ventricular, and pulmonary artery pressures. During apneas, these elevated pressures would rise further due to hypoxic pulmonary vasoconstriction (see Chap. 12).

A tracheostomy is performed. In the recovery room, the patient has severe bronchospasm. Bronchodilators are begun and the patient is transferred to the intensive care unit (ICU). One day later, a fever to 102°F develops. The following arterial blood gases are obtained during the patient's stay in the ICU:

Hospital Day	F_{IO_2}	pH	Pa_{O_2}(mmHg)	Pa_{CO_2}(mmHg)	$[HCO_3^-]$ (mEq/L)
1	0.35	7.38	61	52	30
2	0.28	7.29	51	77	36
3*	0.35	7.46	65	50	33
6	0.26	7.45	64	40	28
9	0.21	7.47	67	36	26

*Patient on mechanical ventilation.

Throughout his hospitalization, the patient's physical examination shows persistent wheezing; however, he does not appear to be in any respiratory distress.

The initial postoperative arterial blood gases show a moderate alveolar–arterial oxygen gradient and hypercapnia; in addition, a compensated respiratory acidosis is present (see Chap. 10). The second specimen shows worsening hypercapnia and respiratory acidosis; hypoxia is evident. A reduced ventilatory drive (e.g., from administration of sedative drugs) may account for the worsening CO_2 retention. When mechanical ventilation was initiated on day 3, the Pa_{CO_2} declined because of increased alveolar ventilation; the pH rose accordingly.

With institution of antibiotics, bronchodilators, and corticosteroids, the patient improves and is eventually discharged.

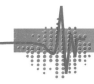

CASE 3

A 63-year-old alcoholic woman is admitted to the hospital after being found stuporous by her husband. She has been on an alcoholic binge for about 10 days before admission to the hospital.

Physical examination shows a thin, dehydrated, delirious woman. Her blood pressure is 110/70 mmHg; her pulse is 114 beats per minute, and her respiratory rate is 30 breaths per minute. Her temperature is 94°F. The chest is clear. Cardiac examination is normal. The liver is enlarged, and its edge is smooth and slightly tender. The spleen is not palpable. No localizing neurologic signs are present.

Laboratory data include a hemoglobin of 11.5 g/dl and a white blood cell count of 19,800 per mm³ (60% polymorphonuclear leukocytes, 5% bands, 6% monocytes, and 20% lymphocytes). The glucose is 55 mg/dl and the [HCO_3^-] is 5 mEq/L. A serum ammonia level is elevated. The electrocardiogram is unremarkable, except for sinus tachycardia. A chest radiograph is normal. Arterial blood gases obtained while the patient is breathing room air reveal a pH of 6.9, a Pa_{O_2} of 69 mmHg, a Pa_{CO_2} of 19 mmHg, and a [HCO_3^-] of 4 mEq/L.

The patient has been drinking heavily and has an altered mental status—factors that may predispose to development of aspiration pneumonia. She is tachycardic, tachypneic, and hypothermic. These are nonspecific signs, but they suggest the possibility of underlying sepsis. The liver enlargement may be secondary to alcohol-related liver disease.

The laboratory data show a mild anemia and marked leukocytosis. The blood glucose is low, perhaps secondary to depleted glycogen stores and ineffective gluconeogenesis in the setting of advanced liver disease. Alternatively, the hypoglycemia may be the result of sepsis. The elevated serum ammonia reflects severe liver disease.

Of particular note is the low bicarbonate concentration, consistent with a metabolic acidosis, as indicated in the arterial blood gas results. The patient's acid–base status is actually that of a mixed disturbance—a metabolic acidosis and a respiratory acidosis (see Chap. 10).

The PaO_2 of 69 mmHg and $PaCO_2$ of 19 mmHg indicate an increased alveolar–arterial oxygen gradient ($[760 - 47] \cdot 0.21 - [1.2 \cdot 19] - 69 = 57$ mmHg), which may be caused by preexisting lung disease or a new, acute process not yet evident radiographically.

The patient is treated for sepsis, severe metabolic acidosis, and hepatic coma with intravenous fluid, sodium bicarbonate, and antibiotics. Her mental status improves. Her temperature rises to 101°F and her respiratory rate slows to 16 breaths per minute. Twelve hours after admission, arterial blood gases obtained while she is breathing room air show a pH of 7.24, a PaO_2 of 63 mmHg, a $PaCO_2$ of 20 mmHg, and a $[HCO_3^-]$ of 13 mEq/L.

The patient's condition stabilizes after 48 hours in the intensive care unit, although her fever continues. On the third hospital day, a right upper lobe pulmonary infiltrate is noted on chest radiography. Physical examination at the time reveals decreased breath sounds over the right upper lobe, but no rales or wheezes. Blood cultures obtained at the time of admission grow *Staphylococcus aureus*.

The repeat arterial blood gases show a persistent metabolic acidosis and further increase in the alveolar–arterial oxygen gradient ($[760 - 47] \cdot 0.21 - [1.2 \cdot 20] - 63 = 62$ mmHg). The chest radiograph now shows a right upper lobe infiltrate, consistent with pneumonia. The pneumonia is probably the basis for the widened alveolar–arterial oxygen gradient.

Over a 48-hour period, tachypnea, dyspnea, and cyanosis develop. A chest radiograph on the fifth hospital day shows diffuse abnormalities (Fig. 20-3). Fifty milliliters of clear, straw-colored fluid are removed by thoracentesis. Gram stain of the fluid shows no organisms. Arterial blood gases obtained while the patient is breathing 60% O_2 reveal a pH of 7.32, a PaO_2 of 40 mmHg, and a $PaCO_2$ of 30 mmHg.

The patient's clinical condition has deteriorated, and her chest radiograph shows diffuse infiltrates, suggesting progression of the pneumonia or a superimposed process. The pleural effusion is a complication of the pneumonia. Although Gram stain of the fluid is negative, a decision on whether the fluid is infected is based, ultimately, on culture results, which take 24 to 48 hours.

The results of arterial blood gases on 60% O_2, once again, demonstrate a metabolic acidosis and marked worsening of the alveolar–arterial oxygen gradient. ($[760 - 47] \cdot 0.6 - [1.2 \cdot 30] - 40 = 352$ mmHg).

The patient is intubated and mechanical ventilation is initiated using 100% O_2. The respiratory rate is 24 per minute. The tidal volume is 800 ml, and the minute ventilation is 19 L/minute. Arterial blood gases show a pH of 7.34, a PaO_2 of 65 mmHg (90% saturation), and a $PaCO_2$ of 30 mmHg. The concentration of inspired O_2 is lowered to 50%.

On the 10th hospital day, positive end-expiratory pressure (PEEP) at 5 cm H_2O is instituted. The patient is given intravenous diuretics.

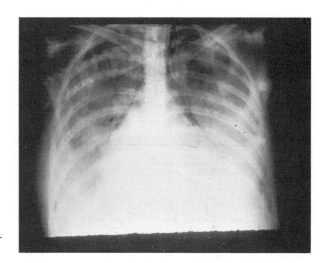

Figure 20-3. Case 3: chest radiograph obtained during hospital course.

Her blood pressure falls from 110/70 mmHg to 90/60 mmHg, and urine output decreases dramatically after an initial diuresis.

One day later, a pulmonary artery flotation catheter and radial arterial line are placed. The following data are obtained:

PEEP (cm/H$_2$O)	F$_{IO_2}$	Pa$_{O_2}$ (mmHg)	Pa$_{CO_2}$ (mmHg)	pH	C.O. (L/min)	$\overline{BP}$ (mmHg)	$\overline{PAP}$ (mmHg)	PAOP (mmHg)
0	0.98	76	36	7.35	4.8	63	21	8
5	0.98	151	—	—	4.5	59	22	9
10	0.98	313	—	—	4.2	54	25	11
15	0.98	481	—	—	2.9	40	27	12
0*	0.98	76	—	—	4.9	62	18	8

$\overline{BP}$, mean arterial blood pressure; $\overline{PAP}$, mean pulmonary arterial pressure; PAOP, pulmonary artery occlusion pressure.
*Second trial at PEEP = 0 cm H_2O.

Based on these data, a decision is made to maintain the patient on a PEEP of 5 cm H$_2$O and an F$_{IO_2}$ of 0.40. The Pa$_{O_2}$ is 102 mmHg and the mean pulmonary artery pressure is 22 cm H$_2$O.

In this patient, the adult respiratory distress syndrome (ARDS) developed in association with staphylococcal septicemia (see Chap. 14). The hypoxemia of ARDS is caused by severe ventilation–perfusion abnormalities and physiologic shunt. The underlying abnormality is probably interstitial and alveolar edema and alveolar collapse.

The patient was initially placed on PEEP in an attempt to improve oxygenation without using potentially toxic levels of inspired O$_2$. However, hypotension developed. The hypotension may have resulted from a significant decrease in cardiac output or from a decrease in blood volume.

Therefore, it was necessary to assess the effect of PEEP on the patient's hemodynamics by inserting the pulmonary artery flotation catheter and measuring cardiac output as PEEP was increased.

Maximal O_2 delivery was achieved with 5 cm H_2O PEEP, making it the optimal choice. The patient's O_2 carrying capacity is: [12 g Hb/dl · 1.34 ml O_2/g Hb] = 16 ml O_2/dl = 160 ml O_2/L of blood. The patient's oxyhemoglobin saturation is 93% at a PEEP of 0 cm H_2O and 100% at PEEP levels of 5, 10, and 15 cm H_2O. With dissolved O_2 added, O_2 content at a PEEP of 5 cm H_2O is [12 g Hb/dl · 1.34 ml O_2/g Hb] + [0.003 ml O_2/dl/mmHg · 151 mmHg] = 16.53 ml O_2/dl. Therefore, O_2 delivery at a PEEP of 5 cm H_2O is 4.5 L/minute · 165.3 ml/L = 743.9 ml/minute or 0.744 L/minute.

During the next week, the patient improves slowly. Her minute ventilation declines to 10 L/minute on the 14th hospital day, when the PEEP is reduced gradually and eventually discontinued. Several days later, the patient is weaned from mechanical ventilation.

APPENDIX 1

Symbols and Terms Used Commonly in Respiratory Physiology

PRIMARY SYMBOLS

Symbol	Definition	Example
C	Concentration of gas in blood	Ca_{O_2} = O_2 concentration in blood
F	Fractional concentration in dry gas	F_{IO_2} = fractional concentration of O_2 in inspired gas
P	Pressure or partial pressure	P_{O_2} = partial pressure of O_2
Q	Volume of blood	
$\dot{Q}$	Volume of blood per unit time (flow)	$\dot{Q}$ = cardiac output (L/min)
R	Respiratory exchange ratio	
S	Saturation in blood	S_{O_2} = saturation of hemoglobin with O_2 (%)
V	Volume of gas	V_A = alveolar volume (L)
$\dot{V}$	Volume of gas per unit time (flow)	$\dot{V}_A$ = alveolar ventilation (L/min)

SECONDARY SYMBOLS

Gas Phase

Symbol	Definition	Example
A	Alveolar	V_A = alveolar volume
B	Barometric	P_B = barometric pressure
D	Dead space	V_D = dead space volume
E	Expired	$\dot{V}_E$ = expired minute ventilation
I	Inspired	$\dot{V}_I$ = inspired minute ventilation
L	Lung	C_L = lung compliance
T	Tidal	V_T = tidal volume
ATPD	Ambient temperature and pressure, dry	
ATPS	Ambient temperature and pressure, saturated with water vapor at these conditions	

APPENDIX 1: *Symbols and Terms Used Commonly in Respiratory Physiology*

Gas Phase

Symbol	Definition	Example
BTPS	Body conditions: body temperature and ambient pressure, saturated with water vapor at these conditions	
STPD	Standard conditions: temperature 0°C, pressure 760 mmHg, and dry (0 mmHg water vapor)	
an	Anatomic	VD_{an} = volume of anatomic dead space
f	Respiratory frequency, per minute	
max	Maximum	$\dot{V}max_{50\%}$ = maximum expiratory flow at 50% of vital capacity
t	Time	FEV_t = volume expired at time t; $FEV_{1.0}$ = volume expired during first second of FVC

Blood Phase

Symbol	Definition	Example
a	Arterial	Pa_{O_2} = partial pressure of O_2 in arterial blood
c	Capillary	Cc_{O_2} = concentration of O_2 in capillary blood
c′	End-capillary	Cc'_{O_2} = concentration of O_2 in end-capillary blood
v	Venous	
v̄	Mixed venous	$C\bar{v}_{O_2}$ = concentration of O_2 in mixed venous blood

TERMS

MECHANICS

Abbreviation	Definition
C	Compliance of the lungs, chest wall, or total respiratory system
Cdyn	Dynamic compliance. Respiratory frequency appears as a qualifier (eg, $Cdyn_{40}$ = dynamic compliance at respiratory frequency of 40 per minute)
Cst	Static compliance
C/V_L	Specific compliance. Compliance divided by the lung volume at which it is determined (usually FRC)
E	Elastance (reciprocal of compliance)
EPP	Equal pressure point

APPENDIX 1: *Symbols and Terms Used Commonly in Respiratory Physiology*

Abbreviation	Definition
Gaw	Airway conductance (reciprocal of Raw)
P_A	Alveolar pressure
Pao	Pressure at airway opening
Paw	Pressure at any point along the airway
Pbs	Pressure at body surface
Pes	Esophageal pressure
Ppl	Pleural pressure
Pst	Static recoil pressure of the lung (at specified lung volume, eg, TLC)
P_A − Pbs	Transthoracic pressure
P_A − Ppl	Transpulmonary pressure
Ppl − Pbs	Pressure across the chest wall
R	Frictional resistance (pressure difference divided by flow)
Raw	Airway resistance (pressure difference between airway opening and alveoli divided by flow)
W	Mechanical work of breathing

LUNG VOLUMES

CC	Closing capacity
CV	Closing volume
ERV	Expiratory reserve volume
FRC	Functional residual capacity
IC	Inspiratory capacity
IRV	Inspiratory reserve volume
RV	Residual volume
TLC	Total lung capacity
VC	Vital capacity
V_T	Tidal volume

SPIROMETRY

$FEF_{x\%-y\%}$	Mean forced expiratory flow between two designated volume points, x and y, in FVC (eg, $FEF_{25\%-75\%}$ = flow between 25% and 75% of the expired vital capacity—previously called maximal mid-expiratory flow rate or MMEFR)
FEV_t	Forced expiratory volume in time interval, t
$FEV_t/FVC\%$	Percentage of FVC expired in time interval, t
$FIF_{x\%-y\%}$	Mean forced inspiratory flow between two designated volume points, x and y, in FIVC (eg, $FIF_{25\%-75\%}$ = flow between 25% and 75% of the inspired vital capacity—previously called maximal mid-inspiratory flow rate or MMIFR)
FIVC	Forced inspiratory vital capacity
FVC	Forced vital capacity (expiratory)
MEFV	Maximum expiratory flow–volume curve
MFSR	Maximum flow–static recoil curve

APPENDIX 1: *Symbols and Terms Used Commonly in Respiratory Physiology*

MIFV	Maximum inspiratory flow–volume curve
MVV	Maximal voluntary ventilation
PEF	Peak expiratory flow
$\dot{V}max_{x\%}$	Maximal expiratory flow at x% of VC

GAS EXCHANGE

D_L	Diffusing capacity of the lung
D_M	Diffusing capacity of the alveolar–capillary membrane
R	Respiratory exchange ratio (ratio of CO_2 output to O_2 uptake in the lungs)
$\dot{V}_{CO_2}$	Carbon dioxide production per minute (STPD)
$\dot{V}_{O_2}$	Oxygen consumption per minute (STPD)

VENTILATION

$\dot{V}_A$	Alveolar ventilation per minute (BTPS)
$\dot{V}_D$	Ventilation of physiologic dead space per minute (BTPS)
V_D	Volume of physiologic dead space
$\dot{V}_{D_A}$	Ventilation of alveolar dead space per minute (BTPS)
V_{D_A}	Volume of alveolar dead space
$\dot{V}_{D_{an}}$	Ventilation of anatomic dead space per minute (BTPS)
$V_{D_{an}}$	Volume of anatomic dead space (BTPS)
$\dot{V}_E$	Expired volume per minute (BTPS)
$\dot{V}_I$	Inspired volume per minute (BTPS)

APPENDIX 2

Useful Equations in Respiratory Physiology

EQUATION	REFERENCE IN TEXT

MECHANICS

Airway Resistance
$R = P/\dot{V}$

P is driving pressure; $\dot{V}$ is flow.

Chapter 2; Equation [2-10]; Page 27

Alveolar Pressure
$Palv = Pel + Ppl$

Pel is elastic recoil pressure; Ppl is pleural pressure.

Chapter 2; Equation [2-3]; Page 19

Equation of Motion of the Lung
$Ptot = (E \cdot \Delta V) + (R \cdot \dot{V}) + (I \cdot \ddot{V})$

Ptot is total pressure across the respiratory system (the difference between mouth and alveolar pressures); V is lung volume; $\dot{V}$ is airflow; $\ddot{V}$ is rate of change of airflow (acceleration); E is elastance; R is resistance; I is inertance. For air, I is very small, and the last term can be ignored.

Chapter 2; Equation [2-4]; Page 19

Laplace Equation
$P = 2T/r$

P is pressure within the sphere; T is surface tension; r is radius. For a structure with two surfaces, eg, a bubble, the relationship becomes $P = 4T/r$.

Chapter 2; Figure 2-8; Page 23

Poiseuille's Law
$\dot{V} = P\pi r^4/8\eta l$

$\dot{V}$ is airflow rate; P is pressure; r is airway radius; η is gas viscosity; l is airway length.

Chapter 2; Equation [2-11]; Page 27

APPENDIX 2: *Useful Equations in Respiratory Physiology*

EQUATION	REFERENCE IN TEXT

Pressure Across Respiratory System

$$Prs = Pl + Pw$$

Pl is pressure across the lung (Palv − Ppl); Pw is pressure across the chest wall (Ppl − Pbs).

Chapter 2; Equation [2-6]; Page 26

Reynolds Number

$$Re = 2rvd/\eta$$

r is airway radius; v is gas linear velocity; d is gas density; η is gas viscosity.

Chapter 2; Equation [2-14]; Page 28

Static Compliance of Respiratory System

$$Crs = \Delta V/Prs$$

ΔV is change in volume of the respiratory system; Prs is pressure across the respiratory system (inflation pressure).

Chapter 2; Equation [2-9]; Page 26

Transdiaphragmatic Pressure

$$Pdi = Pab - Ppl$$

Pab is intraabdominal pressure; Ppl is pleural pressure.

Chapter 2; Equation [2-2]; Page 17

Work of Breathing

$$W = \int P\Delta V$$

P is pressure generated across the respiratory system by respiratory muscles; ΔV is change in volume (inflation volume).

Chapter 2; Equation [2-15]; Page 38

VENTILATION

Alveolar Ventilation

$$\dot{V}A = K \cdot \frac{\dot{V}CO_2}{PaCO_2}$$

$\dot{V}A$ is expressed at BTPS; $\dot{V}CO_2$ is rate of production of CO_2 (L/min) and is expressed at STPD. Under these conditions, K, a constant equal to 0.863, permits conversion from STPD to BTPS.

Chapter 3; Equation [3-10]; Page 46

EQUATION

REFERENCE IN TEXT

Bohr Equation

$$\frac{V_D}{V_T} = \frac{P_{ACO_2} - P_{\bar{E}CO_2}}{P_{ACO_2}}$$

V_D/V_T is the ratio of volume of dead space to tidal volume; P_{ACO_2} is alveolar P_{CO_2}; $P_{\bar{E}CO_2}$ is mixed expired P_{CO_2}. P_{aCO_2} can be used as an approximation of P_{ACO_2}. This permits calculation of physiologic dead space by measuring P_{CO_2} in arterial blood gas and "mixed" expired gas samples.

Chapter 3; Equation [3-9];
Page 45

Minute Ventilation

$$\dot{V}_E = \dot{V}_A + \dot{V}_D = (V_A \cdot f) + (V_D \cdot f)$$

V_A is alveolar volume; V_D is dead space volume. The sum of alveolar and dead space volumes is tidal volume, V_T. Multiplication of V_A and V_D by respiratory rate (f) yields the minute ventilation of each compartment ($\dot{V}_A$ and $\dot{V}_D$).

Chapter 3; Equation [3-3];
Page 42

GAS EXCHANGE

Alveolar Gas Equation

$$P_{AO_2} = P_{IO_2} - P_{ACO_2}\left[F_{IO_2} + \frac{1 - F_{IO_2}}{R}\right]$$

Alveolar P_{O_2} (P_{AO_2}) equals inspired P_{O_2} (P_{IO_2}) minus alveolar P_{CO_2} (P_{ACO_2}) "corrected" for the rate of exchange of CO_2 with O_2 (R) and F_{IO_2}. In the steady state, R equals the metabolic respiratory quotient (RQ).

Chapter 3; Equation [3-11];
Page 47

Boyle's Law

$$P_1V_1 = P_2V_2$$

P_1 and V_1 represent pressure and volume, respectively, under initial set of conditions; P_2 and V_2 represent pressure and volume, respectively, under altered set of conditions. Temperature is constant.

Chapter 4; Equation [4-3];
Page 62

EQUATION   **REFERENCE IN TEXT**

Charles' Law

$$\frac{V_1}{V_2} = \frac{T_1}{T_2}$$

Pressure is constant. T_1 and T_2 represent initial and subsequent temperatures.

Dalton's Law

$$P_x = P \cdot F_x$$

The partial pressure of gas x (P_x) in a mixture of gases is the pressure that the gas would exert if it occupied the same volume as the mixture *in the absence of the other components*. P_x is the product of the total *dry* gas pressure (ie, with water vapor pressure subtracted) and the fractional concentration of the gas. Within alveoli, the sum of the partial pressures of alveolar gases (O_2, CO_2, N_2, and water vapor) equals barometric pressure (P_B): $P_B = P_{O_2} + P_{CO_2} + P_{N_2} + P_{H_2O}$.

Chapter 9; Equation [9-1]; Page 139

Diffusing Capacity of the Lung

$$(1) \quad D_L = \frac{\dot{V}_G}{P_1 - P_2}$$

$$(2) \quad \frac{1}{D_L} = \frac{1}{D_M} + \frac{1}{\Theta V_c}$$

Chapter 9; Equation [9-7]; Page 145

The first equation is Fick's law (see below). D_L is diffusing capacity of the lung; D_M is diffusing capacity of the alveolar–capillary membrane; Θ is reaction rate of CO with hemoglobin; V_c is capillary blood volume.

Fick's Law for Diffusion

$$\dot{V}_G = D_M \cdot (P_1 - P_2)$$

Chapter 9; Equation [9-3]; Page 139

The volume of gas moving across the alveolar–capillary membrane per unit time ($\dot{V}_G$) is proportional to the diffusing capacity of the membrane (D_M) and the difference in partial pressures of the gas across the membrane ($P_1 - P_2$).

EQUATION

Henry's Law

$$C_x = K \cdot P_x$$

C_x, the concentration of gas x dissolved in a liquid, is proportional to the partial pressure of x (P_x).

Respiratory Exchange Ratio

$$R = \frac{\dot{V}_{CO_2}}{\dot{V}_{O_2}}$$

$\dot{V}_{CO_2}$ is rate of CO_2 elimination (L/min); $\dot{V}_{O_2}$ is rate of O_2 uptake (L/min).

GAS TRANSPORT

Fick Principle

$$\dot{Q} = \frac{\dot{V}_{O_2}}{Ca_{O_2} - C\bar{v}_{O_2}}$$

$\dot{Q}$ is cardiac output; Ca_{O_2} is arterial O_2 content; $C\bar{v}_{O_2}$ is mixed venous O_2 content.

Chapter 10; Equation [10-9]; Page 158

Oxygen Carrying Capacity

$$O_2 \text{ carrying capacity} = [Hb] \cdot 1.34 \text{ ml } O_2/g \text{ Hb/dl blood}$$

1.34 ml O_2/g Hb/dl represents the amount of O_2 that each gram of hemoglobin (per deciliter of blood) can carry when fully saturated.

Chapter 10; Equation [10-1]; Page 153

Oxygen Content

$$C_{O_2} = (Sol. \cdot Pa_{O_2}) + ([Hb] \cdot S_{O_2} \cdot 1.34 \text{ ml } O_2/g \text{ Hb/dl blood})$$

O_2 content (C_{O_2}) is equal to the sum of dissolved O_2, which is the product of O_2 solubility in plasma (Sol. = 0.0031 ml/dl/mmHg) and Pa_{O_2}, and hemoglobin-bound O_2, which is the product of hemoglobin concentration ([Hb]), hemoglobin saturation (S_{O_2}), and O_2-binding capacity per gram of hemoglobin (1.34 ml O_2/g Hb/dl blood).

Chapter 10; Equation [10-6]; Page 154

APPENDIX 2: *Useful Equations in Respiratory Physiology*

EQUATION

REFERENCE IN TEXT

Oxygen Saturation

$$SaO_2 = \frac{O_2 \text{ bound to Hb}}{O_2 \text{ carrying capacity}} \cdot 100\%$$

O_2 bound to hemoglobin is expressed as ml O_2 per gram of hemoglobin per deciliter of blood. O_2 carrying capacity (see above) represents the total volume of O_2 that the hemoglobin in each deciliter of blood can bind (ie, at 100% hemoglobin saturation with O_2).

Chapter 10; Equation [10-2]; Page 153

Systemic Oxygen Delivery

$$DO_2 = \dot{Q} \cdot [([Hb] \cdot 1.34 \cdot SO_2) + (0.0031 \cdot PaO_2)]$$

DO_2 is systemic O_2 delivery, which is the product of cardiac output ($\dot{Q}$) and O_2 content.

Chapter 10; Equation [10-8]; Page 158

ACID–BASE BALANCE

Henderson–Hasselbalch Equation

$$pH = pK_A + \log \frac{[HCO_3{}^-]}{[H_2CO_3]}$$

The pK_A for the bicarbonate buffer system is 6.1. The equilibrium between H_2CO_3 and CO_2 strongly favors CO_2. [CO_2] can be substituted for [H_2CO_3] and expressed as the product of PCO_2 (mmHg) and 0.03 ml/dl/mmHg, the solubility coefficient of CO_2.

Chapter 10; Equation [10-17]; Page 164

HEMODYNAMICS

Pulmonary Vascular Resistance

$$PVR = \frac{\bar{P}pa - \bar{P}la}{\dot{Q}} \cdot 79.9$$

$\bar{P}pa$ is mean pulmonary artery pressure; $\bar{P}la$ is mean left atrial pressure; $\dot{Q}$ is cardiac output. Multiplication by the factor, 79.9, converts Wood units to dyne · sec · cm^{-5}.

Chapter 12; Table [12-5]; Page 192

Systemic Vascular Resistance

$$SVR = \frac{\bar{P}a - \bar{P}ra}{\dot{Q}} \cdot 79.9$$

$\bar{P}a$ is mean systemic arterial pressure; $\bar{P}ra$ is mean right atrial pressure.

Chapter 12; Table [12-5]; Page 192

EQUATION	REFERENCE IN TEXT

Venous-to-Arterial Shunt

$$\frac{\dot{Q}_s}{\dot{Q}_T} = \frac{Cc'o_2 - Cao_2}{Cc'o_2 - C\bar{v}o_2}$$

Chapter 12; Table [12-5]; Page 193

Venous-to-arterial shunt ($\dot{Q}_s/\dot{Q}_T$) is also called shunt fraction. $Cc'O_2$ is end-capillary O_2 content; Cao_2 is arterial O_2 content; $C\bar{v}o_2$ is mixed venous O_2 content. When inspired O_2 content (CIo_2) is substituted for end-capillary O_2 content, physiologic shunt is calculated.

FLUID EXCHANGE

Starling Equation

$$Q_f = K_f[(P_{mv} - P_i) - \sigma(\Pi_{mv} - \Pi_i)]$$

Chapter 14; Equation [14-1]; Page 215

Q_f is fluid filtration rate; K_f is filtration coefficient; P_{mv} and P_i are hydrostatic pressures in the microvasculature and interstitial space, respectively; σ is the reflection coefficient; Π_{mv} and Π_i are colloid oncotic pressures in the microvasculature and interstitial space, respectively.

EXERCISE

Oxygen Pulse

$$\frac{\dot{V}o_2}{HR} = SV \cdot (Cco_2 - C\bar{v}o_2)$$

Chapter 19; Equation [19-2]; Page 285

Oxygen pulse is the ratio of O_2 uptake to heart rate. It equals the product of stroke volume (SV) and the difference between capillary and mixed venous O_2 contents (Cco_2 and $C\bar{v}o_2$, respectively).

Age-Predicted Maximal Heart Rate

$$\text{Maximal HR} = 210 - [0.65 \cdot \text{Age (yr)}]$$

Chapter 19; Equation [19-3]; Page 286

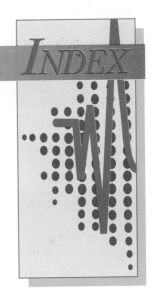

Page numbers followed by *t* and *f* indicate tables and figures, respectively.